VARIATION IN WORKING

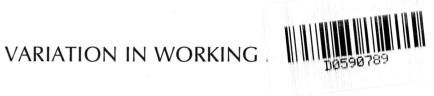

Variation in Working Memory

Edited by

Andrew R. A. Conway
Christopher Jarrold
Michael J. Kane
Akira Miyake
John N. Towse

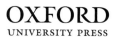

UNIVERSITY PRESS

2007

OXFORD

UNIVERSITY PRESS

Oxford University Press, Inc., publishes works that further
Oxford University's objective of excellence
in research, scholarship, and education.

Oxford New York
Auckland   Cape Town   Dar es Salaam   Hong Kong   Karachi
Kuala Lumpur   Madrid   Melbourne   Mexico City   Nairobi
New Delhi   Shanghai   Taipei   Toronto

With offices in
Argentina   Austria   Brazil   Chile   Czech Republic   France   Greece
Guatemala   Hungary   Italy   Japan   Poland   Portugal   Singapore
South Korea   Switzerland   Thailand   Turkey   Ukraine   Vietnam

Copyright © 2007 by Oxford University Press, Inc.

Published by Oxford University Press, Inc.
198 Madison Avenue, New York, New York 10016

www.oup.com

Oxford is a registered trademark of Oxford University Press

Library of Congress Cataloging-in-Publication Data
Variation in working memory / edited by Andrew Conway ... [et al.].
    p.   cm.
Includes bibliographical references.
ISBN-13: 978-0-19-516863-1
ISBN-10: 0-19-516863-1
1. Short-term memory.   I. Conway, Andrew (Andrew R. A.)
BF378.S54V37 2006
153.1'3—dc22   2006009858

9 8 7 6 5 4 3 2 1

Printed in the United States of America
on acid-free paper

Dedicated to our families

Preface

Working memory — the ability to keep important information in mind while comprehending, thinking, and doing — changes dramatically over the life span and varies considerably from person to person at a given age. Understanding such individual and developmental differences is crucial because working memory is a key contributor to general intellectual functioning. It has been demonstrated to be relevant to many everyday tasks, such as reading, making sense of spoken discourse, problem solving, and mental arithmetic. As such, it is the focus of considerable research efforts in cognitive psychology and cognitive neuroscience. This research has wide-ranging implications for our general understanding of cognitive processes in a variety of populations and settings.

Since Baddeley and Hitch (1974) introduced their seminal model of working memory, there has been growing interest in this area. As a testament to the importance of this work, the work by Baddeley and Hitch was identified in a discipline-wide poll as one of the 100 most influential works in cognitive science

(http://www.cogsci.umn.edu/OLD/calendar/past_ events/millennium/top100.html). It has also served as a catalyst for active research and theoretical development, as reflected by the large number of edited books and monographs currently available on working memory (including several edited volumes that originated as special issues of academic journals), some of which have documented recent theoretical developments in the area (e.g., Cowan, 2005; Miyake & Shah, 1999).

Despite the existence of various edited volumes and monographs on working memory, no previous publication has properly explored the issue of the causes and consequences of *variation* in working memory, the focus of this volume and an issue of particular importance in the field (e.g., see Jarrold & Towse, 2006). Since Daneman and Carpenter (1980) developed the first useful measure of working memory capacity as an individual-differences construct among adults (for a seminal developmental perspective on working memory capacity, see Case, Kurland, & Goldberg, 1982), research on working memory variation has made critical contributions to theory on working memory in general. Indeed, individual- and group-differences research has had more impact on the development of working memory theory than on any other cognitive construct. Working memory research thus represents a most successful integration of the experimental and correlational traditions or what Cronbach (1957) called "the two disciplines of scientific psychology." It also serves as an exemplary instantiation of Underwood's (1975) notion that individual differences may act as a "crucible" in which to test general theory (see also Kosslyn et al., 2002).

In addition, there are a number of other reasons why a focus on individual differences is especially important and timely. First, in the last few years, new techniques developed in individual-differences research, cognitive science and neuroscience have been applied to the issue of variation in working memory. These new techniques include the statistical approach of latent variables analysis (e.g., Conway, Cowan, Bunting, Therriault, & Minkoff, 2002; Miyake et al., 2000) and functional neuroimaging techniques (e.g., Braver et al., 1997; Jonides, Smith, Marshuetz, Koeppe, & Reuter-Lorenz, 1998). Second, there has been a growing realization that the dominant theoretical conceptualization of working memory that depends solely on the ability to share resources between information processing and storage demands may be limited in explanatory power. In particular, researchers are highlighting the need to also consider long-term memory constraints (e.g., Baddeley, 2000; Ericsson & Kintsch, 1995) and additional if not alternative theoretical mechanisms and processes for working memory performance (e.g., Barrouillet, Bernadin, & Camos, 2004; Lustig, May, & Hasher, 2001; Saito & Miyake, 2004; Towse, Hitch, & Hutton, 1998). Third, despite the centrality of sentence comprehension research for understanding the nature of individual differences in working memory (Daneman & Merikle, 1996; Just & Carpenter, 1992), there has been controversy regarding the nature of working memory implicated during language comprehension (e.g., Caplan & Wa-

ters, 1999). Finally, this growth in interest in variation in working memory has been matched by growth in the scope of the practical application of this approach. Recent studies have applied an individual-differences analysis to examine the importance of working memory variance in predicting learning disability (see discussion in Jarrold, 2001) as well as intellectual functioning in typically developing children (e.g., Bayliss, Jarrold, Gunn, & Baddeley, 2003; Fry & Hale, 1996) and adults (e.g., Engle, Kane, & Tuholski, 1999; Miyake, Friedman, Rettinger, Shah, & Hegarty, 2001). Moreover, advances in the understanding of the neural basis of individual and age-related variation in working memory (e.g., Kane & Engle, 2003; Munakata, 2004; Oberauer & Kliegl, 2001; Reuter-Lorenz et al., 2001; Roberts & Pennington, 1996) have also been important in shaping the present research field.

There is clearly a need to bring this recent work together in a comprehensive yet cohesive volume, particularly because existing models and theories of working memory variation are quite diverse and straddle so many research areas. Although some theories provide sophisticated and well-developed accounts of certain aspects of working memory variation, they also tend to have different theoretical orientations and at the same time leave unspecified some important aspects of working memory. In addition, we view progress in this field as being hindered by a prototypical research strategy of proposing one particular underlying source of working memory variation and confirming predictions based on that idea, without parallel consideration of other mechanisms. Likewise, researchers often focus their empirical efforts on working memory variation within one particular target population, without considering how research with other populations might complement or conflict with their findings. In short, there is a lack of overall cohesion among different research findings, and this problem inhibits the ability to compare and contrast different proposals about the nature of working memory variation.

The present volume attempts to offer an integrative yet thorough approach by focusing on explicit, detailed comparisons of current major theoretical proposals on working memory variation. Research groups have been drawn from both the United States and Europe to ensure that the rather different research perspectives that operate on the two sides of the Atlantic are well represented. A particular strength of the book is its coverage of working-memory research on a wide variety of populations, such as healthy adults, children with and without learning difficulties, older adults, and neurological patients.

Another major feature of the volume is that each research group has explicitly addressed the same set of important theoretical questions—from the perspective of their own theoretical and applied research, and from the perspective of competing views from within and beyond this volume. We believe that this common-question approach was adopted successfully in Miyake and Shah's (1999) edited volume *Models of Working Memory: Mechanisms of Active Maintenance and Executive Control* and ensured that book had a coherent focus. We hope this approach serves as a useful device to elucidate the commonalities and differences among different theoretical proposals on the nature of working memory variation. The questions to be addressed by each research team are as follows:

QUESTION 1: OVERARCHING THEORY OF WORKING MEMORY

What is the theory or definition of working memory that guides your research on working memory variation?

QUESTION 2: CRITICAL SOURCES OF WORKING MEMORY VARIATION

What is your view on the critical source(s) of working memory variability within your target population(s) of study? Why do you focus on the specific source(s) of variability in your research?

QUESTION 3: CONSIDERATION OF OTHER SOURCES OF WORKING MEMORY VARIATION

Do you find other sources of working memory variability proposed in this volume to be applicable to your target population of study? Are these sources of working memory variation compatible or incompatible with your view of your target population?

QUESTION 4: CONTRIBUTIONS TO GENERAL WORKING MEMORY THEORY

What does the variability within your target population of study tell us about the structure, function, and/or organization of working memory in general?

These questions were carefully chosen (through extensive discussions among the five editorial team members) not only to help each contributing team clearly outline their main theoretical position in a larger theoretical context but also to maximize the possibility of successfully elucidating the commonalities and differences among the different theoretical proposals. More specifically, Question 1 was included to encourage each contributing team to articulate their theoretical background directly (particularly some underlying assumptions that are not always made explicit and, hence, often hinder comparisons among different theoretical proposals). Question 2 is perhaps the most central one of the four common questions in that it asks each contributing team to specify their theoretical proposals about the nature of variation in working memory in the target population(s) the team focused on. Question 3 was designed specifically to alleviate the problem noted earlier of researchers often focusing on a single theoretical construct or mechanism in their work and not considering other constructs or mechanisms proposed in the literature. This question essentially led each contributing team to reflect upon other related theoretical proposals and clearly articulate the relationship to those alternative proposals by either arguing against them or offering a theoretical synthesis. Finally, Question 4 raised a metatheoretical issue and asked each contributing team to discuss the theoretical benefits (or even the necessity of) studying variation in working memory. Answers to this final question provided by different researchers in the volume will help us to better understand the strengths (and likely weaknesses) of the individual-differences approach and, as a whole, offer an interesting case study (in the context of working memory research) of how studies of interindividual and intraindividual variation in general can inform or guide theory development and practical applications.

References

Baddeley, A. (2000). The episodic buffer: a new component of working memory. *Trends in Cognitive Sciences, 4*, 417–423.

Baddeley, A. D., & Hitch, G. J. (1974). Working memory. In G. H. Bower (Ed.), *The psychology of learning and motivation: Advances in research and theory* (Vol. 8, pp. 47–89). New York: Academic Press.

Barrouillet, P., Bernadin, S., & Camos, V. (2004). Time constraints and resource sharing in adults' working memory span. *Journal of Experimental Psychology: General, 133*, 83–100.

Bayliss, D. M., Jarrold, C., Gunn, D. M., & Baddeley, A. D. (2003). The complexities of complex span: Explaining individual differences in working memory in children and adults. *Journal of Experimental Psychology: General, 131*, 71–92.

Braver, T. S., Cohen, J. D., Nystrom, L. E., Jonides, J., Smith, E. E., & Noll, D. C. (1997). A parametric study of prefrontal cortex involvement in human working memory. *NeuroImage, 5*, 49–62.

Caplan, D., & Waters, G. S. (1999). Working memory and sentence comprehension. *Behavioral and Brain Sciences, 22*, 77–126.

Case, R., Kurland, M., & Goldberg, J. (1982). Operational efficiency and the growth of short term memory span. *Journal of Experimental Child Psychology, 33*, 386–404.

Conway, A. R. A., Cowan, N., Bunting, M. F., Therriault, D., & Minkoff, S. (2002). A latent variable analysis of working memory capacity, short-term memory capacity, processing speed, and general fluid intelligence. *Intelligence, 30*, 163–183.

Cowan, N. (2005). *Working memory capacity*. Hove, UK: Psychology Press.

Cronbach, L. J. (1957). The two disciplines of scientific psychology. *American Psychologist, 12*, 671–684.

Daneman, M., & Carpenter, P. A. (1980). Individual differences in working memory and reading. *Journal of Verbal Learning and Verbal Behavior, 19*, 450–466.

Daneman, M., & Merikle, P. M. (1996). Working memory and language comprehension: A meta-analysis. *Psychonomic Bulletin & Review, 3*, 422–433.

Engle, R. W., Kane, M. J., & Tuholski, S. W. (1999). Individual differences in working memory capacity and what they tell us about controlled attention, general fluid intelligence, and functions of the prefrontal cortex. In A. Miyake & P. Shah (Eds.), *Models of working memory* (pp. 102–134). New York: Cambridge University Press.

Ericsson, K. A., & Kintsch, W. (1995). Long-term working memory. *Psychological Review, 102*, 211–245.

Fry, A. F., & Hale, S. (1996). Processing speed, working memory, and fluid intelligence. *Psychological Science, 7*, 237–241.

Jarrold, C. (2001). Applying the working memory model to the study of atypical development. In J. Andrade (Ed.), *Working memory in perspective* (pp. 126–150). Hove, UK: Psychology Press.

Jarrold, C., & Towse, J. N. (2006). Individual differences in working memory. *Neuroscience, 139*, 39–50.

Jonides, J., Smith, E. E., Marshuetz, C., Koeppe, R. A., & Reuter-Lorenz, P. A. (1998). Inhibition in verbal working memory revealed by brain activation. *Proceedings of the National Academy of Sciences USA, 95*, 8410–8413.

Just, M. A., & Carpenter, P. A. (1992). A capacity theory of comprehension: Individual differences in working memory. *Psychological Review, 99*, 122–149.

Kane, M. J., & Engle, R. W. (2003). Working memory capacity and the control of attention: The contributions of goal neglect, response competition, and task set to Stroop interference. *Journal of Experimental Psychology: General, 132*, 47–70.

Kosslyn, S. M., Cacciopo, J. T., Davidson, R. J., Hugdahl, K., Lovallo, W. R., Spiegel, W. R., et al. (2002). Bridging psychology and biology: The analysis of individuals in groups. *American Psychologist, 57*, 341–351.

Lustig, C., May, C. P., & Hasher, L. (2001). Working memory span and the role of proactive interference. *Journal of Experimental Psychology: General, 130*, 199–207.

Miyake, A., Friedman, N. P., Emerson, M. J., Witzki, A. H., Howerter, A., & Wager, T. D. (2000). The unity and diversity of executive functions and their contributions to complex "frontal lobe" tasks: A latent variable analysis. *Cognitive Psychology, 41*, 49–100.

Miyake, A., Friedman, N. P., Rettinger, D. A., Shah, P., & Hegarty, M. (2001). How are visuo-spatial working memory, executive functioning, and spatial abilities related? A latent-variable analysis. *Journal of Experimental Psychology: General, 130*, 621–640.

Miyake, A., & Shah, P. (Eds.). (1999). *Models of working memory: Mechanisms of active maintenance and executive control.* New York: Cambridge University Press.

Munakata, Y. (2004). Computational cognitive neuroscience of early memory development. *Developmental Review, 24*, 133–153.

Oberauer, K., & Kliegl, R. (2001). Beyond resources: Formal models of complexity effects and age differences in working memory. *European Journal of Cognitive Psychology, 13*, 187–215.

Reuter-Lorenz, P. A., Marshuetz, C., Jonides, J., Smith, E. E., Hartley, A., & Koeppe, R. (2001). Neurocognitive ageing of storage and executive processes. *European Journal of Cognitive Psychology, 13*, 257–278.

Roberts, R. J., & Pennington, B. F. (1996). An interactive framework for examining prefrontal cognitive processes. *Developmental Neuropsychology, 12*, 105–126.

Saito, S., & Miyake, A. (2004). On the nature of forgetting and the processing-storage relationship in reading span performance. *Journal of Memory and Language, 50*, 425–443.

Towse, J. N., Hitch, G. J., & Hutton, U. (1998). A reevaluation of working memory capacity in children. *Journal of Memory and Language, 39*, 195–217.

Underwood, B. J. (1975). Individual differences as a crucible in theory construction. *American Psychologist, 30*, 128–134.

Acknowledgments

We would like to thank those who helped stage the Variation in Working Memory Conference held at the University of Illinois at Chicago, July 24–26, 2003.

Sponsors of that meeting included the following:

University of Illinois at Chicago, Department of Psychology

University of Illinois at Chicago, Office of the Vice Chancellor for Research

University of Illinois at Chicago, Center for the Study of Learning, Instruction, and Teacher Development

University of Colorado at Boulder, Department of Psychology

University of North Carolina at Greensboro, Department or Psychology

Jim Pellegrino (University of Illinois at Chicago) and Alan Baddeley (University of York) attended the conference and acted as discussants; they offered wise and constructive reflections on the contributions, and they helped to give a context and framework for the issues that emerged.

We thank Greg Colflesh for maintaining the Web site where drafts of chapters were made available for review and circulation.

The book has benefited from an extensive review process. Each of the contributors' chapters has been studied by relevant experts and by graduate students, as well as by the editorial team. They were asked to assess a chapter in terms of coherence and cogency, and they also had a specific brief to reflect on the readability of the work (for a non-expert audience), and the extent to which the text addressed the book questions. We are grateful to the following reviewers: Ivan Ash, Phil Beaman, Greg Colflesh, Rick Cooper, Margaret Cousins, Dale Dagenbach, Eddy Davelaar, Rik Henson, Elizabeth Jeffries, Robert Kail, Susan Kemper, Alycia Kubat-Silman, Monica Luciana, Denis Mareschal, Murray Maybery, Candice Morey, Tim Nokes, Harry Purser, Sarah Ransdell, Alastair Smith, Craig Thorley, and Geoff Ward.

In addition, the book benefited from important advice given by Nelson Cowan, who acted as an overall reviewer.

Assembling a volume with five editors and over 30 contributors has presented its own challenges, but it has also been fun. The ability to communicate by e-mail has been crucial; one editor alone has a collection of over 1700 messages connected with this book, and the camaraderie among the editors has helped to ensure the success of the project. In this context, we are grateful to Catharine Carlin at OUP for her steadfast belief in the idea from its beginning. We appreciate the work of all the OUP staff who have helped, especially Nancy Wolitzer, who has coordinated production.

Contents

PART III Working memory variation due to normal and pathological aging

Contributors

Donna M. Bayliss
School of Psychology
University of Western Australia
Crawley WA, Australia
E-mail: donna@psy.uwa.edu.au

Todd S. Braver
Department of Psychology
Washington University
St. Louis, MO
E-mail: tbraver@artsci.wustl.edu

Gregory C. Burgess
Department of Psychology
University of Colorado at Boulder
Boulder, CO
E-mail: greg.burgess@colorado.edu

David Caplan
Neuropsychological Laboratory
Massachusetts General Hospital
Boston, MA
E-mail: caplan@helix.mgh.harvard.edu

Andrew R. A. Conway
Department of Psychology
Princeton University
Princeton, NJ
E-mail: aconway@Princeton.edu

Gayle DeDe
Department of Communication Disorders
Sargent College of Health and
Rehabilitation Sciences
Boston University
Boston, MA
E-mail: gdede@bu.edu

Carolyn Dufault
Department of Psychology
Washington University
St. Louis, MO
E-mail: cdufault@wustl.edu

Lisa J. Emery
Department of Psychology
North Carolina State University
Raleigh, NC
E.mail: ljemery@ncsu.edu

Randall W. Engle
School of Psychology
Georgia Institute of Technology
Atlanta, GA
E-mail: re23@prism.gatech.edu

Jeremy R. Gray
Department of Psychology
Yale University
New Haven, CT
E-mail: jeremy.gray@yale.edu

Sandra Hale
Department of Psychology
Washington University
St. Louis, MO
E-mail: sshale@artsci.wustl.edu

David Z. Hambrick
Department of Psychology,
Michigan State University
East Lansing, MI
E-mail: hambric3@msu.edu

Lynn Hasher
Department of Psychology
University of Toronto
Toronto, Ontario, Canada
E-mail: hasher@psych.utoronto.ca

Graham J. Hitch
Department of Psychology
University of York
York, UK
E-mail: g.hitch@psychology.york.ac.uk

Christopher Jarrold
Department of Experimental
Psychology
University of Bristol
Bristol, UK
E-mail: C.Jarrold@bristol.ac.uk

John Jonides
Department of Psychology
University of Michigan
Ann Arbor, MI
E-mail:jjonides@umich.edu

Michael J. Kane
Department of Psychology
University of North Caroline at
Greensboro
Greensboro, NC
E-mail: mjkane@uncg.edu

Bonnie M. Lawrence
Department of Psychology
Case Western Reserve University
Cleveland, OH
E.mail: bonnie.Lawrence@case.edu

Cindy Lustig
Department of Psychology,
University of Michigan
Ann Arbor, MI
E-mail: clustig@umich.edu

Akira Miyake
Department of Psychology
University of Colorado at Boulder
Boulder, CO
E-mail: akira.miyake@colorado.edu

J. Bruce Morton
Department of Psychology
University of Western Ontario
London, Ontario, Canada.
E-mail: bmorton3@uwo.ca

Yuko Munakata
Department of Psychology
University of Colorado at Boulder
Boulder, CO
E-mail: munakata@psych.colorado.edu

Joel Myerson
Department of Psychology
Washington University
St. Louis, MO
E-mail: jmyerson@wustl.edu

Klaus Oberauer
Department of Experimental Psychology
University of Bristol
Bristol, UK
E-mail: K.Oberauer@bristol.ac.uk

Randall C. O'Reilly
Department of Psychology
University of Colorado at Boulder
Boulder, CO
E-mail: oreilly@psych.colorado.edu

Patricia A. Reuter-Lorenz
Department of Psychology
University of Michigan
Ann Arbor, MI
E-mail: parl@umich.edu

Nicolas Sander
University of Mannheim
Projekt Auswahlverfahren
Mannheim, Germany
E-mail: sander@tnt.psychologie
.uni-mannheim.de

Heinz-Martin Süß
Institute of Psychology
University of Magdeburg
Magdeburg, Germany
E-mail: heinz-martin.suess@gse-w.uni-
magdeburg.de

John N. Towse
Department of Psychology
Fylde College
Lancaster University
Lancaster, UK
E-mail: j.towse@lancaster.ac.uk

Gloria Waters
Department of Communication Disorders
Sargent College of Health and
Rehabilitation Sciences
Boston University
Boston, MA
E-mail: gwaters@bu.edu

Oliver Wilhelm
Institute of Psychology
Humboldt University Berlin
Berlin, Germany
E-mail: oliver.wilhelm@rz.hu-berlin.de

Rose Zacks
Department of Psychology
Michigan State University
East Lansing, MI
E-mail: ZacksR@msu.edu

VARIATION IN WORKING MEMORY

1

Variation in Working Memory: An Introduction

ANDREW R. A. CONWAY, CHRISTOPHER JARROLD,
MICHAEL J. KANE, AKIRA MIYAKE,
and JOHN N. TOWSE

Individual differences have been an annoyance rather than a challenge to the experimenter. His goal is to control behavior, and variation within treatments is proof that he has not succeeded. Individual variation is cast into that outer darkness known as "error variance." For reasons both statistical and philosophical, error variance is to be reduced by any possible device. . . . The correlational psychologist is in love with just those variables the experimenter left home to forget. He regards individual and group variation as important effects of biological and social causes. All organisms adapt to their environments, but not equally well. His question is: what present characteristics of the organism determine its mode and degree of adaptation? (Cronbach, 1957, p. 674)

Neither group nor individual differences research alone is sufficient; researchers need to combine the two. Indeed, by combining the two, one may discover that the group results reflect the combination of several strategies, each of which draws on a different (or partially different) system. Thus, the group and individual differences findings mutually inform each other, with the synergy be-

tween them illuminating the complex relations between psychology and biology. (Kosslyn et al., 2002, p. 348)

The ability to mentally maintain information in an active and readily accessible state, while concurrently and selectively processing new information, is one of the greatest accomplishments of the human mind; it makes possible planning, reasoning, problem solving, reading, and abstraction. Of course, some minds accomplish these goals with more success than do others. *Working memory* (WM) is the term that cognitive psychologists use to describe the ability to simultaneously maintain and process goal-relevant information. As the name implies, the WM concept reflects fundamentally a form of memory, but it is more than memory, for it is memory *at work*, in the service of complex cognition. As well, WM is a system with multiple components, or a collection of interrelated processes, that carries out several important cognitive functions. Most WM theories argue that the system comprises mechanisms devoted to the storage of information and mechanisms for cognitive control (see Miyake & Shah, 1999a). These mechanisms of active maintenance and executive control are thought to be involved in most complex cognitive behaviors and so WM has become a central construct in psychology.

A fundamental characteristic of WM is that it has a limited capacity, which constrains cognitive performance, such that individuals with greater capacity typically perform better than individuals with lesser capacity on a range of cognitive tasks. For example, older children have greater capacity than younger children, healthy adults have greater capacity than patients with frontal-lobe damage or disease, younger adults have greater capacity than elderly adults, and in all such cases, those individuals with greater WM capacity outperform individuals with lesser capacity in several important cognitive domains, including complex learning, reading and listening comprehension, and reasoning. In short, we know that variation in WM capacity exists and that this variation is important to everyday cognitive performance.

The central goal of this volume is to advance understanding of WM variation and its consequences. In recent years, several theories and empirically based arguments have been proposed to explain some form of inter- or intraindividual variation or another, yet no comprehensive account of variation in WM has emerged. Instead, the literature is cluttered with competing claims and data sets that are inadequate at leveraging support for one theory or another. This state of affairs is the result of several unfortunate, yet not surprising, aspects of research on WM variation. First, no consensus has yet emerged regarding nomothetic WM theories or models (see Miyake & Shah, 1999a), and so variation researchers start with different assumptions about what WM is, how it plays a role in complex cognition, and how best to measure its capacity. Second, variation researchers study a variety of subject populations—some are primarily interested in individual differences in young adults, others are interested in child development, while others are interested in cognitive aging, and so on. Not only does this create divisions within the WM literature, but it also complicates theories of variation because the

sources of variation in one research population may not be the same as the sources of variation in another. Third, specific investigations often entertain only one or two potential sources of WM variation, often pitting them against one another (e.g., processing speed vs. attentional inhibition), when many other mechanisms or processes are potentially at play. Finally, much of the research in this area has been plagued by poorly operationalized constructs, and so the mapping from constructs to mechanisms to measures is often weak.

In this book we take a more comprehensive look at variation in WM. Multiple models of WM are considered, data from different subject populations are presented, multiple sources of variation are discussed, and close attention is paid to the relation between constructs, mechanisms, and measurement. We hope that such a comprehensive, diversified approach to one common issue will result in both a convergence and a divergence of ideas. Ideally, some consensus can be achieved, while at the same time this synthesis of perspectives should illuminate current points of contention within the field, which should inspire investigation of the most important empirical and theoretical questions.

To properly contextualize the chapters that follow, this Introduction will begin with a brief historical overview of WM research, paying close attention to the role played by *variation research*, such as studies of individual differences, child development, aging, and neuropsychology. In that spirit, this chapter will also highlight the importance of combining the experimental and differential disciplines in psychology and the benefits of converging operations. Finally, we will introduce and discuss the four questions that were posed to each contributing research group in this volume.

HISTORICAL OVERVIEW

The concept of a limited-capacity immediate memory system has a long history in psychology. Ebbinghaus (1885/1964) reported that he could perfectly recall lists of 7 or fewer nonsense syllables upon a single presentation, but that lists of 8, 9, and 10 syllables required approximately 5, 9, and 12 repetitions, respectively (and the learning curve continued to grow steeply for still longer lists). However, in light of modern views that distinguish immediate memory from long-term memory, it is interesting that Ebbinghaus had so little to say about this dramatic finding. He certainly proposed no special mental state or faculty associated with immediate recall of short sequences.

Others soon did. In a review of Ebbinghaus's (1885/1964) book, Jacobs (1885) predicted that the objective study of memory would allow for the assessment of people's mental abilities: "If this be visionary, we may at least hope for much of interest and practical utility in the comparison of the varying powers of different minds which can now be laid down to scale" (p. 456). Moreover, in his subsequent call for the formation of a Society for Experimental Psychology, Jacobs (1886) cited Ebbinghaus's immediate-memory findings to argue that a high priority for psychology should be to understand variation in immediate memory:

There is, I submit, a certain number of syllables up to which each person can repeat a nonsense word like *borg-nap-fil-trip* after only once hearing; and it is probable, though we cannot know for certain, that this number varies with different persons, giving a sort of test of their linguistic capacity. . . . But this law, if it is a law, has at present only been deduced from the observation of one man's mind, and is therefore obviously not a law of mind in general, but at best a law of Dr. Ebbinghaus's mind. (p. 53)

The following year, Jacobs (1887) reported the first empirical paper on the memory span task and one of the first systematic individual-differences studies of memory. Students between the ages of 8 and 20 years were presented with lists of auditory nonsense syllables, letters, or digits to repeat. The largest set that each student perfectly reproduced was termed his or her *span of prehension*. Jacobs found that span increased not only with chronological age but also with higher school grades. In a supplemental report to Jacobs, Galton (1887) noted that the spans among institutionalized children and young adults (then classified as "idiots") were quite limited, averaging only three to four

items. The capacity of immediate memory, as reflected by prehension span, thus appeared to be a source of intellectual ability:

Under these circumstances we might expect that "span of prehension" should be an important factor in determining mental grasp, and its determination one of the tests of mental capacity. (Jacobs, 1887, p. 79)

Following such reports, it may not be surprising that span tasks soon became a part of intelligence test batteries (e.g., Binet & Simon, 1905; Burt, 1909; Cattell & Galton, 1890; Ebbinghaus, 1897). At about the same time, William James (1890) drew a theoretical distinction between "primary" memory and "secondary" memory, or memory proper. According to James, primary memory is equated with the current contents of consciousness and the "rearward portion of the present space of time," and therefore suffers from a severe capacity limit. Secondary memory, in contrast, is thought to consist of memories of the distant past and to be unlimited in capacity. James Mark Baldwin (1894), who was jointly influenced by Wundt's experimental psychology (see below) and Darwin's theory of evolution, similarly argued that immediate memory is capacity limited and that the development of this capacity is central to the development of intelligence and cognitive abilities.

But what did this capacity represent? Although span tasks clearly required remembering and were soon referred to as "memory span" tasks (e.g., Bennett, 1916; Humpstone, 1917), and although James used the phrase "primary memory" to describe the underlying construct, it is quite clear that most early theorists considered the span task to reflect the contents of consciousness or the capacity of *attention*. Jacobs (1887, p.79) described it as an index of what could be "taken on" by the mind. Cattell and Galton (1890, p. 377) considered the span task to test "memory and attention." Bolton (1892) argued that span tested "the power of concentrated and sustained attention" (p. 364), and Humpstone (1919) viewed it as "the ability to grasp a number of discrete units in a single moment of attention." In Wundt's classic (1912/1973) text, he viewed the span of memory and the span of apprehension as reflecting a common limit to focus of attention, thus foreshadowing Miller's (1956) famous haunting by the magical number 7 as a general limit to cognitive capacity.[1] Moreover, much like the modern theory of Cowan (1988, 1995, 2001), Wundt used the findings from span tasks to argue for a limited-capacity attentional focus of six or fewer impressions (termed *apperception*), and a larger and more variably limited "field of consciousness" (termed *apprehension*).

The historical perspectives we have discussed thus far can all be categorized as "capacity" theories of immediate memory, for each of them embraced, to one degree or another, the notion of an "amount" of information that can be actively maintained at once (for a review, see Blankenship, 1938). Other, subsequent theorists offered time-based or interference-based perspectives on the limits on immediate memory, and so they also more firmly brought "memory span" from the conceptual realm of attention into that of memory (see Cowan, 1995). For example, Hebb (1949) introduced the concept of transient "cell assemblies" by which incoming stimuli form a distributed pattern of activation across neurons that quickly dissipates with time, resulting in the quick loss of information. Similarly, Thorndike (1914) proposed the "law of disuse," arguing that memories are quickly lost over time if they are not used, or retrieved. McGeoch (1932), partly in rejection of Thorndike, argued that memory traces do not decay over time but become unavailable for retrieval due to the forces of retroactive and proactive interference. In fact, McGeoch and subsequent interference theorists argued that there is no distinction between immediate memory and other forms of memory and so the quest to understand the capacity of immediate memory is misguided (Crowder, 1982; Melton, 1963; Nairne, 2002).

Neuropsychological case studies, however, do suggest a distinction between short-term and long-term memory. Perhaps the most famous of these investigations involve the temporal lobectomy patient H.M., who demonstrated normal short-term memory capacity but was unable to form new long-term memories (Milner, 1966). The opposite pattern of deficits has also been demonstrated, i.e., normal long-term memory performance accompanied by verbal short-term memory deficits (Baddeley & Warrington, 1970; Shallice & Warrington, 1970; Warrington, Logue, & Pratt, 1971). Patients with long-term memory damage, such as H.M., typically have acquired damage to temporal-lobe structures, such as the hippocampus, whereas patients with short-term memory damage typically suffer from more frontal and left parietal damage, suggesting different memory systems for the short- and long-term retention of information.

Despite the obvious influences upon, and connections to, contemporary research on WM, most of the references we have discussed so far actually predate the introduction of the concept of WM to the field of psychology. The first reference to WM memory, as it is conceived today, was in the influential book *Plans and the Structure of Behavior* (Miller, Galanter, & Pribram, 1960).[2] In sharp contrast to the behavioral psychologists that came before them, Miller et al. argued that a theory was needed to capture the processes that occur *between* the presentation of a stimulus and the execution of a response. In their terms, they were interested in how knowledge is translated into action. They argued that human beings are capable of forming, hierarchically structuring, and executing *plans*. Importantly, plans were considered to be internal knowledge representations that could be retrieved, or activated, *into* WM. According to Miller et al.,

> When we have decided to execute some particular Plan, it is probably put into some special state or place where it can be remembered while it is being executed. Particularly if it is a transient, temporary kind of plan that will be used today and never again, we need some special place to store it. The special place may be a sheet of paper. Or (who knows?) it may be somewhere in the frontal lobes of the brain. Without committing ourselves to any specific machinery, we should like to speak of the memory we use for the execution of our Plans as a kind of quick-access, "working memory." (p. 65)

The connection between this definition of WM and earlier concepts of capacity-limited immediate memory is obvious,[3] yet it also represents an important departure. Note two key phrases in the passage: a "special state or place where it [a plan] can be remembered while it is being executed," and "the memory we use for the execution of our Plans." These phrases imply a unique system responsible not only for the storage of plans but also for their implementation. Prior discussions of a limited-capacity immediate memory system generally emphasized storage more than anything else. Here, the emphasis is on storage and processing in the service of a complex cognitive goal.

While *Plans, and the Structure of Behavior* can be credited with the first mention of WM, Baddeley and Hitch (1974) are duly credited with launching the empirical investigation of WM that continues today. Baddeley and Hitch famously started their seminal chapter with the following complaint:

> Despite more than a decade of intensive research on the topic of short-term memory (STM), we still know virtually nothing about its role in normal human information processing. (p. 47)

Baddeley and Hitch acknowledged that a considerable amount of important research had been conducted to address fundamental questions about STM itself, such as how information is coded in STM (Conrad, 1964; Conrad & Hull, 1964; Wickelgren, 1966), what the capacity of STM is (Miller, 1956; Waugh & Norman, 1965), how information is retrieved from STM (Sternberg, 1966, 1969), and whether forgetting from STM is due to decay or interference (Brown, 1958; Keppel & Underwood, 1962; Petersen & Petersen, 1959; Reitman, 1971, 1974; Waugh & Norman, 1965). However, they also lamented the fact that very little research had addressed the role of STM in more complex cognitive behavior. This was indeed a strange state of affairs, especially considering the primary role granted to STM in the most influential information-processing models of the time (e.g., Atkinson & Shiffrin, 1968; Broadbent, 1958).

Baddeley and Hitch proposed a multicomponent WM model that consisted of domain-specific storage buffers (later referred to as the

"slave systems"; Baddeley, 1986) as well as a central executive. They provided empirical evidence from dual-task studies showing that the mental juggling required by complex cognitive behaviors, such as reasoning, can be achieved by coordinated storage and processing between the slave systems and the central executive. A certain amount of information can be held at bay in the slave systems while the executive works on new information.

As the influence of the Baddeley and Hitch study took hold in the late 1970s, a related thread of research started to emerge from developmental psychology (see Case, 1978; Pascual-Leone, 1970). Particularly relevant here is the work of Robbie Case (1978, 1985) on the development of memory capacity in young children. Like Baddeley and Hitch (1974), he conceived of a limited-capacity mental workspace that was required in the service of complex cognition. He referred to this mental workspace as *M-space* and argued that the development of M-space is essential to the development of cognitive abilities in general. Importantly, Case developed an objective measure of M-space, called the *counting span task* (see Case, Kurland, & Goldberg, 1982). In the task, children are presented with displays (index cards in the original version) consisting of an array of colored objects (e.g., green and yellow circles) and are instructed to count a particular object-type (e.g., green circles) and remember the count-total for later recall. A number of displays are presented in succession and at the end of the series the child is expected to recall all the count-totals in that series. This task is thought to tap M-space, or WM capacity, because it requires storage (remember the digits) in the face of processing (count the objects in the display).

Daneman and Carpenter (1980) developed a similar task to measure WM capacity in adults. In their *reading span task*, the subject is presented with sentences and must read each sentence aloud and remember the last word of the sentence for later recall. After a series of sentences the subject is expected to recall all the sentence-end words. Thus, like counting span, the reading span task requires storage (remember the words) in the face of concurrent processing (read the sentences aloud). Importantly, Daneman and Carpenter (1980) demonstrated that scores on the reading span task predicted measures of reading comprehension better than span tasks that did not have the secondary processing component (e.g., simple word span).

Several WM span tasks have been developed over the years (see Kane et al., 2004; Shah & Miyake, 1996; Turner & Engle, 1989) and they consistently show better predictive validity with respect to complex cognitive behaviors, such as reasoning, reading comprehension, and problem solving, than do simple span tasks thought to just tap the capacity of a short-term store, à la Miller (1956). In this respect, WM span tasks are thought to be a success. That is, they say something about how well people perform real-world cognitive tasks and they explain real-world variation in performance. Working-memory span tasks therefore directly address the frustration evident in the Baddeley and Hitch (1974) quote above.

In addition, the development of tasks designed specifically for the measurement of WM capacity allowed for a surge in variation research. WM span tasks, and similar measures of WM function, have now been extensively used to examine individual differences in cognitive abilities in young adults, the development of WM and cognitive functioning in children, the declines in cognitive performance associated with aging, and the deficits experienced by patients with brain damage or disease.

Despite this progress, several important questions remain and the chapters in this book will address them. For instance, it still is not entirely clear why WM span tasks, such as counting span and reading span, predict complex cognitive behavior better than simple span tasks do. Furthermore, the relation between span tasks and other measures of WM (such as the "n-back" task, used often in neuroimaging studies) has not been properly investigated. As a result, the mechanisms underlying performance of these tasks are not completely understood. Finally, and most imperative here, the sources of variation in WM performance—among children, among healthy young adults, among the elderly, and among patients—have not been identified, hence the need for a comprehensive review of current research on WM variation.

VARIATION

> The approach proposed here, the approach which makes individual-differences variables crucibles in theory construction, will identify the process variables as a fallout from nomothetic theory construction. (Underwood, 1975, p. 134)

All of the research presented in the subsequent chapters is influenced by classic experimental psychology; indeed, many sophisticated experimental manipulations are presented and discussed. At the same time, each of these chapters takes seriously and attempts to provide a theoretical account of variation in performance. This combination of experimental and differential psychology is an answer to Cronbach's (1957) largely unheeded call for a unification of "the two disciplines of scientific psychology." Cronbach argued that a comprehensive account of human behavior could only be achieved through the synergy of experimental and differential approaches to studying psychology. He claimed:

> A true federation of the disciplines is required. Kept independent, they can only give wrong answers or no answers at all regarding certain important problems. It is shortsighted to argue for one science to discover the general laws of mind or behavior and for a separate enterprise concerned with individual minds. (p. 673)

Sadly, despite Cronbach's call for unification, most experimental psychologists still disregard individual differences as error variance; indeed, a similar plea for integration was deemed necessary, yet again, this decade (Kosslyn et al., 2002). A perusal of most mainstream cognitive psychology and neuroscience journals will reveal that individual differences analyses are still few and far between. Even more rare are studies that successfully combine experimental and differential approaches as Cronbach suggested. Fortunately, the contributors to this volume are a welcome exception.

These contributors recognize that individual-differences data can be used in combination with experimental data to test theories and suggest hypotheses (Kosslyn et al., 2002; Underwood, 1975). More specifically, most models or theories of WM make either explicit or implicit claims about individual differences in performance and therefore a differential approach can provide supportive or problematic data for a theory, whether that theory concerns primarily behavioral or neural mechanisms. As this volume attests, the strategy of exploiting individual differences to test theory can of course be applied beyond individual differences in healthy adults, but also to normal and atypical development and aging, and even to interspecies variation.

As well, an understanding of how experimental manipulations impact individual differences can lead to better measurement of psychological constructs. Bindra and Scheier (1954) called upon psychometricians to make use of experimental design for this reason:

> The knowledge of what experimental conditions do change a property may enable the psychometrician to control such conditions in future measurements of that property, and it also may lead to the discovery of new properties not affected by these conditions. Thus, the use of experimental variation in psychometric research may be of considerable help both in making psychometric measurement more exact, that is, reliable, and in suggesting ways of experimentally changing the organism's "invariant" properties. (Bindra & Scheier, 1954, p. 70)

In sum, investigations of variation benefit both the experimentalist and the psychometrician. Theories of the general laws of mind and behavior are enhanced by a consideration of individual-differences data, and individual-differences investigations are enhanced by knowledge of experimental outcomes.

CONVERGING OPERATIONS

> The necessary condition which makes possible the determination of particular characteristics of any concept . . . is the use of what have been called converging operations. Converging operations may be thought of as any set of two or more experimental operations which allow the selection or elimination of alternative hypotheses or concepts

which could explain an experimental result. They are called converging operations because they are not perfectly correlated and thus can converge on a single concept. (Garner, Hake, & Eriksen, 1956, pp. 150–151)

One of the primary strengths of each of the research groups contributing to this volume is their use of converging operations to test hypotheses and compare theories. Rather than rely on one particular methodological approach, such as computational modeling, neuroimaging, or structural equation modeling, each of the research programs represented here employs a combination of methods. Some combine imaging and modeling, others combine imaging and patient data, still others combine multivariate statistical techniques and modeling, and so on. Just as Underwood (1975) recognized the theoretical leverage to be gained from a consideration of individual-differences data, the contributing chapters illustrate the force of argument gained by considering data garnered from different methodological approaches. For example, jointly considering neuroimaging and neuropsychological data yields at least two benefits:

> (1) Neuroimaging and neuropsychological studies should provide converging information about the locus of brain regions that contribute to a particular task; failures to find convergence can direct attention to new brain regions and cognitive processes that contribute to task performance, and they can provide important challenges to the theoretical assumptions of each methodology; and (2) . . . neuroimaging and neuropsychology should provide converging information about associations and dissociations between tasks; failures to find convergence can direct attention to alternative theoretical accounts of cognition, while unexpected associations can direct attention to cognitive processes that cross traditional domains of study. (Fiez, 2001, p.20)

As another example, consider the benefits of using computational modeling to complement behavioral work:

> Such models can be crucial for helping us to understand complex, nonlinear interactions of the

sort that characterize brain–behavior relations. Moreover, such models assist in theory comparison and evaluation by requiring theories to be specific and plausible enough that they can lead to working models, and by generating testable predictions. For these reasons and others, many researchers argue that such modeling work is essential for advancing theorizing about cognitive functioning. (Munakata, Morton, & O'Reilly, Chapter 7, this volume)

Similar statements can be made about other combinations of methodologies as well. Generally speaking, the more converging operations the better. Sternberg and Grigorenko (2001, p. 1069) recently referred to this approach as "unified psychology," which is "the multiparadigmatic, multidisciplinary, and integrated study of psychological phenomena through converging operations." Sternberg and Grigorenko argue that the vast majority of contemporary psychologists are specialists and fail to consider research questions from multiple perspectives. They further argue that such specialization thwarts real progress in psychological science and produces scientists who might be productive but not provocative in their research.

The project presented here is an attempt to put WM variation in the crosshairs of unified psychology. Across the subsequent chapters, multiple paradigms are presented, converging operations are used to test and contrast theories, and scientists from different subdisciplines are required to address a common set of theoretical questions. Furthermore, the common set of questions forces each contributing research group to consider the responses of the other contributors, thus enhancing the degree of integration across chapters. It is to this set of shared questions that we now turn our attention.

THE FOUR DESIGNATED QUESTIONS FOR THIS VOLUME

Each contributing research group was asked to address the same set of important theoretical questions in an attempt to make plain the basic tenets that guide their current research on WM

variation. Through these common questions, each research group explicitly addressed the theories and subject populations at the focus of "competing" research programs, presented in this volume's other chapters.

By adopting this common-question approach, we are following the successful example set by Miyake and Shah (1999a). In their edited book, *Models of Working Memory: Mechanisms of Active Maintenance and Executive Control*, each contributing research group addressed eight theoretical questions about their particular model or theory of WM. We believe that this is an extremely fruitful approach because it allows the reader to compare and contrast alternative answers to the same questions, in turn allowing for a synthesis of information across chapters. This is especially helpful for students, or researchers new to the field, who are struggling to understand fundamental differences and similarities among competing or complementary theories.

QUESTION 1: OVERARCHING THEORY OF WORKING MEMORY

What is the theory or definition of working memory that guides your research on working memory variation? Miyake and Shah (1999) demonstrated that there are currently at least a dozen nomothetic theories of WM that are competing in the intellectual marketplace. Our first question therefore encourages each contributing research group to articulate their theoretical framework and to make explicit any fundamental assumptions that underlie their approach. As it turns out, some aspects of different models that might appear at to be odds with one another at first glance are actually compatible (Kintsch, Healy, Hegarty, Pennington, & Salthouse, 1999; Miyake & Shah, 1999b). Other aspects of different models, however, are indeed in opposition to one another. By making explicit the fundamental aspects of different definitions of WM, these points of convergence and divergence will more easily be revealed. Most current theories of WM differ in their approach to a limited number of key issues, which we address in turn below.

Cognitive Control

One of the most contentious issues with respect to WM is the nature of cognitive control and the characterization of the "central executive." Several of the current chapters eschew the notion of a central executive altogether in favor of models that view cognitive control as an emergent property of a dynamic interactive network (see Chapters 3, 4, and 7). For example, Munakata et al. (Chapter 7) claim that their model "has the elements in place for a fully self-contained theory of both maintenance and control of WM, without relying on unexplained 'homunculi' such as a central executive." Other chapters seem to accept at face value the existence of a central executive in their model of WM, perhaps revealing the influence of the original Baddeley and Hitch (1974; Baddeley, 1986) model (see Chapters 8 and 11). Still others place executive processes and attention at the center of their research program, thus not eliminating an "executive" system, but also not accepting the original conception of a central executive (see Chapters 2, 5, 6, 9, and 10).

Unitary vs. Multifaceted Approach

Each of the WM models endorsed in this book embraces the idea that WM is a multicomponent system, or that it represents a multiplicity of mental and neurological processes, including interactive mechanisms of information storage and cognitive control. As well, each chapter recognizes the contribution to WM function of both domain-general and domain-specific processes. However, the chapters differ in the extent to which they take a unitary or a multifaceted approach to the characterization of variation in WM and with respect to their emphasis on domain-general vs. domain-specific sources of variation in performance. For example, Braver et al. (Chapter 4), Hasher et al. (Chapter 9), Kane et al. (Chapter 2), and Munakata et al. (Chapter 7) take primarily a unitary approach, their emphasis being on domain-general mechanisms of cognitive control. In contrast, Hale et al. (Chapter 8), Jarrold and Bayliss (Chapter 6), and Caplan et al. (Chapter 11) take a much more multifaceted approach, elucidating all the components of the WM system and suggesting multiple sources of variation in performance.

The Nature of Capacity Limitations in Working Memory

Each of the chapters recognizes that WM is a limited-capacity system. However, the chapters differ in how they conceptualize this limit. Some models are consistent with the original notion of capacity, as an amount of information (e.g., Jacobs, 1887; Miller, 1956; Woodworth, 1938; Wundt, 1912/1973). For example, Oberauer et al. (Chapter 3) argue that *capacity* refers to the number of simultaneous bindings of independent chunks of information that can be achieved at once. Other researchers attribute the capacity limitation to an "attentional" system, such as executive attention (Kane et al., Chapter 2) or attentional inhibition (Hasher et al., Chapter 9). Others argue that the capacity limit is simply a natural property of a highly interactive biological system (Braver et al., Chapter 4; Munakata et al., Chapter 7; Reuter-Lorenz & Jonides, Chapter 10). Yet another set of researchers advocates the notion of a limited pool of "resources" available for the storage and processing of information (Hale et al., Chapter 8; Jarrold & Bayliss, Chapter 6; Towse & Hitch, Chapter 5).

QUESTION 2: CRITICAL SOURCES OF WORKING MEMORY VARIATION

What is your view on the critical source(s) of working memory variation within your target population(s) of study? Why do you focus on the particular source(s) of variation in your research? This is perhaps the most central question of the four and is the one that motivated the current volume. Here we ask each contributing chapter to specify a theoretical proposal about the nature of variation in WM in some target population(s). Several different theoretical sources of variation are proposed throughout the book, including mental speed (Hale et al., Chapter 8); attentional inhibition (Hasher et al., Chapter 9); reduction in the fidelity of memory when engaged in process-ing (Towse & Hitch, Chapter 5); executive atten-tion processes of goal maintenance and conflict resolution (Kane et al., Chapter 2); the isolation and strength of representations (Munakata et al., Chapter 7); the capacity of simultaneous binding of independent chunks (Oberauer et al., Chapter 3); the relative contributions of proactive and reactive cognitive control (Braver et al., Chapter 4); and the nature of domain-specific content (Jarrold & Bayliss, Chapter 6; Reuter-Lorenz & Jonides, Chapter 10). Some of these proposals are more in agreement than others. For example, there are rather subtle differences between Kane et al.'s executive attention, Hasher et al.'s atten-tional inhibition, and Braver et al.'s proactive control. Yet there are substantial differences here as well. In particular, Hale et al.'s speed account, Oberauer et al.'s binding theory, and the multi-ple attentional approaches mentioned above are certainly at odds with one another.

The chapters also differ with respect to whe-ther they view WM variation as coming from primarily one source or multiple sources. Some chapters clearly argue in favor of the notion that there is a primary source, such as executive at-tention (Chapter 2), attentional inhibition (Chap-ter 9), or binding (Chapter 3), while others argue for multiple sources of variation, all of equal importance (Chapters 6 and 10).

QUESTION 3: CONSIDERATION OF OTHER SOURCES OF WORKING MEMORY VARIATION

Do you find other sources of working memory variation proposed in this book to be applicable to your target population of study? Are these sources of working memory variation compatible or incompatible with your view of your target population? The purpose of posing this ques-tion was to encourage each contributing re-search group to carefully consider sources of WM variation proposed by "competing" con-tributors to this volume. This question addresses our concern that research in this area is too often narrowly focused on a single construct or mech-anism. This question also requires researchers to consider directly the sources of variation in re-

search populations other than their own. That is, the main sources of variation in WM may differ across subject populations. For instance, it is possible that processing speed accounts for more variation in the development of WM in children than it does in variation among healthy young adults (see Chapters 2 and 8). As well, it is possible that abnormalities in domain-specific memory representations may account for more variation among patient populations than among normals (see Chapter 6). Similarly, strategic allocation of resources may account for varia-tion associated with aging more than it does for normal variation among younger adults (see Chapters 2 and 10). In essence, the subsequent chapters unmistakably illustrate that there is no single source (mechanism, process, or resource) that can account for all WM variation.

QUESTION 4: CONTRIBUTIONS TO GENERAL WORKING MEMORY THEORY

What does the variability within your target pop-ulation of study tell us about the structure, func-tion, and/or organization of working memory in general? How has the investigation of variation contributed to WM theory in general? As the question implies, variation research has contrib-uted to knowledge about the structure of WM and its role in successful complex cognition. In terms of structure, experimental, psychometric, neuroimaging, and neuropsychological data have supported (1) the distinction between a memory system responsible for retention of information in the short term and a system responsible for long-term retention, and (2) domain-specific as well as domain-general components of the WM system. In terms of function, variation researchers have made several important discoveries about when and where WM does and does not play a role in other cognitive processes or functions (see Chap-ters 2 and 11).

Variation research has also exposed the dif-ficulty in operationalizing psychological con-structs and the importance of measurement to any scientific pursuit. Psychometric studies in particular (Chapters 2, 3, and 11) have dem-onstrated the importance of having valid and reliable measures of WM functioning. Similarly, neuropsychological, developmental, and aging studies have demonstrated that validity and reliability can vary across research populations—i.e., a measure that is valid and reliable for one group of subjects may not be for another group of subjects.

ORGANIZATION OF THE BOOK

The book is organized into three parts pertaining to the type of WM variation under investigation. The first part is devoted to variation reflected by normal inter- and intra-individual differences. The second part covers variation due to normal and atypical development and the third section reviews variation due to normal and pathological aging. As a result of this organizational structure, chapters within a part tend to have more in common with each other than do chapters across sections. However, there are several points of contact across parts as well. For example, Kane et al.'s approach to individual differences in young adults has much in common with Hasher et al.'s theory of cognitive aging. Also, Munakata et al.'s developmental work has a great deal of theoretical overlap with Braver et al.'s program of research on young adults. Readers will undoubtedly discover more subtle points of convergence across chapters as well. Below we review the key points made by subsequent chapters.

Working-Memory Variation Reflecting Normal Inter- and Intra-individual Differences

The first part deals primarily with individual differences in young adults. Perhaps due to the influence of Daneman and Carpenter (1980), or perhaps because college students are more readily available as research subjects than children, the elderly, or neuropsychological patients, investigations of individual differences in young adults have dominated the variation landscape for the last two and a half decades (see Miyake, 2001). In Chapter 2, Kane et al. present their executive-attention theory of WM capacity, which is largely based on investigations of individual differences in WM capacity among healthy young adults. Kane et al. argue for multiple sources of variation in performance of WM tasks, including domain-specific skills and strategies as well as a domain–general attention capability. It is this latter attention factor, they argue, that accounts for the predictive validity of WM span tasks and drives the strong relationship between WM capacity and a range of important cognitive abilities, including general fluid intelligence. In Chapter 3, Oberauer et al. review their psychometric research on WM and reasoning ability. From this work they argue that individual differences in WM capacity are primarily driven by a general factor and this factor is strongly related to reasoning. They further argue that the mechanism underlying this general ability is a mechanism that simultaneously binds independent chunks of information in the focus of attention. They also argue that some measures of executive function, such as task-set switching, are not related to WM capacity, and therefore conclude that WM capacity cannot be equated with executive attention. Chapter 4 presents Braver et al.'s dual-mechanism theory, according to which there are two modes of cognitive control: proactive and reactive. They argue that performance in most cognitive tasks involves a mixture of these two modes of control and that individual differences in WM capacity may be associated with the extent to which subjects are able to engage proactive control and/or the extent to which they are able to efficiently move from one mode of control to another.

Working Memory Variation Due to Normal and Atypical Development

The second part is primarily concerned with the development of WM capacity. As mentioned above, the investigation into the development of immediate memory has a long history in psychology, dating back to the work of Jacobs (1887) and Baldwin (1894), and was continued by prominent developmental psychologists, such as Pascual-Leone (1970) and Case (1985). The chapters in this section follow in that tradition.

Specifically, in Chapter 5, Towse and Hitch consider in some detail contemporary theoretical accounts of the development of children's

WM capacity. They review data that have led them to propose their own view of WM in children; their task-switching model emphasizes the temporal dynamics of span tasks, and they argue that there are multiple sources of variation in WM. Moreover, they attempt to illustrate how experimental data can be used in conjunction with the analysis of individual differences to marshal theoretical arguments, i.e., how each approach can complement the other. In Chapter 6, Jarrold and Bayliss look at the constraints on performance in the complex-span paradigm, to determine the causes of individual and developmental differences in WM. They present evidence to suggest that both storage capacity and processing efficiency are separable determinants of WM performance, and that a third, potentially executive, source of variance arises from the need to combine these two requirements of the complex span task. They go on to argue that variation in rate of reactivation of to-be-remembered material and variation in speed of processing underlie the first two of these constraints, and that the third may reflect variation in the rate at which individuals forget information while occupied by processing activities. In Chapter 7, Munakata et al. present a biologically plausible computational model to account for the development of WM and cognitive control in young children. They focus their work on the complementary processes of maintenance and updating and argue that these simple processes can account for a range of phenomena related to WM (e.g., "executive" processes, such as inhibition). In Chapter 8, Hale et al. review a long line of research on the development of cognitive abilities in children and adolescents. According to their perspective, mental processing speed accounts for a large portion of developmental variance in WM, and the development of more efficient (i.e., faster) processes in turn results in greater capacity.

Working Memory Variation Due to Normal and Pathological Aging

The third part covers variation due to aging. In Chapter 9, Hasher et al. present an "inhibitory" view of cognitive aging and WM. According to their perspective, performance on tasks designed to measure WM is largely influenced by an individual's ability to cope with the effects of proactive interference. Hasher et al. argue that individuals differ in a general inhibitory ability to cope with interference. This ability accounts for a large portion of developmental and intraindividual variance, and is a primary source of WM variation in general. In Chapter 10, Reuter-Lorenz and Jonides emphasize the role of the executive processes in all measures of immediate memory and argue that the distinction between measures of storage only and storage + processing is overstated. They take a multifaceted approach to the sources of variation in WM associated with age and argue that several factors are at play. Specifically, they illustrate how the elderly may allocate resources differently than younger adults as they perform tests of WM. In Chapter 11, Caplan et al. review their work on the relation between WM capacity and language comprehension. Based on evidence of a disconnect between traditional measures of WM and critical aspects of comprehension, such as the assignment of syntactic structure, Caplan et al. argue against a general factor in WM (cf., Kane et al., Chapter 2; Oberauer et al., Chapter 3). Instead, they consider the role that long-term memory plays in the performance of WM and suggest skill and experience as potential sources of variation in WM (cf., Ericsson & Delaney, 1999).

In summary, the ability to process new information while simultaneously holding onto the previous results of processing is essential in many domains of higher-level cognition, such as language comprehension and production, mental arithmetic, spatial thinking, complex reasoning, and problem solving. The cognitive mechanism that supports this essential human capability is WM. Reflecting its important role in human cognition, WM has become a central topic in cognitive psychology, cognitive science, and cognitive neuroscience. In this volume we explore variation in WM, broadly construed to include individual differences in healthy adults, age-related changes due to normal development and aging, and the effects of cognitive pathologies. We hope that this diversified approach, which unites the experimental and differential approaches to psychology and uses the philosophy of converging operations, will result in a more comprehensive account of variation in WM.

Notes

1. The *span of apprehension* refers to the number of simultaneously presented stimuli, as opposed to sequentially presented stimuli, that a person can mentally grasp.

2. At least this seems to be the first use of the phrase "working memory." A similar idea was expressed earlier by Johnson (1955):

> Whatever the items of the problem to be organized, manipulated, or otherwise dealt with, there is a limit to the number of separate items that can be thus grasped, retained, and manipulated, and that limit is the span of immediate memory. If remote memory is the storehouse of ideas, immediate memory is the workshop wherein ideas are processed. (p. 82)

3. Indeed, 4 years earlier, Miller (1956) published his famous *Psychological Review* report on memory capacity, and all three of these authors were largely influenced by James and Woodworth, among others.

References

Atkinson, R. C., & Shiffrin, R. M. (1971). The control of short-term memory. *Scientific American, 225,* 82–90.

Baddeley, A. D. (1986). *Working memory.* New York: Oxford University Press.

Baddeley, A. D., & Hitch, G. (1974). Working memory. In G. H. Bower (Ed.), *The psychology of learning and motivation: Advances in research and theory* (Vol. 8, pp. 47–89). New York: Academic Press.

Baddeley, A. D., & Warrington, E. K. (1970). Amnesia and the distinction between long- and short-term memory. *Journal of Verbal Learning and Verbal Behavior, 9,* 176–189.

Baldwin, J. M. (1894). *Mental development in the child and the race.* New York: Macmillan.

Bennett, F. (1916). The correlations between different memories. *Journal of Experimental Psychology, 1,* 404–418.

Bindra, D., & Scheier, I. H. (1954). The relation between psychometric and experimental research in psychology. *American Psychologist, 9,* 69–71.

Binet, A., & Simon, T. (1905). Méthodes nouvelles pour le diagnostic du niveau intellectuel des anormaux. *L'Année Psychologique, 11,* 191–244.

Blankenship, A. B. (1938). Memory span: A review of the literature. *Psychological Bulletin, 35,* 1–25.

Bolten, T. L. (1892). The growth of memory in school children. *American Journal of Psychology, 4,* 362–380.

Broadbent, D. E. (1958). *Perception and communication.* New York: Pergamon Press.

Brown, J. (1958). Some tests of the decay theory of immediate memory. *Quarterly Journal of Experimental Psychology, 10,* 12–21.

Burt, C. (1909). Experimental tests of general intelligence. *British Journal of Psychology, 3,* 94–177.

Case, R. (1978). Intellectual development from birth to adulthood: A neo-Piagetian interpretation. In R. S. Siegler (Ed.), *Children's thinking: What develops?* (pp. 37–71). Hillsdale, NJ: Lawrence Erlbaum Associates.

Case, R. (1985). *Intellectual development: Birth to adulthood.* New York: Academic Press.

Case, R., Kurland, M. D., & Goldberg, J. (1982). Operational efficiency and the growth of short-term memory span. *Journal of Experimental Child Psychology, 33,* 386–04.

Cattell, J. M., & Galton, F. (1890). Mental tests and measurements. *Mind, 15,* 373–381.

Conrad, R. (1964). Acoustic confusion in immediate memory. *British Journal of Psychology, 55,* 75–84.

Conrad, R., & Hull, A. J. (1964). Information, acoustic information and memory span. *British Journal of Psychology, 55,* 429–432.

Cowan, N. (1988). Evolving conceptions of memory storage, selective attention, and their mutual constraints within the human information processing system. *Psychological Bulletin, 104,* 163–191.

Cowan, N. (1995). *Attention and memory: An integrated framework.* Oxford, UK: Oxford University Press.

Cowan, N. (2001). The magical number 4 in short-term memory: A reconsideration of mental storage capacity. *Behavioral and Brain Sciences, 24,* 87–185.

Cronbach, L. J., (1957). The two disciplines of scientific psychology. *American Psychologist, 12,* 671–684.

Crowder, R. G. (1982). The demise of short-term memory. *Acta Psychologica, 50,* 291–323.

Daneman, M., & Carpenter, P. A. (1980). Individual differences in working memory and reading. *Journal of Verbal Learning and Verbal Behavior, 19,* 450–466.

Ebbinghaus, H. (1885/1964). *Memory: A contribution to experimental psychology.* New York: Dover Publications, Inc.

Ericsson, K. A., & Delaney, P. (1999). Long-term working memory as an alternative to capacity models of working memory in everyday skilled performance. In A. Miyake & P. Shah (Eds.), *Models of working memory: Mechanisms of active maintenance and executive control* (pp. 257–297). New York: Cambridge University Press.

Fiez, J. A. (2001). Bridging the gap between neuroimaging and neuropsychology: Challenges and potential benefits. *Journal of Clinical and Experimental Neuropsychology, 23,* 19–31.

Galton, F. (1887). Supplementary notes on "prehension" in idiots. *Mind, 12,* 79–82.

Garner, W. R., Hake, H. W., & Eriksen, C. W. (1956). Operationism and the concept of perception. *Psychological Review, 63,* 149–159.

Hebb, D. O. (1949). *Organization of behavior.* New York: Wiley.

Humpstone, H. J. (1917). *Some aspects of the memory span test: A study in associability.* Philadelphia: Psychological Clinic Press.

Humpstone, H. J. (1919). Memory span tasks. *The Psychological Clinic, 12,* 196–200.

Jacobs, J. (1885). Ueber das Gedachtnis [Review of Ebbinghaus (1885) Memory: A contribution to experimental psychology]. *Mind, 10,* 454–459.

Jacobs, J. (1886). The need of a society for experimental psychology. *Mind, 11,* 49–54.

Jacobs, J. (1887). Experiments on "prehension." *Mind, 12,* 75–79.

James, W. (1890). *The principles of psychology.* New York: Henry Holt.

Johnson, D. M. (1955). *The psychology of thought and judgment.* New York: Harper & Brothers.

Kane, M. J., Hambrick, D. Z., Tuholski, S. W., Wilhelm, O., Payne, T. W., & Engle, R. W. (2004). The generality of working memory capacity: A latent-variable approach to verbal and visuospatial memory span and reasoning. *Journal of Experimental Psychology: General, 133,* 189–217.

Keppel, G., & Underwood, B. J. (1962). Proactive inhibition in short-term retention of single items. *Journal of Verbal Learning and Verbal Behavior, 1,* 153–161.

Kintsch, W., Healy, A. F., Hegarty, M., Pennington, B. F., & Salthouse, T. A. (1999). Models of working memory: Eight questions and some general issues. In A. Miyake & P. Shah (Eds.), *Models of working memory: Mechanisms of active maintenance and executive control* (pp. 412–441). New York: Cambridge University Press.

Kosslyn, S. M., Cacioppo, J. P., Davidson, R. J., Hugdahl, K., Lovallo, W. R., Spiegel, D., & Rose, R. (2002). Bridging psychology and biology: The analysis of individuals in groups. *American Psychologist, 57,* 341–351.

McGeoch, J. A. (1932). Forgetting and the law of disuse. *Psychological Review, 39,* 352–370.

Melton A. W. (1963). Implications of short-term memory for a general theory of memory. *Journal of Verbal Learning and Verbal Behavior, 2,* 1–21.

Miller, G. A. (1956). The magical number seven, plus or minus two: Some limits on our capacity for processing information. *Psychological Review, 63,* 81–97.

Miller, G. A., Galanter, E., & Pribram, K. H. (1960). *Plans and the structure of behavior.* New York: Holt.

Milner, B. (1966). Amnesia following operation on the temporal lobes. In C. W. M. Whitty & O. L. Zangwill (Eds.), *Amnesia.* London: Butterworths.

Miyake, A. (2001). Individual differences in working memory: Introduction to the special section. *Journal of Experimental Psychology: General, 130,* 163–168.

Miyake, A., & Shah, P. (1999a). *Models of working memory: Mechanisms of active maintenance and executive control.* New York: Cambridge University Press.

Miyake, A., & Shah, P. (1999b). Toward unified theories of working memory: Emerging general consensus, unresolved theoretical issues, and future research directions. In A. Miyake & P. Shah (Eds.), *Models of working memory: Mechanisms of active maintenance and executive control* (pp. 442–482). New York: Cambridge University Press.

Nairne, J. S. (2002). Remembering over the short-term: The case against the standard model. *Annual Review of Psychology, 53,* 53–81.

Pascal-Leone, J. (1970). A mathematical model for the transition rule in Piaget's developmental stages. *Acta Psychologica, 32*, 301–345.

Peterson, L. R., & Peterson, M. J. (1959). Short-term retention of individual verbal items. *Journal of Experimental Psychology, 58*, 193–198.

Reitman, J. (1971). Mechanisms of forgetting in short-term memory. *Cognitive Psychology, 2*, 185–195.

Reitman, J. (1974). Without surreptitious rehearsal, information in short-term memory decays. *Journal of Verbal Learning and Verbal Behavior, 13*, 365–377.

Shah, P., & Miyake, A. (1996). The separability of working memory resources for spatial thinking and language processing: An individual differences approach. *Journal of Experimental Psychology: General, 125*, 4–27.

Shallice, T., & Warrington, E. K. (1970). Independent functioning of verbal memory stores: A neuropsychological study. *Quarterly Journal of Experimental Psychology, 22*, 261–273.

Sternberg, S. (1966). High-speed scanning in human memory. *Science, 153*, 652–654.

Sternberg, S. (1969). The discovery of processing stages: Extensions of Donders' method. *Acta Psychologica, 30*, 276–315.

Sternberg, R. J., & Grigorenko, E. L. (2001). Unified psychology. *American Psychologist, 56*, 1069–1079.

Thorndike, E. L. (1914). *The psychology of learning.* New York: Teachers College.

Turner, M. L., & Engle, R. W. (1989). Is working memory capacity task dependent? *Journal of Memory and Language, 28*, 127–154.

Underwood, B. J. (1975). Individual differences as a crucible in theory construction. *American Psychologist, 30*, 128–134.

Waugh, N. C., & Norman, D. A. (1965). Primary memory. *Psychological Review, 72*, 89–104.

Warrington, E. K., Logue, V., & Pratt, R. T. C. (1971). The anatomical localisation of selective impairment of auditory verbal short-term memory. *Neuropsychologia, 9*, 377–387.

Wickelgren, W. A. (1966). Distinctive features and errors in short-term memory for English consonants. *Journal of the Acoustical Society of America, 39*, 388–398.

Woodworth, R. S. (1938). *Experimental psychology.* New York: Holt.

Wundt, W. (1912/1973). *An introduction to psychology.* Originally published by G. Allen, London. Reprinted by Arno Press, New York.

I

Working Memory Variation
Reflecting Normal Inter- and
Intra-individual Differences

2

Variation in Working Memory Capacity as Variation in Executive Attention and Control

MICHAEL J. KANE, ANDREW R. A. CONWAY,
DAVID Z. HAMBRICK, and RANDALL W. ENGLE

If, as many psychologists seem to believe, immediate memory represents a distinct system or set of processes from long-term memory (LTM), then what might it be for? This fundamental, functional question was surprisingly unanswerable in the 1970s, given the volume of research that had explored short-term memory (STM), and given the ostensible role that STM was thought to play in cognitive control (Atkinson & Shiffrin, 1971). Indeed, failed attempts to link STM to complex cognitive functions, such as reading comprehension, loomed large in Crowder's (1982) obituary for the concept.

Baddeley and Hitch (1974) tried to validate immediate memory's functions by testing subjects in reasoning, comprehension, and list-learning tasks at the same time their memory was occupied by irrelevant material. Generally, small memory loads (i.e., three or fewer items) were retained with virtually no effect on the primary tasks, whereas memory loads of six items consistently impaired reasoning, comprehension, and learning. Baddeley and Hitch therefore argued that "working memory" (WM)

is a flexible and limited-resource system with storage and processing capabilities that are traded off as needed. In this system, small memory loads are handled alone by a peripheral phonemic buffer, leaving central processing unaffected, whereas larger loads require additional resources of a central executive. Thus, WM was proposed to be a dynamic system that enabled active maintenance of task-relevant information in support of the simultaneous execution of complex cognitive tasks.

As we will detail below, there are certainly aspects of our theoretical perspective that can be traced to Baddeley and Hitch's (1974) views. But our approach to conducting WM research is also strongly influenced by another article that appeared at about the same time, entitled "Individual differences as a crucible in theory construction." In this report, Underwood (1975) argued that psychological theories should be subjected promptly to an individual-differences test as a means of falsification. Most nomothetic theories in psychology make predictions about individual differences, even if only implicitly, and so testing these predictions is an efficient means to determine whether a theory merits further pursuit. Although Baddeley and Hitch (1974) formulated and pursued WM theory based on experiment, the question of WM function obviously lent itself to individual-differences predictions. Quite simply, if WM were a central mechanism to higher-order cognition, then individuals with greater WM capacity should perform better on complex cognitive tasks than those with lesser WM capacity.

These important predictions became testable a half-decade later, when Daneman and Carpenter (1980) created the "complex span" tasks that initiated an individual-differences approach to WM research. These span measures were dual tasks, requiring information storage in the context of simultaneous processing of other information. They therefore reflected Baddeley and Hitch's (1974) idea that the executive component of WM must be measured in a dual processing and storage context. Most importantly, scores on complex span tasks correlated strongly with measures of language comprehension, and this provided important validation for WM theory. Indeed, subsequent individual-differences research has led the way in fulfilling the theory's greatest promise—to elucidate the function of immediate memory—by linking variation in WM to diverse aspects of higher-order cognition, including language learning (e.g., Baddeley, Gathercole & Papagno, 1998), comprehension (e.g., Daneman & Merikle, 1996), reasoning (e.g., Kyllonen & Christal, 1990), and cognitive control (e.g., Miyake, Friedman, Rettinger, Shah, & Hegarty, 2001). These correlational findings have indicated that WM plays an important role in a host of complex cognitive capabilities and that WM measures have practical value in assessing intellectual ability.

However, the magnitude and breadth of the correlations between WM span and other cognitive measures do not necessarily illuminate the psychological source of those correlations. We suggest that individual-differences research will have its greatest impact on basic WM theory only when it pursues questions of mechanism simultaneously with questions of function. Our research program has therefore addressed both mechanism and function, in the spirit of Cronbach's (1957) call to align the "two disciplines of scientific psychology" and his argument that scientific psychology should aim to understand *individual* minds as well as the general, nomothetic principles of mind. To do so, we use both experimental and correlational methodologies and examine individual-by-treatment interactions. The central question that drives our research, then, which is unapologetically tied to individual differences, has clear ramifications for general WM theory: *Why do WM capacity (WMC) measures so successfully predict performance across a range of cognitive abilities?*

OVERVIEW OF AN "EXECUTIVE ATTENTION" THEORY OF WORKING MEMORY CAPACITY

Our approach to understanding WMC and its variation emphasizes the synergy of "attentional" and "memorial" processes in maintaining and recovering access to information that is relevant to ongoing tasks and in blocking access to task-irrelevant information (e.g., Engle & Kane, 2004; Engle, Kane, & Tuholski, 1999; Kane & Engle, 2002; Kane, Hambrick, & Conway, 2005). Our theory, which follows in part from Cowan (1995), is depicted in Figure 2.1. We view STM as a metaphorical "store" represented by LTM traces activated above threshold. These traces may be maintained in the limited focus of attention (conscious awareness) or kept active and accessible through domain-specific rehearsal and coding processes (e.g., inner speech, chunking, imagery). Domain-general executive attention processes may also be engaged to sustain activation of information beyond attentional focus, or to retrieve no-longer active information from outside of conscious focus. These executive processes will be particularly useful when rehearsal or coding routines are relatively unpracticed or not useful in a particular context (e.g., with novel visuospatial materials, or in dual-task situations). These same executive attention mechanisms may also be deployed to block or inhibit goal-irrelevant representations or responses elicited by the environment.

We propose that the extent to which executive attention is engaged by a task, for maintenance,

Any given WMC or STM task reflects all components to some extent

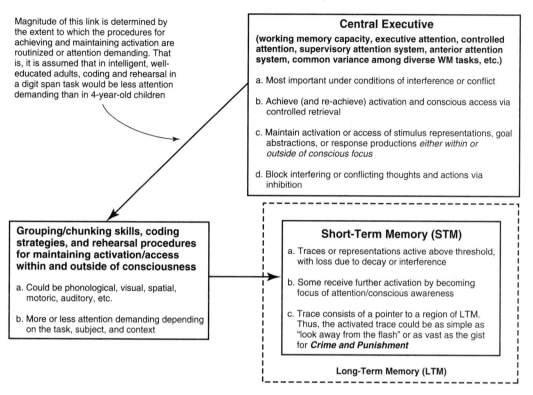

Figure 2.1. Measurement model of the working memory system, version 1.2. (Adapted from Engle, Kane et al., 1999 [version 1.0], and Engle & Kane, 2004 [version 1.1].)

retrieval, or for blocking, is critically determined by the degree of interference or conflict presented by the context. Proactive interference from prior events may, for example, slow the search for one's car in a familiar parking lot. Or, the environment may induce competition between habitual responses and more novel ones when the context is ambiguous or unusual, such as when an American drives on the wrong side of the road in Dublin. Our view is that the presence of such interference or conflict makes the executive functions of WM most helpful and readily measurable (Norman & Shallice, 1986). Thus, when we use the term *working memory capacity*, we refer to the attentional processes that allow for goal-directed behavior by maintaining relevant information in an active, easily accessible state outside of conscious focus, or to retrieve that information from inactive memory, under conditions of interference, distraction, or conflict.

Working Memory Capacity, Executive Attention, and Working Memory Span Tasks

Our perspective is closely tied to the complex span tasks we have used to measure WMC, which show good reliability by internal-consistency and test-retest measures (e.g., Klein & Fiss, 1999; Turner & Engle, 1989; but see Chapter 11, this volume).[1] These WM span tasks present subjects with the traditional memory span demand to immediately recall short lists of unrelated stimuli. Additionally, and critically, WM span tasks challenge memory maintenance by presenting a secondary processing task in alternation with each memory item. Reading span (Daneman & Carpenter, 1980), for example, requires subjects to read series of sentences for comprehension and then recall the sentence-ending words from the series (or sometimes, to recall an isolated word or letter that followed each sentence); operation span, in contrast, presents subjects with series of equations to verify, with each equation followed by an unrelated word to memorize (Turner & Engle, 1989). Less verbal tasks include counting span, which presents series of arrays in which to-be-counted target items are surrounded by distractors and subjects must recall the count from each array in the series (Case, Kurland, & Goldberg, 1982), and spatial (rotation) span, which presents series of rotated letters that subjects judge to be normal or reversed while memorizing the letters' original orientations (e.g., Shah & Miyake, 1996).

Working memory span tasks are obviously complex and multiply determined tasks, and so none of them can be considered a process-pure measure of "executive function." Instead, WM span tasks measure, in part, executive attention processes that we believe are domain general and contribute to WM span performance irrespective of the skills or stimuli involved. In addition, WM span tasks reflect the contributions of rehearsal, coding, storage, processing skills, and strategies that are domain specific and vary with the component tasks and stimuli presented (see also Chapters 5 and 6). Our view is that WM span tasks reflect primarily general executive processes and secondarily, domain-specific rehearsal and storage processes. Moreover, the broad predictive utility of WM span tasks derives from the general, executive attention contributions to performance. Short-term memory span tasks, in contrast, reflect domain-specific storage and rehearsal skills and strategies primarily and executive attention processes only secondarily. That said, we should emphasize that we do not claim that STM tasks are pure measures of storage and rehearsal, without any influence of attention processes; nor do we claim that WM span tasks measure or correlate with all possible aspects of attentional processing. Instead, we think that WM span tasks are reasonably good measures of a domain-general attentional capability that is involved in the control of behavior and thought and is important to many cognitive abilities. Thus WM span tasks are generally better measures of the executive attention construct than STM span tasks (see Kane et al., 2005).

Working memory span tasks tap into executive attention by requiring subjects to maintain or recover access to target information under proactive interference from prior trials (e.g., Lustig, May, & Hasher, 2001), while that access or retrieval is challenged by intermittently shifting attentional focus between the memory and secondary processing tasks (e.g., Barrouillet, Bernadin, & Camos, 2004; Hitch, Towse, & Hutton, 2001). That is, interference encourages subjects to rely on sustained, active access to the memoranda, rather than on LTM retrieval, but subjects cannot easily maintain that access because the processing task prevents them from keeping target items in the focus of attention (the processing task also limits use of rehearsal or chunking strategies). Executive processes thus help maintain or recover access to the target items in the absence of focal attention and effective rehearsal procedures.

EXECUTIVE ATTENTION AS THE CRITICAL SOURCE OF WORKING MEMORY CAPACITY VARIATION

Our proposal, that WMC variation is driven largely by individual differences in executive attention processes, represents a web of inference across correlational and experimental studies. Some of these studies, which we have described as "macroanalytic" (Engle & Kane, 2004; see Salthouse & Craik, 2001), have examined the relations between WMC and other hypothetical constructs, such as general fluid intelligence, using large subject samples and multiple tasks to identify each construct. Two other kinds of studies, which we term "microanalytic," take a more focused approach to analyzing span–ability relations. One line of microanalytic work combines correlational and experimental designs by manipulating variables within WM span tasks to determine how those manipulations affect the span–ability correlation. These are essentially task analyses of WM span that consider not only the processes required by span tasks but also the processes shared between span and other measures. The second line of microanalytic research, using quasi-experimental designs, tests for WM span–related differences by comparing individuals with high WM span scores (*high spans*, from the upper quartile of a university student distribution) to those with low scores (*low spans*, from the lower quartile) in the performance of "elementary" cognitive tasks from the memory and attention literatures. We discuss these three sets of macro- and microanalytic findings in detail below.

Macroanalytic Studies of Working Memory Capacity

The use of large-scale, structural equation modeling studies in WMC research has increased recently, influenced by the growing confluence of the WMC and intelligence literatures (for reviews, see Conway, Kane, & Engle, 2003; Kane et al., 2005). An advantage of these techniques is that they permit the use of latent variables, which reflect the shared variance among a number of tasks hypothesized to reflect the same construct (e.g., WMC). As such, latent variables are free from the measurement error associated with any one multiply determined task. Through use of latent variables and structural equation modeling, research conclusions can be shifted from the level of observed variables, which always reflect some measurement error, to the theoretical constructs of interest.

The Relation of Working Memory Capacity to Short-Term Memory and Fluid Intelligence

Engle, Tuholski, Laughlin, and Conway (1999) tested 135 university subjects in WMC tasks (operation span, reading span, counting span), STM tasks (backward and forward word span), and tests of fluid intelligence, or psychometric Gf (novel figural and spatial reasoning). Our questions for this study were whether WMC and STM were dissociable constructs and, if so, whether WMC was the better predictor of Gf. In fact, WMC and STM were separable: the two latent variables correlated substantially (.68), but a model forcing a single factor onto the span data did not fit well. We believe that the correlation between STM and WMC was driven primarily by the shared requirement among span tasks to immediately recall short lists of verbal items—that is, it reflected primarily "storage" (although some shared variance between STM and WMC will also reflect executive attention). The unique residual variance in WMC reflected the dual-task demand in the WMC tasks only, that is, the increased demand they made on executive attention for active maintenance outside of conscious focus.

Given that WMC and STM reflected both shared and unique variance, which might contribute to general intellectual ability? We found that the WMC factor, but not STM, predicted unique variance in Gf, suggesting that the greater executive demands of WM span tasks are the source of WMC–Gf correlations, rather than the "simple" storage demands shared by STM and WM tasks. However, as a further test of this idea, we constructed a hierarchical model of our span data (illustrated in Fig. 2.2). Here, separate factors were derived for WMC and STM, but in addition, the considerable variance shared between WMC and STM was modeled as a second-order factor. This second-order "common" factor ostensibly represented the storage, coding, and rehearsal (and some executive) processes involved in both WMC and STM tasks, and it shared significant, unique variance with Gf. However, the residual, unique variance from WMC (i.e., WMC with STM factored out) predicted Gf more strongly. Whatever WM span tasks demand beyond simple storage seems to account primarily for the WM–Gf correlation. We interpret this residual WMC variance to reflect the relatively strong executive attention demands of WM span tasks, elicited by their dual-task requirements.

Processing Speed and Working Memory Capacity–Gf Association

Conway, Cowan, Bunting, Therriault, and Minkoff (2002) replicated these findings while additionally testing the contribution of processing speed to predicting Gf and accounting for the WMC–Gf correlation. Developmental research clearly shows that speeded measures of

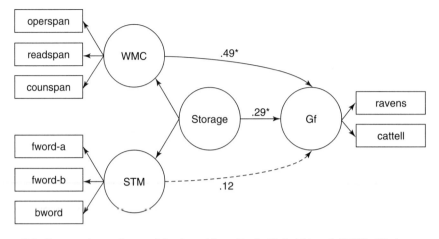

Figure 2.2. Structural-equation model, adapted from Engle, Tuholski et al. (1999). Circles represent latent variables and boxes represent individual tasks. Solid arrows with path coefficients with asterisks represent significant shared variance between constructs. Counspan = Counting span task; Fword-a = Forward Word span task, version a; Fword-b = Forward Word span task, version b; bword = Backward word span task. Gf = general fluid intelligence; Operspan = Operation span task; Readspan = Reading span task; WMC = working memory capacity; STM = short-term memory.

simple cognitive processes often account for a lion's share of age-related variance in higher-order cognition, overwhelming the contribution of WMC (Kail & Salthouse, 1994). Much less clear, however, is whether processing-speed variation within an age group can account for the relation between WMC and intelligence. To find out, we tested 113 university subjects in the WM span and Gf tasks used by Engle, Tuholski et al. (1999), along with several STM and speed tasks. The latter were paper-and-pencil tasks requiring subjects to copy or compare lists of stimuli quickly and accurately. Because correlations between processing speed and Gf measures typically increase with the complexity of speeded tasks (e.g., Jensen, 1998), thus clouding the interpretation of what "processing speed" reflects, we chose simple speed tasks as a most stringent test of their importance.

In order to examine the independent contributions of executive attention and storage, coding, and rehearsal to the association between WMC and Gf, we used a nested structure in which all the span tasks loaded onto a common "STM–storage" factor to represent their shared storage, coding, and rehearsal variance. WMC tasks also loaded onto a residual factor, reflecting the additional executive attention processes en-

gaged by the dual-task nature of the WM span tasks. As shown in Figure 2.3, the shared "storage" variance was a relatively weak predictor of Gf, and the residual WMC variance was stronger. These findings support the idea that "executive" variance, tapped by WMC tasks to a greater degree than by STM tasks, drives the WMC–Gf relationship. It is also worth noting here that not only did speed fail to predict Gf while controlling for WMC, but speed also correlated more strongly with STM–storage than WMC–executive processes. Among young adults, then, with relatively "simple" tests of processing speed and with untimed measures of WMC, the two constructs share little variance, and only WMC is a significant source of variation in general ability.

Domain Generality of Working Memory Capacity and Short-Term Memory

Our latent-variable research shows strong correlations between WMC and Gf, therefore suggesting WMC to be an important mechanism of general cognitive ability. Moreover, our WMC latent variables were derived from *verbal, symbolic* WM span tasks and the Gf latent

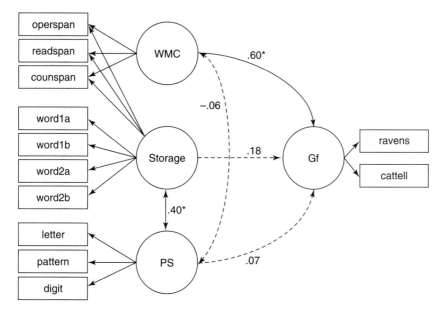

Figure 2.3. Structural-equation model, adapted from Conway et al. (2002). WMC = working memory capacity; STM = short-term memory; PS = processing speed; Gf = general fluid intelligence; Operspan = Operation span task; Readspan = Reading span task; Counspan = Counting span task.

variables were created from *nonverbal, figural* reasoning tasks. This cross-domain generality indicates that the variance common to WM span tasks cannot be substantially verbal. Instead, we submit that the executive attention variance that is shared among WM span tasks reflects domain-general processes.

However, a few studies indicate domain specificity in WM span, with low correlations between individual verbal and visuospatial WM span tasks, low cross-domain correlations between WM span and ability, or both (e.g., Shah & Miyake, 1996). We suspect that restricted ranges of general ability and measurement error biased these studies toward finding exaggerated domain specificity in WMC. All were derived from samples of university students, some from prestigious schools, that might represent a narrow range of general intellectual ability relative to the population at large. Without suitable variation in general ability in a sample, any variability in cognitive performance must result from something else, such as domain-specific abilities, skills, or strategies. (Because universities are more likely to select students

from a narrow range of general ability than from a narrow range of any one specific ability, samples drawn from these populations are more likely to represent restricted ranges of general ability.) Moreover, with respect to measurement error, these "domain-specific" studies used only one measure each of verbal and spatial WMC. With only one task per construct, the low correlations might result from dissociable constructs (i.e., verbal and spatial WMC), or instead from other, non-WMC abilities, skills, and processes tapped by complex span tasks.

To address these possibilities, Kane et al. (2004) tested 236 subjects from both competitive and comprehensive universities, as well as from two urban community samples, in multiple tests of verbal and spatial WM and STM span. We thus ensured some degree of variation in domain-general ability in our sample and used latent-variable models to factor out sources of measurement error. We first contrasted the fit of two kinds of models for the WM span data: unitary models derived from all six WM span tasks and two-factor models with separate verbal and spatial WMC factors.

Depending on the technical details of these models, verbal and spatial WMC factors shared 70%–85% of their variance (correlations from .84 to .93), demonstrating that WM span measures tap primarily general processes and abilities. In contrast, verbal and spatial STM measures shared only 40% of their variance, consistent with our view that complex WM span tasks measure primarily the contribution of general executive processes and simple STM span tasks measure primarily the contributions of domain-specific ones. We also tested whether the domain generality of WMC and STM varied with the range of Gf in the sample, by dividing our subjects into different groups on the basis of their matrix-reasoning performance: a high-Gf group, a low-Gf group, and two groups representing the full range of Gf. We found that both WMC and STM were much more domain specific in our high-Gf group than they were among our low-Gf subjects or our full Gf–range sample. Thus, as we suspected, prior findings of domain-specific

WMC may have resulted from testing subjects from a restricted range of high general ability.

Like Engle, Tuholski et al. (1999) and Conway et al. (2002), we also tested whether the general executive contributions to span, or domain-specific STM–storage contributions, were the primary source of the WMC–Gf correlation. In our nested-factor model, depicted on the left side of Figure 2.4, all 12 of the verbal and spatial WMC and STM tasks loaded onto a common factor reflecting their shared variance. Additionally, the six verbal and spatial span tasks each loaded onto a domain-specific residual factor. The logic, again, was that both WM and STM span tasks reflect joint contributions of general executive attention and domain-specific STM and storage. At the same time, WM span taps primarily general executive attention processes and STM span taps primarily domain-specific storage, coding, and rehearsal processes. However, in contrast to the Engle and Conway models, note that we interpreted the common factor to represent general executive attention variance and

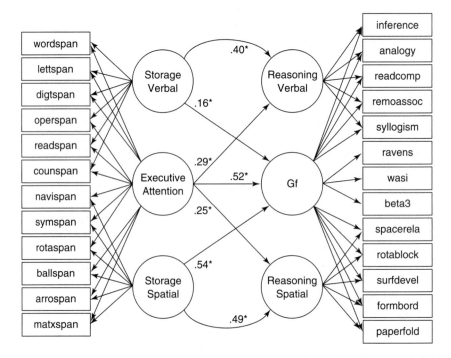

Figure 2.4. Structural-equation model, adapted from Kane et al. (2004). Gf = general fluid intelligence. For descriptions of the individual span and reasoning tasks, see Kane et al. (2004).

the residual factors to represent domain-specific STM–storage variance, rather than the reverse.

Our interpretation of these factors had rational and empirical grounding. First, given the substantial dissociability between verbal and spatial STM span in our data and in others' (see Jonides et al., 1996, for a review), it is unlikely that shared variance among verbal and spatial span measures reflected *domain-specific* storage and rehearsal abilities. Second, the WMC and STM tasks loaded differently onto the "executive" and "STM–storage" factors. The WMC tasks all had higher loadings on the common "executive" factor than did the STM tasks, and they had higher loadings on the executive factor than on their respective "storage" factors. The STM tasks showed the opposite pattern. Thus, the executive attention factor captured more variance from WMC than STM tasks, and the storage factors showed the opposite pattern. In this data set, then, the common span variance reflected domain-general executive attention and the domain-specific residual variance reflected STM storage and rehearsal processes. Of most importance, the executive attention factor strongly predicted Gf (path coefficient = .52), with a similar magnitude to our previous studies. Moreover, it was similar to the correlation we found in a separate model where Gf was predicted by a WMC factor derived from only the six WM span tasks (.64). This consistency across models and studies is compelling, given that we defined WMC and Gf much more broadly here than in our prior work, with Gf reflecting shared variance among verbal and visuospatial reasoning tests. Indeed, in a separate article we reanalyzed all the published latent variable data on the WMC–Gf correlation and found that WMC accounted for approximately 50% of the variance in Gf (i.e., the median correlation between WMC and Gf constructs across studies was .72; Kane et al., 2005). This shared variance is not strong enough to claim that WMC and Gf are synonymous. However, we submit that WMC, which reflects primarily a general executive construct, is one critical source of Gf variation. Short-term memory, in contrast, reflects more domain-specific storage and rehearsal processes that are less important to general aspects of ability.[2]

Summary of Macroanalytic Research

As measured by a variety of span tasks, WMC and STM are strongly correlated constructs. However, despite this close relationship, the attentional processes engaged primarily by WM span tasks (and to a lesser extent by STM tasks) are responsible for WM span's general and superior predictive utility. The executive attention processes that contribute to WM span tasks are an important mechanism of fluid intelligence, and furthermore, these executive attention processes are domain general. In contrast, variance associated with simple storage and rehearsal activities, captured primarily by STM tasks, is relatively domain specific (for alternative views on WMC's domain generality, see Chapters 6 and 8).

Microanalytic Studies of Working Memory Capacity

Two lines of "microanalytic" research, using smaller scale quasi-experiments and regression- or ANOVA-based analytic approaches, have addressed the mechanisms of span task performance and its relation to complex cognitive abilities. One line has clarified which processes are *not* important to WMC variation and covariation. We discuss this work first. We then review research that more closely and specifically links WMC to the constructs of attention and executive control.

Ruling out Some Mechanisms of Variation and Covariation in Working Memory Capacity

Task skill and processing efficiency The idea that individual differences in task-specific skills affect the correlations between WM span and higher-order cognitive measures is an old one. Daneman, Carpenter, and colleagues (e.g., Daneman & Carpenter 1980) proposed that good comprehenders could devote fewer WM resources to the reading and listening component of the span task than could poor comprehenders, thereby relieving more resources for the simultaneous task of memory storage. Thus, strong language skills lead to a larger functional WMC for language, rather than a larger WMC leading to stronger language skills. In a similar vein, MacDonald and Christiansen (2002) claimed that "the reading span task is simply a measure of language processing skills" (p. 39). However, our research (Conway & Engle, 1996; Engle, Cantor, & Carullo, 1992) demonstrates that partialing out subjects' processing speed during span tasks does not diminish the correlation between WM span and verbal ability, nor does tailoring the difficulty of the span task processing demand to each subjects' individual skill level. If partialing out processing speed and matching processing skills do not reduce span–ability correlations, then the relationship must reflect more than domain-specific processing skills.

Strategy use   Given the complexity of WM span tasks, individual differences in strategies might contribute to WM span scores, as well as to the general patterns of WMC covariation with other constructs. In fact, when McNamara and Scott (2001) trained subjects to use a semantic "chaining" strategy during simple word span tasks, they found that it substantially increased subsequent reading span (WMC) scores. Moreover, subjects who initially reported using a semantic strategy to remember the STM task words had higher reading span and verbal Scholastic Aptitude Test (VSAT) scores than those of subjects who reported using only rehearsal or no strategies.

However, despite the effects of strategy use on WM span scores overall, we believe that McNamara and Scott's (2001) data actually argue against the importance of strategy variables to WMC variation and covariation. First, standard deviations in WM span were generally larger after training than before training, indicating that training *increased*, rather than reduced, span variability. Second, initially high-strategic subjects benefited more from strategy training than did initially low-strategic subjects, and so WMC seems to determine how effectively people learn and use demanding strategies. Third, higher WM span scores were associated with higher VSAT and math SAT (MSAT) scores, but high strategy use was asso-

ciated only with higher VSAT and not with MSAT. Strategy use therefore cannot account for the *general* predictive power of reading span. Finally, McNamara and Scott did not report what should be critical evidence concerning a strategy hypothesis—if individual differences in strategy use account for WM–ability correlations, then a span–ability correlation should be weaker after strategy instruction than before it.

The few studies that have directly tested whether indices of strategy use might account for the covariation between WMC and complex cognition have been negative. In two different WM span tasks, Engle et al. (1992) allowed subjects to control their study time for each to-be-recalled word. Those subjects with high spans studied the target words for more time than those with low spans, but when Engle et al. partialed out study time from the span–VSAT correlations, they actually *increased* nonsignificantly. Thus, strategic allocation of study time did not drive covariation between WMC and verbal ability; if anything, strategy use suppressed measurement of the relationship (see also Friedman & Miyake, 2004).

A series of training studies by Turley-Ames and Whitfield (2003) also found strategy use to suppress correlations between WMC and verbal ability. Following a pretest on operation span, subjects were instructed to engage in rehearsal, imagery, or semantic chaining to help them remember the target words. Instructed subjects greatly improved their span scores relative to uninstructed control subjects, but scores following strategy instruction were more *strongly* correlated with verbal ability than were control scores. That is, matching subjects in their knowledge and encouragement of effective WM strategies did not make the span–ability correlation go away, as it should have if strategic differences accounted for the correlation. Instead, normal variation in strategy use (as reflected by control subjects) actually worked against finding correlations between WM span and verbal ability. Variation in strategy use during WM span tasks, even if substantial, does not account for shared variance between WMC and ability measures.

Summary   Microanalytic studies have not found the contributions of processing efficiency, processing skill, or strategy use to be compelling; they either fail to account for performance of WM span tasks or, if they do affect WM span scores, they do not contribute to the correlations between WM span and higher-order abilities. Something else drives the predictive power of WMC measures. We can rule out STM storage and rehearsal as well, because macroanalytic studies find that STM tasks are not as good predictors of general ability as WM tasks, and the demands made by WM span tasks, beyond STM storage and rehearsal, drive their association with complex cognition.

We think the studies described in this section serve as good examples of the importance of combining experimental and correlational approaches to WM research. Experimental task analyses of WM span tasks may suggest any number of variables that serve to either increase or decrease span scores. Such findings may be interesting in their own right, but it is a mistake to infer from them that any of these variables must contribute to the correlations between WM span and other tasks. At least some variables that affect span scores clearly have no influence on WM span correlations.

Variation in Working Memory Capacity and Individual Differences in Executive Attention

With the elimination of processing skill or efficiency, strategy use, and STM storage as causes of the WMC–ability relationship, we infer that the attentional demands made by WM span tasks are most important in producing that relationship. Moreover, our second line of microanalytic work, discussed below, provides direct evidence for an association between WMC and executive attention capabilities. First we review evidence linking individual differences in WMC to the attentional control of interference in memory. We then discuss evidence from relatively low-level attention tasks, not involving memory retrieval, that WMC predicts control over goal-directed behavior. Specifically, we find that WMC is associated with successful maintenance of task goals and the attendant blocking of strong but contextually inappropriate

responses, mechanisms that may be analogous to the "proactive" and "reactive" control modes, respectively, proposed by Braver et al. (Chapter 4).

Working memory capacity and executive attention in resolving memory interference   Our executive attention theory holds that the control of memory retrieval in the face of interference is central to the attentional construct measured by WM tasks. The supporting evidence—a strong connection between WMC and interference vulnerability—comes from a variety of experimental preparations that pose different types of interference and competition (e.g., retroactive, fan-type, output). In these studies, extreme (quartile) groups of high– and low–WM span subjects, identified via operation span, differ in recall accuracy or latency under high-interference but not low-interference conditions (e.g., Conway & Engle, 1994).

Proactive interference, for example, affects low- more than high-WMC individuals. Kane and Engle (2000) tested subjects in a delayed free-recall task presenting three consecutive lists of 10 words each, with recall preceded by a 15 s rehearsal prevention task. To maximize interference, the words from all three lists belonged to one semantic category (e.g., animals). On List 1, in the absence of interference, the two span groups showed equivalent free recall. However, by List 3, under proactive interference from prior lists, low-span subjects' recall dropped more precipitously than that of high-span subjects ($Ms \approx -50\%$ vs. -30%, respectively). Rosen and Engle (1998) demonstrated span differences in interference susceptibility during learning of paired associates. In List 1, all subjects learned 12 compound word pairs (e.g., *bird-bath*). In List 2, control subjects learned 12 pairs of semantically related words that were unrelated to the List 1 pairs (e.g., *eye-tear*), while interference subjects learned pairs using the List 1 cues (e.g., *bird-dawn*). High and low spans reached learning criterion equally quickly for List 1, where interference was absent. However, in List 2, low spans required an average of two more learning trials than did high spans overall, and low spans' impairment was especially evident in the interference condition. Low spans under interference also committed more overt List 1 intrusions during List 2 learning than did high spans.

These studies additionally yielded evidence that WMC-related variation in interference arises from attention-control variation, consistent with theories linking interference resistance to attentional inhibition (e.g., Anderson & Neely, 1996; Hasher & Zacks, 1988). Most directly, Kane and Engle (2000) tested some subjects under dual-task conditions, in which they continuously maintained a complex finger-tapping sequence during either study or recall of each list. Under both these dual-task conditions, the span groups showed *equivalent* interference. The secondary task had no effect on the low-span group's interference vulnerability but it increased the high-span group's interference vulnerability to that of the low-span group. These counterintuitive findings indicate that span differences in proactive interference normally result from high spans' superior use of controlled processes to combat it (e.g., via inhibition, blocking, source monitoring, etc.). Thwarting high spans' control by imposing a secondary task increased their interference susceptibility. In contrast, low span subjects were less effective in engaging controlled processing to limit interference in the first place, so dividing their attention was irrelevant—they could not lose what they were not already using.

Rosen and Engle (1998) inferred a role for attention in interference differences more indirectly. Their subjects attempted to relearn List 1 (e.g., *bird-bath*) after learning List 2 (e.g., *bird-dawn*). The critical dependent measure here was cued-recall latency following the very first learning trial for each list. Note that if high spans under interference conditions had blocked their List 1 associations in learning List 2 via an inhibitory process, then these pairs should subsequently suffer some residually impaired accessibility. Accordingly, high span subjects under interference should be slower to recall List 1 than they had been in originally learning them, and they should be slower to recall List 1 than control subjects. Low span subjects, by contrast, should show no evidence of inaccessibility for List 1. This is precisely what was found. High spans' relearning latencies in the interference

condition were significantly longer than those in the control condition. In contrast, low-span individuals' response times (RTs) were actually *shorter* in the interference than in the control condition. Moreover, high spans' relearning latencies were significantly slower than their own List 1 learning latencies; low spans' latencies were statistically equivalent to one another. Thus, only high spans showed something analogous to a negative priming effect in relearning a list that had previously been a source of interference, and so was inhibited.

High- and low-span subjects recall information from LTM equivalently quickly and accurately in the absence of interference. Thus, WM span does not predict variability in *all* aspects of remembering. Instead, WMC appears important for learning and retrieval only when the environment presents a substantial source of interference and competition. Moreover, our dual-task and RT results strongly suggest that high spans' relative invulnerability to interference stems from a superior executive attention capability, whereby potentially competing information is blocked or inhibited. Only high spans show an effect of divided attention on their interference susceptibility, and only high spans show impaired access to initially learned but subsequently interfering associations.

Working memory capacity and executive attention in resolving response competition. If WMC reflects an attentional construct, as we claim, then WMC differences should be observable in contexts that make no explicit memory-retrieval demands. That is, variation in WMC should be associated with variation not only in memory-interference tasks but also in simpler indices of attention control. In fact, high spans (as measured by operation span) are less vulnerable to salient distractors in dichotic listening than are low spans. Conway, Cowan, and Bunting (2001) had subjects shadow a list of unrelated words presented to their right ear while distractor words were presented to their left ear. Either 4 or 5 min into the task, the subject's name was presented in the distractor channel. Prior research indicated that approximately 33% of subjects report hearing their name in such contexts (e.g., Wood & Cowan,

1995). Here, only 20% of the high span subjects, but 65% of the low span subjects, reported hearing their name.

WMC-related differences also arise in the arguably simpler "antisaccade" task of attention control. In two experiments, Kane, Bleckley, Conway, and Engle (2001) tested high and low spans in prosaccadic and antisaccadic versions of a letter-identification task. Each trial briefly displayed a letter to the right or left of fixation for identification. In prosaccade trial blocks the target location was always cued by a flashing stimulus near its upcoming location, so subjects could allow reflexive orienting responses to guide, or "pull," their attention and eyes to the target. Here, both high- and low-span subjects identified targets equivalently quickly. In contrast, antisaccade trial blocks always cued the target by presenting the flash to the *opposite* screen location, and so subjects had to block, or quickly recover from, the orienting response to the flash and endogenously "push" their attention and eyes toward the target. In both experiments, high spans identified antisaccade targets more quickly than did low spans. Moreover, Experiment 2 measured eye movements across hundreds of antisaccade trials, and high span subjects showed fewer saccades toward the cue, faster recovery from these saccade errors, and faster correctly guided saccades than did low span subjects.

Both the dichotic-listening and antisaccade tasks make few demands on subjects beyond blocking a habitual orienting response in the service of a novel goal. How do subjects actually succeed? We hypothesize that a critical aspect of preventing elicited but inappropriate response tendencies from controlling behavior is to actively maintain access to the novel goal. That is, to successfully block a prepotent response, such as looking toward a flash, one must keep this goal especially accessible. Although it may be trivial to recall from LTM the rules of a task, the rules of decorum, or the laws of the land, it is often quite a bit more challenging to behave, *in the moment*, according to these rules. Our view is that active goal maintenance and the resolution of response competition are interdependent processes of

executive control, therefore, "memory" is an important determinant of "attentional" behavior (see also Chapter 4, this volume; De Jong, 2001; for an alternative view, see Butler, Zacks, & Henderson, 1999).

To explicitly test the idea that WMC may be tied to the executive acts of goal maintenance and competition resolution, Kane and Engle (2003) tested subjects with high and low spans in several versions of the Stroop color-word task. The Stroop task is a paradigmatic example of an executive attention task—a habitual, over-learned reading response must be held in check to allow the novel color-naming goal to control behavior. In order to manipulate the requirement to actively maintain access to task goals, we varied the proportion of *congruent* trials in the task. In high-congruency contexts, most trials presented words that matched their colors (e.g., *RED* appearing in red), so the task environment did not reinforce the goal of ignoring the word. Because the automatically elicited response to most stimuli was correct, it should have been easy to slip into word reading rather than color naming. Here, then, accurate responding on the rare incongruent trials, which presented conflicting color words (*BLUE* appearing in red), required that subjects maintained adequate access—in the moment—to the task goal. Failures of executive control should therefore be evident in accuracy.

In contrast, in Stroop contexts that presented few congruent trials and mostly incongruent trials, the stimuli reinforced subjects' goal. When every trial demands that the word be ignored, it may be unnecessary to do the mental work required to actively maintain goal access; the task environment acts as an external "executive." Just as Americans are helped to drive on the correct side of the road in London by road signs, traffic patterns, and the ergonomics of the car's controls, so too may subjects be kept on the desired path to color naming by a preponderance of incongruent Stroop trials. Under these circumstances, Stroop interference is unlikely to reflect goal maintenance to any great degree, and it is also unlikely to be reflected primarily in overt errors. Instead, interference in low-congruency contexts should reflect primarily the effectiveness of the competition resolution processes carried out by the externally cued goal, and should therefore be evident primarily in response latencies—that is, in slow but correct responses.

In fact, when 75% or 80% of the trials were congruent, Kane and Engle (2003) found that low spans had substantially larger error-interference effects than did high spans. These effects, across four samples in three experiments, indicate a low-span deficit in goal maintenance. Although low-span subjects understood the goal of the task, and in some experiments even received accuracy feedback after every trial, they nonetheless often "zoned out" and made word-reading errors on incongruent trials (low-span subjects also responded faster to congruent trials than high-span subjects, a finding suggesting that they periodically read the words aloud on these trials). In contrast, when only 0% or 20% of the trials were congruent, we found modest span effects in RT interference, requiring large samples to reach statistical significance. WMC-related differences were not found in errors indicative of goal neglect but rather in latencies, suggesting a slowed resolution of conflict between elicited and desired responses.

Summary Evidence from dichotic listening, antisaccade, and Stroop tasks converges to suggest that WMC predicts action control in deceptively "simple" attention tasks. Low spans are less able than high spans to act according to novel goals when that action conflicts with well-learned, if not reflexive, response tendencies. Our view is that executive attention processes largely determine performance of both WM span and these attention-control tasks, and so WM per se does not cause attention differences. Instead, a third variable, representing a low-level executive attention capability, influences functioning on all of these selective-attention, WM-span, and memory-retrieval tasks (and, presumably, on indices of Gf as well). Moreover, this executive attention capability has two aspects, one engaged to keep goals of novel tasks accessible in the face of conflict, and the other to resolve the conflict presented by habitual and goal-directed responses, or, in memory-retrieval contexts, to resolve interference between memories for similar events.

We see these goal-maintenance and competition-resolution functions of executive control as being quite similar to the proactive and reactive control modes, respectively, proposed by Braver et al. (Chapter 4) in their dual-process theory of cognitive control. Like Braver et al., we are not yet sure how these dissociable systems of control may interact with one another. On one hand, we propose that goal maintenance is necessary for the proactive blocking of competition, as in high-congruency Stroop tasks, and so here blocking or inhibition is dependent upon maintenance. On the other hand, the more reactive resolution of conflict seems to be accomplished independently of goal maintenance, and these mechanisms may also be the ones required for the resolution of memory interference (e.g., Conway & Engle, 1994; Kane & Engle, 2000; Rosen & Engle, 1998).

CHALLENGES FOR AN EXECUTIVE ATTENTION VIEW OF VARIATION IN WORKING MEMORY CAPACITY

Evidence from a variety of macroanalytic and microanalytic studies indicates that normal variation in WMC reflects primarily the function of executive attention processes. We propose that these executive processes keep representations of goal-relevant plans, responses, and stimuli in a highly accessible state in the presence of interference from prior events and distraction or conflict from the task environment. However, in the sections that follow, we discuss some current challenges for our theory of WMC variation. We first discuss two recent findings from our laboratories that may pose constraints on our conceptualization of executive attention. We then consider several complications that surround the measurement of the executive attention construct.

Boundary Conditions to the Relation between Memory Capacity and Executive Attention?

When we began investigating the connection between WMC and attention control, we had the naïve sense that most cognitive processes widely agreed to be "controlled" or "executive" would be sensitive to individual differences in WMC. However, two lines of research on visual search and task-set switching have shown that simplistic view to be incorrect.

The Problem

Following the seminal work of Treisman and Gelade (1980), visual search for targets among perceptually similar distractors has been widely considered a controlled process. That is, failing the automatic "pop out" of a unique visual feature from an array, attention is required to serially integrate the independently processed features into coherent object representations. We therefore reasoned that subjects with high spans should locate visual targets more quickly than those with low spans when attention-demanding search is required to find a target sharing features with its surround. We were wrong. After a pilot study indicated no span differences in visual search for either "automatic" or "controlled" search targets, Kane, Poole, Tuholski, and Engle (2006) replicated this span equivalence in larger samples across several different tasks. In one experiment, high- and low- span subjects searched for a target letter **F** among either **O**s (allowing more automatic, or *efficient* search) or **E**s (forcing more controlled, or *inefficient* search). Displays presented 1, 4, or 16 stimuli, arranged either in a regular matrix or psuedorandomly on-screen. Regardless of the array characteristics, the span groups showed identical search latencies and slopes across display sizes. In a second experiment, subjects searched for targets defined by a conjunction of features (**F**s among **E**s and horizontally tilted **T**s in one block, red vertical bars amidst red horizontal and green vertical bars in another); here, again, high- and low-span subjects demonstrated equivalently large search slopes. Whatever attentional processes are engaged by typical instantiations of visual search are not linked to those captured by WM span.

Inefficient search may be commonly considered a "controlled" task, but it is not nearly the gold-standard measure of executive control that task-set switching is thought to be (see Monsell & Driver, 2001). In these tasks, sub-

jects regularly or unpredictably switch back and forth between two or more response sets for ambiguous stimuli; in either case, task-switch sequences elicit an RT "switch cost" compared to task-repeat sequences. We have so far failed to demonstrate a connection between WMC and switch cost in two prototypical preparations (see also Chapter 3). In our first three experiments, Kane, Poole, Tuholski & Engle (2003) tested high and low spans in a numerical Stroop task where subjects either identified or enumerated the digits in a horizontal string (e.g., 2222 = "two" or "four"). Within a cued prime-probe procedure, half the trial pairs repeated the task between displays and half switched the task. High and low spans showed equivalent RT switch costs in all three experiments. We were surprised by these findings, but also concerned that the prime-probe procedure might be measuring something different than the more typical "alternating-runs" preparation (e.g., Rogers & Monsell, 1995). So, in a fourth experiment we tested subjects in one of four different versions of the alternating-runs task (differing from each other in task-cuing and response-mapping details). Each trial displayed a letter and number, and subjects classified either the letter as vowel or consonant or the number as odd or even. In pure-trial blocks, the same task repeated over trials; in mixed-trial bocks, the tasks alternated in an AABB sequence. In all four versions of the task, high- and low-span subjects showed equivalent RTs in all of the pure- and mixed-trial conditions.

Clearly, we find no evidence for a deficit in visual search or task-set switching in low spans. What should we conclude from these findings? Oberauer et al. (Chapter 3) suggest that our executive attention view of WMC is falsified. We disagree, in part because we find robust WMC differences in a variety of other attention-control tasks. However, it may be that the attentional processes engaged by WM span tasks are related only to "inhibitory" attention tasks requiring prepotent responses to be withheld, as in Stroop and antisaccade tests (see Chapter 9). This idea does not appeal to us either, for a number of reasons. First, as we conceive it, goal maintenance and competition resolution should be quite generally important executive capabilities.

Second, the higher-order cognitive abilities that WMC predicts, such as reading comprehension and inductive reasoning, do not necessarily involve much response conflict or restraint of habit. Third, we do find WMC-related differences in several visual-attention tasks that do not seem to fundamentally measure control of habit or prepotency. For example, Tuholski, Engle, and Bayliss (2001) found that subjects with high spans could count the number of objects presented in a disorganized visual array faster than subjects with low spans when the tally exceeded the "subitizing" (pattern recognition) range of one to four items. Here there was no obvious prepotent response to keep in check (which also suggests a problem for a purely inhibitory view of WMC variation). Likewise, in a very different visual task, Bleckley, Durso, Crutchfield, Engle, and Khanna (2003) asked high- and low-span subjects to identify a letter presented briefly at central fixation. At the same time, another letter appeared in one of 24 locations along three concentric rings around fixation, and subjects tried to identify its location. The ring on which the second letter would appear was cued (with 80% validity) as "close," "medium," or "distant." As expected from "spotlight" or "zoom lens" theories of visual attention (e.g., Eriksen & Murphy, 1987), letters appearing outside the cued ring on invalid trials (i.e., outside the spotlight) were localized more poorly than letters appearing along the cued ring. More interestingly, for high spans only, letters appearing *interior* to the cued ring were also localized more poorly than letters along the cued ring. These findings suggest that high-span subjects flexibly configured attention discontiguously, focusing on the letter at fixation and on a ring beyond fixation, at the exclusion of intermediary rings of space. This pattern suggests that high spans adopted an object-based attentional focus. Low-span subjects, in contrast, showed a benefit for any location along or interior to a cued ring, indicative of a spotlight configuration and a space-based attentional focus.

A Solution?

Given these visual-attention findings that are not obviously inhibitory in nature, how should we reconcile our failures to link WMC to search and switching? We suggest that, unlike the tasks that have yielded WMC correlations, prototypical search and switching methods do not tap volitional, executive-control processes. Of course, if we want to avoid circularity in defining "executive attention" as simply anything that correlates with WMC, we must consider more closely what search and switching actually entail.

With respect to visual search, "guided search" theory (Wolfe, 1994) proposes that attention is pulled across a master map of visual locations, based on activation flowing preattentively from multiple feature maps. That is, attention is probabilistically guided from the highest activation peak to successively lower peaks, with activation summed from "bottom-up" and "top-down" sources. Bottom-up activation accrues from physical differences among stimuli: the more an object differs from its surround, the greater the bottom-up activation to that location. In contrast, the top-down signal represents the subject's knowledge of the features that specify the desired target, expressed as a verbal category (e.g., "red"). If the subject knows the target is red amidst blue and yellow objects, then red features will prompt top-down activation to their locations on the master map.

Despite the "top-down" label, we see little relation between this use of advance knowledge and the attention-control processes we think are central to WMC, because search is proposed here to be passively "pulled" rather than endogenously "pushed." However, there may be some contexts in which top-down control is, in fact, more controlled. Wolfe (1994) proposes that top-down effects may sometimes act to reduce bottom-up contributions to the activation map. For example, if the target is a red horizontal bar amidst many red vertical bars and few green horizontal bars, then color is less diagnostic of the target than is orientation. Based on this knowledge, the bottom-up contribution of orientation could be amplified or that of color reduced. As evidence for this kind of volitional modulation, when experimenters manipulate the proportions of particular non-target features, subjects use this information to speed their search (e.g., Bacon & Egeth, 1997). We wonder whether this top-down ability to amplify or dampen bottom-up influences might vary with WMC, whereas typical conjunction search prevents its expression by presenting equal numbers of non-target types.

With respect to task-set switching, we had many reasons to expect an association with WMC. For example, De Jong (2001) argues that switch costs result largely from periodic failures to engage and maintain goal-related preparation (a parallel to our "goal maintenance" idea). This failure-to-engage hypothesis is supported by findings that variables expected to affect subjects' ability to sustain goals in active memory also affect switch costs. Moreover, mixture models that assume switch trials to produce a distribution of fast RTs on one hand (due to adequate goal maintenance) plus a distribution of slow RTs on the other (due to engagement failures) provide a good fit to the cumulative RT functions from switch trials. As another reason to expect an association with WMC, Allport and Wylie (2000) propose that a proactive interference–like perseveration of task set contributes to switch costs. Using Stroop-like stimuli, they find asymmetrical switch costs that depend more on the difficulty of the task to be switched *from* than the task to be switched *to*: for example, the cost of switching from color naming to word reading is larger than the reverse. Our findings of WMC span differences in proactive interference might therefore suggest WMC-related differences in switching.

At the same time, however, there are growing concerns that task-set switching may not be the "executive" measure it is widely assumed to be (e.g., Altmann, 2002). To discuss just one specific issue, most switching studies cue the task set for each trial by presenting either its name or an abstract symbol, and this cuing allows ostensibly non-executive encoding and retrieval processes to contaminate measurement of switch cost. Specifically, cuing paradigms confound task and cue switches (Logan & Bundesen, 2003). That is, when subjects switch tasks, the new task is signaled by a cue that is different from the immediately preceding one, whereas task-repeat trials always repeat the cue. Logan and Bundesen argue that these switch costs actually reflect a *benefit of repeating the cue on task-repeat trials*. Their idea is that the cue-plus-stimulus compound, by itself, provides all the information needed to determine a response. No executive process is needed to switch task set, so task-switching paradigms actually require only *one* task: identify the cue and target and use them to retrieve prior stimulus and cue episodes. Critically, when cues repeat, cue identification and retrieval are facilitated, and so task-repeat trials yield faster responses than those of task-switch trials.

Evidence for these ideas comes from experiments in which cues and tasks repeated or switched independently (e.g., Logan & Bundesen, 2003). For example, subjects were cued to make digit-magnitude judgments following the cues *Magnitude* or *HighLow* and parity judgments following the cues *Parity* or *Even-Odd*. When both the cue and task repeated across trials (e.g., *Parity → Parity*), RTs were substantially faster than when the cue switched but the task repeated (e.g., *EvenOdd → Parity*), indicating a cue-switch cost in the absence of a task switch. Moreover, RTs for cue-switch trials were virtually identical to actual task-switch RTs (e.g., *Magnitude → Parity*). Data like these suggest that cue switches are responsible for most of the switch cost observed in cued procedures. Thus, in order to tap truly volitional and executive processes (and to be sensitive to WMC variation), task-switching procedures must eliminate the roles of cue encoding and cue-based retrieval processes.

Summary

It may be surprising, initially, that WMC is unrelated to search slopes and switch costs. And, taken at face value, these null findings may seem to call our "executive attention" theory of WMC into question (see Chapter 3). However, we suggest that our null effects are less surprising when we appreciate the complexity of visual search and task switching. Most task-switching and visual-search paradigms are simply not good indices of executive control, and just because researchers label search and switching tasks as "controlled" or "executive" does not make them so. More broadly, given the number of WMC–attention associations we have observed, we submit that the mere failure to find a correlation between WMC and any particular executive task does not necessarily falsify our view. However, such failures do point to obviously important questions for future research on the nature of both WMC and executive control, and the *tasks that we use to measure them.*

Measuring Working Memory Capacity and Executive Attention

We view WM span tasks as reasonably good measures of executive attention (along with a host of other processes) because their dual-task requirements challenge subjects to maintain access to information outside of conscious awareness, recover access to information that was outside of awareness, or both, all in the face of proactive interference. However, a WMC measure need not be a dual task in order to tax attention control. Indeed, Oberauer and colleagues have shown that a latent factor derived from various "coordination" tasks can be indistinguishable from a "storage-plus-processing" WM span factor (see Chapter 3). These coordination tasks generally require subjects to keep track of a large number of stimuli at the same time, or to rapidly switch attention among these active stimuli, and so they also require maintained access to information that is momentarily outside the focus of attention.

Indeed, prototypical STM span tasks should also make non-negligible demands on executive control, particularly when routinized rehearsal techniques are made ineffective or when the lists are too long to be maintained entirely in conscious focus. In fact, spatial STM tasks, which do not afford phonological rehearsal, seem to be quite good measures of the WMC–executive construct and correlate strongly with general ability (e.g., Kane et al., 2004; see also Chapters 3 and 8, this volume). Moreover, Unsworth and Engle (2006) found that long lists from verbal STM span tasks correlate strongly with all list lengths from verbal WMC span tasks, and long STM lists predict similar variance in Gf, as do long and short WMC lists. Because the focus of attention comprises

only about 4 ± 1 items (Cowan, 2001), and because the phonological loop can hold only what can be spoken in about 2 s (Baddeley, 1986), verbal STM lengths larger than four items or so will require some degree of executive attention to be maintained or recovered from outside conscious focus.

By this view, span tasks (or any other memory tasks) cannot be dichotomized as reflecting either STM or WMC, or either storage or executive control, because all immediate memory tasks are complex and determined by a host of factors, including both storage and executive attention. The challenge for researchers of WM variation is to assess the contributions of these various processes to the associations between memory tasks and measures of higher-order cognition (or between these memory tasks and age, or personality, or psychopathology, etc.). We have focused our research on WM span because these tasks have undergone more parametric and task-analytic work than the alternatives, and we suggest that researchers conduct similar explorations of other candidate WMC tasks to move the field forward.

Before leaving a consideration of WMC measurement, we must accept a shortcoming of our view, pointed out in Chapter 3. Our research has demonstrated a strong association between WMC and Gf on one hand, and statistically significant differences between high- and low-span subjects in attention performance on the other hand. From these findings, we have inferred that executive attention processes tapped by WMC tasks are responsible for its covariation with Gf and cognitive ability. Note, however, that there are two important inferences here that require more explicit support, preferably from a latent-variable approach. First, we have not yet established the strength of the correlation between WM span and attention-control measures; our extreme-group designs testing high- vs. low-span subjects may overestimate the WMC effect size. Second, if executive attention is responsible for the covariation between WMC and cognitive ability, then a latent factor comprised of *the shared variance among WMC and attention-control tasks* should predict substantial variance in Gf. At the same time, any remaining, unique WMC and attention-control variance should not correlate with Gf as strongly. If WMC and attention-control constructs correlate weakly, or if shared WMC–attention variance is not a strong predictor of cognitive ability, then our theory is in trouble.

OUR EXECUTIVE ATTENTION VIEW IN RELATION TO OTHER THEORIES

General Theories of Working Memory

Our view is that WM span tasks are complex and determined by many general and domain-specific processes, skills, and strategies. However, variation in WMC, as measured by individual differences in WM span, reflects primarily executive attention capabilities. These executive activities are general and important to a range of intellectual functions, from controlling inappropriate actions, to learning and recalling information amidst competing memories, to solving complex verbal and nonverbal problems. Before we reflect upon particular "competing" perspectives on WMC variation, we first consider our views in light of important nomothetic WM theories, such as Baddeley's "multiple-component" WM theory (Baddeley, 1986, 2000), and Nairne's very different, more process-oriented approach (Nairne, 2002).

The Multiple-Component Working Memory Model

Our theory of WM variation is inspired by Baddeley and Hitch's (1974) demonstration that the cognitive problem of balancing memory storage and ongoing mental activity is central to a range of intellectual capabilities. Moreover, our distinction between general attention processes and domain-specific storage processes is consistent with Baddeley's (1986, 2000) separation of the central-executive (attentional) component from the phonological-loop and visuospatial-sketchpad (storage/rehearsal) components of the WM system.

However, our view differs from the multiple-component model in emphasizing function and process over structure. That is, we view the domain specificity of "STM storage" to reflect different perceptual bases of, and rehearsal activities afforded by, different stimuli. As we stated earlier, our process-oriented view is more akin to Cowan's (1995) conception of immediate memory. "STM" is represented by graded activation of LTM traces (with "focal attention" representing the limited, conscious portion of activated LTM), along with routinized and executive processes that maintain activation. Cowan's model, in turn, closely resembles Wundt's (1912/1973) conception of consciousness. Wundt distinguished *apprehension*, the graded entrance of objects into consciousness, from *apperception*, the entrance of apprehended objects into awareness. In today's terms, Wundt argued that information could remain accessible (or activated) outside attentional focus. Moreover, Wundt claimed, like Cowan, that the focus of attention is strictly limited, whereas above-threshold activation is more broad and variable in scope. These ideas resonate with our claims regarding WMC, particularly that executive processes maintain or recover access to "apprehended" representations of goals, response productions and stimuli in the absence of focal attention or skilled rehearsal routines, and in the presence of interference or conflict.

The Baddeley (1986, 2000) model is most obviously characterized by its structural focus, that is, by its separation of WM into distinct components with different attributes and functions. In general, we are unenthusiastic about such neo-structuralist approaches to memory theorizing. Although Baddeley has been more restrained in proposing structures to account for new dissociations than have LTM researchers, WM structures have begun to proliferate. Theorists now pose separate buffers for semantic information (e.g., Haarmann, Davelaar, & Usher, 2003), visual imagery vs. visual rehearsal (Pearson, 2001), and assigning syntactic structures (Caplan, Waters, and DeDe, Chapter 11). As in LTM research, consensual and specific criteria for proposing new immediate-memory systems are lacking, and we therefore envision an undisciplined explosion of WM buffers as "explanations" for behavior.

Baddeley's (2000, 2001) most recent incarnation of the WM model makes a structural claim that is most relevant to our work. A new subsystem, the "episodic buffer," is proposed to handle some problems for the model, such as how verbal material is maintained under articulatory suppression. The episodic buffer is essentially an immediate-memory version of episodic memory, a mnemonic store for maintenance of integrated, multidimensional representations of objects and events. Of primary concern here, Baddeley (2001) speculates that the episodic buffer underlies performance of WM span tasks: by the multiple-component view, the phonological loop cannot support verbal WM span when the processing-task stimuli are read aloud (and thus provide articulatory suppression). From our perspective, however, the episodic buffer currently offers little to research on WM variation. Baddeley has not yet clarified the buffer's importance to the predictive power of WM span: is it incidental, with the executive driving the correlations, or does the buffer's multimodal nature make it critical to cognition broadly? Furthermore, the "constrained-sentence span" task, designed to measure the capacity of the episodic buffer (Baddeley, 2001), seems a minor variation on the reading span task. We are therefore skeptical that individual-differences research will soon clarify the nature or utility of this new WM component, or vice versa.

Functionalist and Process-Oriented Approaches to Immediate Memory

Our view of immediate memory is less structural than Baddeley's (1986, 2000) model. Nonetheless, we do identify the executive attention processes tapped by WM span tasks with particular brain systems, particularly the circuitry of the dorsolateral prefrontal cortex (dPFC; Kane & Engle, 2002). Moreover, like many cognitive psychologists, we retain a conceptual distinction between immediate memory and LTM, regarding the former as an activated portion of the latter.

Our comfort with the dichotomy of active and inactive memory is not for lack of a good alternative. Research deriving from the verbal-learning and functionalist traditions generally assumed a unitary memory, and neofunctionalist and proceduralist views draw upon this heritage (e.g., Crowder, 1982; Melton, 1963; Toth & Hunt, 1999). According to these accounts, one set of processing rules governs remembering: memory is an activity, not a thing, and remembering over the "short term" and "long term" is identical, despite the phenomenological and folk-psychological distinction. Most recently, Nairne (2002) questioned the activation metaphor of immediate memory, arguing that evidence is wanting for such a special memory state, its loss through decay, and its protection via rehearsal. By Nairne's view, which is widely agreed upon in the study of LTM, memories have no special status outside of a given constellation of cues. Remembering is not determined by the strength of a trace, but rather by the discriminability of the target event amidst competitors, given a specific task environment. In Nairne's "feature model," specifically, all retrieval is governed by the match between environmental cues and the fragile (non-conscious) "processing records" of recent events that are vulnerable to interference. Forgetting thus occurs when the cue and/or processing records fail to uniquely prompt recollection of the target event.

The activation and decay of representations are appealing metaphors for WM research, including that on WM variation. Indeed, our research relies heavily on the activation metaphor to describe the heightened accessibility of information, resulting from rehearsal or executive attention processes, which contributes to various complex cognitive tasks. Nairne (2002) provides compelling arguments and evidence against decay and the protective powers of rehearsal, but we still find the activation concept useful. Heuristically, it provides language with which to describe the ways in which goals may control behavior in the face of conflict, as in Stroop tasks, as well as to conceive of the relation between measures of WM span and attention control more broadly. The feature model, emphasizing cue-driven discrimination among stored processing records, is not easily extended into the domain of WM variation. If WMC reflected such memory-discrimination processes, even if closely tied to interference, we do not yet see how they should relate to reading comprehension, spatial visualization, or moving one's eyes away from a flash. In contrast, the idea that WMC reflects an ability to maintain information in an activated or accessible state during ongoing processing is more easily applied across simple and complex cognitive tasks.[3]

Moreover, recent research suggests a strong link between WMC and dPFC functioning, and in the realm of neuroscience, the activation metaphor is less of a metaphor. For example, individual dPFC cells that are "tuned" to particular locations, objects, rules, or their combinations maintain a pattern of sustained firing over memory delays for their preferred stimuli. What's more, these dPFC cells, unlike those in posterior brain areas, maintain their activity when distracting stimuli are presented during the delay (for a review, see Kane & Engle, 2002). Such target-specific, delay-related activity is difficult to interpret from a neo-functional perspective that denies a special state of activity tied to immediate memory. It fits quite well, however, with our view that executive attention involves the active maintenance of goal-relevant information in the face of interference and distraction.

As an "attentional" example, sustained dPFC activity that is related to goal maintenance predicts Stroop interference. Under functional magnetic resonance imaging (fMRI), MacDonald, Cohen, Stenger, and Carter (2000) presented subjects with word-reading and color-naming Stroop tasks, unpredictably cued 11 s before each stimulus. Fifty percent of the trials were congruent, and so in combination with the frequent word-reading demand, the overall task environment did not reinforce the color-naming goal. On color-naming trials, which demanded an anti-habitual response, dPFC activity increased steadily over the cue-to-target delay and this increase correlated negatively with interference magnitude ($r = -.63$). Subjects who were better able to activate and sustain the "ignore-the-word" goal were also better able to resist interference from the words.

Across memory and attention studies in the neuroscience literatures, then, we see a parallel

between neural activity and WM maintenance, and we view these more literal demonstrations of activation as license to use the activation metaphor in describing normal behavioral variation in WMC.

Theories of Variation in Working Memory Capacity

The most popular alternative views of WMC variation that we analyze below, processing-speed and attentional-inhibition theories, have been most widely and successfully applied to studies of life span cognitive development. Indeed, we will claim that, whereas processing speed seems to be important to age-related variation in WMC, it has yet to prove its mettle in accounting for within-age variation. Our discussion of attentional inhibition will be more nuanced and less decisive because, in our view, the inhibition approach is only subtly different from our own. First, however, we briefly consider the overlapping, recently developed views of Oberauer et al. (Chapter 3) and Cowan (2004).

Capacity of Attentional Focus and Region of Direct Access

Although Oberauer et al. (Chapter 3) accept Cowan's (1995) conceptualization of the WM system, as do we, our view of WMC variation is distinguishable from both of these views. Cowan (2005a, 2005b) recently suggested that WMC variation and covariation may reflect the size, or capacity, of attentional focus. Thus, WMC is a true "capacity" by Cowan's view, corresponding to a structural limit in the amount of material that can be held in a particular state, in parallel to the 7 ± 2 capacity limit for STM proposed by Miller (1956). Our view, in contrast, is that high-WMC individuals are not necessarily able to hold more discreet representations in consciousness than are low-WMC individuals, but high spans are better able to actively maintain task-relevant information outside of consciousness and to do the mental work necessary to quickly recover information from inactive memory despite interference.

We see evidence against Cowan's view in two findings of WMC equivalence in ostensible signatures of focused-attention capacity: subitizing and primary memory. Tuholski et al. (2001) found that high- and low-span subjects could enumerate in parallel (or "subitize") an equal number of visual objects (3.35 and 3.25, respectively), but low spans showed a much steeper counting slope *beyond* the subitizing range than that of high spans. Engle, Tuholski et al. (1999) tested subjects in an immediate free-recall task, and their derived estimates of primary memory capacity did not correlate with WMC; only estimates of secondary memory capacity did. Both results suggest that high and low spans can keep a similar number of representations available in the conscious focus of attention. Where they differ, instead, is in processing and recovering representations *outside* attentional focus. Because Oberauer et al. (Chapter 3) equate their "direct-access" component of WM with Cowan's focus of attention, their view that individual differences in WMC and reasoning ability centrally reflect variation in direct access also seems to be contradicted by our findings.

General Processing Speed

General processing-speed (PS) theories broadly propose to account for variation in higher-order cognition via the measurement of latencies from simple cognitive tasks (e.g., Jensen, 1998). The idea is that people with low PS complete fewer mental operations per unit time, and this leads to a failure in completing some critical operations, a greater likelihood of losing the products of processing through decay, or a reduced ability to keep multiple processing streams active via rehearsal or switching. With respect to life span cognitive development, a key finding is that age-related variance in complex cognitive activity, and in WMC, is reduced dramatically after statistically controlling for variance in mean PS (Kail & Salthouse, 1994; see also Chapters 6 and 8, this volume).

However, we have already reported findings from our research indicating that PS is not a promising mechanism for WMC variation among young adults. First, PS measures neither correlate strongly with WMC nor account for the shared variance between WMC and Gf (Conway et al., 2002). Second, studies of retrieval interference find that high and low spans' recognition latencies are equivalent in the absence, but not the presence, of response competition (Conway & Engle, 1994). Indeed, high-span subjects' recall latencies are actually *longer* than those of low-span subjects when the target information had previously been suppressed when related information was learned (Rosen & Engle, 1998). Third, high and low spans' letter-identification latencies are equivalent in the prosaccade task when it was presented before antisaccade (Kane et al., 2001), and span differences in baseline Stroop RTs come and go across experiments independently of interference differences (Kane & Engle, 2003). Fourth, and finally, in visual search and task switching, high and low spans show equivalent RTs in relatively complex conditions with long mean latencies.

Processing-speed theory cannot accommodate these results. However, even if it could be modified to do so without incorporating our theoretical premises, we would remain unenthusiastic because PS theory has yet to provide a reasonably specific *psychological* account for its variation or covariation. Conway, Kane, and Engle (1999) suggested that researchers consider the role of variation in attention control in producing variation in PS within and across age groups (see also Chapter 9). For example, increases in PS–ability correlations with PS task complexity and decreases in PS–ability correlations with task practice seem fit for an attentional explanation. Furthermore, in studies of young adults, individuals' *variability* in RT is often more strongly correlated with cognitive ability than is median RT (Jensen, 1998). Given that RT variability may reflect failures of sustained attention, RT variability may reflect executive-control difficulties. At least among young adults, then, WMC–attention variation might drive PS variation, rather than the reverse.

Attentional Inhibition

Finally, an influential research program by Hasher, Zacks, and colleagues suggests that WM variation derives from the operation of inhibitory attentional mechanisms (e.g., Hasher & Zacks, 1988; see Chapter 9). Their claim is that what appears to be a structurally reduced WMC in some individuals (e.g., the elderly, or young adults at their off-peak hours) actually reflects a *functional* reduction due to the intrusion and persistence of irrelevant information. Inhibitory attention mechanisms, which control cognition by restricting access to and deleting information from WM, often fail with aging and circadian variation. Thus, individuals with ineffective inhibition due to aging, normal individual differences, variation in circadian arousal, or what have you, suffer disproportionately from memory interference, language production and comprehension difficulties, and contextually inappropriate responding. Interference and distraction are thus central problems of control and WM variation.

These ideas have significantly influenced our view of WMC variation, and indeed, the difference between the inhibitory view and ours is quite subtle. Hasher and colleagues argue that WMC variation is driven largely by variation in inhibitory control. As evidence, their microanalytic work has investigated the role of proactive interference in determining WM span scores. In typical "ascending" administrations of reading span, large sets are encountered only after interference from prior trials builds up. Thus, interference-vulnerable individuals, such as the elderly, are disadvantaged on the large sets that are most critical to the span score. Lustig et al. (2001) therefore tested some subjects with an ascending task, proceeding from set-size 2 to 4, and others in a descending task, proceeding from size 4 to 2. Additional young subjects were tested on a descending task with filled breaks between every set to reduce interference further. Lustig et al. found significant age differences in WM span in the ascending but not the descending condition—reducing proactive interference reduced age differences. Furthermore, within age groups, the span condition with the least interference (descending for older adults, descending-with-breaks for younger adults) showed no correlation with reading comprehension. Thus, interference resistance, assumed to reflect inhibition, mediated span correlations with age and ability (see also Bunting, 2006).

We have characterized the executive-attention and attentional-inhibition views as providing a "chicken–egg" dilemma, where one assumes WMC to determine inhibitory control and the other, the reverse (Kane et al., 2001). However, upon further reflection we do not think this is quite right. Instead, whereas the inhibitory view assumes inhibition to determine WMC, we submit that a third variable causes both. Our view is that executive attention processes block sources of interference and competition, as well as keep information active in interference- and conflict-rich contexts and in the service of ongoing cognitive processes. Thus, WMC and inhibition are strongly linked, but indirectly through a more basic attentional construct.

Although interference clearly contributes to particular tests of reading comprehension, WM span predicts performance in many tasks where interference or inhibition are not obviously relevant but active maintenance should be, such as mental rotation, verbal analogies, or counting visual objects (Kane et al., 2004; Tuholski et al., 2001). In addition, our Stroop findings, as well as those reviewed from the neuroscience literature, suggest that PFC maintenance of stimuli and goals allows for effective inhibition under some conditions. We are unsure how inhibition might account for sustained memory-related activity of dPFC cells, increasing dPFC activation prompted by Stroop-task cues, or congruency effects on span differences in Stroop interference. Moreover, if resistance to proactive interference actually reflects inhibition (but for alternative views, see Hasher & Johnson, 1975; Underwood & Ekstrand, 1967), we find that high spans' inhibitory control is impaired by secondary tasks, which suggests that some more fundamental control process governs inhibition (Kane & Engle, 2000). Thus, we believe our more general, "executive attention" view to be more comprehensive than the inhibitory view in accounting for the breadth of the cognitive and neuroscience findings regarding the covariation of WMC with other cognitive activities and abilities.

BOX 2.1. SUMMARY ANSWERS TO BOOK QUESTIONS

1. THE OVERARCHING THEORY OF WORKING MEMORY

Following Cowan (1995), we view WM as an integrated memory and attention system, comprised of long-term memory representations (for stimuli, goals, or action plans) activated above threshold, procedural skills for rehearsal and stimulus coding, and executive attention processes. Activated representations represent the contents of "short-term memory," and a very limited subset of these are experienced as the focus of conscious awareness, or "focused attention." Procedural skills and executive attention are engaged to maintain activation or access to goal-relevant representations, particularly those outside of focused attention, which would otherwise return to baseline as a result of decay or interference.

2. CRITICAL SOURCES OF WORKING MEMORY VARIATION

Variation may occur in any WM component. However, in healthy adults, WM capacity's covariation with general cognitive ability stems from variation in executive attention. Executive attention maintains activation to goal-relevant representations outside of conscious focus, recovers access to non-active representations against interference, and resolves competition between co-active representations or between habitual and goal-appropriate actions. *Macroanalytic*, latent-variable studies suggest that WMC and Gf share substantial variance while controlling for STM. As well, *microanalytic*, quasi-experimental studies indicate that WMC variation predicts individual differences in a variety of memory-interference and attention-control tasks.

3. OTHER SOURCES OF WORKING MEMORY VARIATION

Our executive attention view, emphasizing goal maintenance and competition resolution, parallels the dual mechanisms of cognitive control proposed by Braver et al. (Chapter 4), and is only subtly different from the inhibitory view of Hasher et al. (Chapter 9), who suggest that inhibition drives WMC. We argue that a common attention-control capability underlies WMC and inhibition. However, our view is incompatible with those of others. Although measures of processing speed account for age-related variance in WMC and cognitive ability (see Chapter 8), they do not account for WMC–ability covariation in young adults. In addition, WMC differences do not correspond to measures of focused-attention capacity, but rather to processing beyond conscious focus, contradicting proposals by Cowan (2005a,b) and Oberauer et al. (Chapter 3).

4. CONTRIBUTIONS TO GENERAL WORKING MEMORY THEORY

The study of WMC variation has led the way in fulfilling WM theory's original and greatest promise—to illuminate the *functions* of immediate memory. This work shows that the domain-general, executive components of the WM system support a broad range of cognitive abilities, and may even provide the scaffolding for a cognition-based understanding of intelligence. Correlational research also provides support for the dissociability of domain-specific storage and rehearsal processes and for the idea that domain-specific memory processes and domain-general attention processes are intimately linked (if not synthesized) within the WM system.

Notes

1. Demonstrations of low reliability reported by Caplan et al. (Chapter 11) are troubling. However, Turley-Ames and Whitfield (2003) showed operation span to be reliable over minutes ($rs = .7 - .8$), Klein and Fiss (1999) showed it to be reliable over weeks and months ($rs = .7 - .8$), and an automated version of operation span had a test-retest reliability of .83 with an average lag of 13 days (Unsworth,

Heitz, Schrock, & Engle, 2005). Of course, strong correlations between WM and cognitive ability measures, reported throughout the literature, also indicate their reliability.

2. In the Kane et al. (2004) model (Fig. 2.4), verbal storage correlated substantially with only verbal reasoning, but spatial storage strongly predicted both spatial and general reasoning. Indeed, the storage–Gf correlation appeared despite the model's controlling for the executive–Gf association. Spatial storage processes thus accounted for as much unique variance in Gf as did executive attention, consistent with correlational evidence that spatial STM tasks are good measures of general ability (see also Chapters 3 and 8).

3. Nairne's approach could be made somewhat more compatible with ours by assuming that executive attention were involved in cue-driven retrieval under interference.

References

Allport, D. A., & Wylie, G. (2000). Task switching, stimulus–response bindings, and negative priming. In S. Monsell & J. Driver (Eds.), *Attention and performance XVIII: Control of cognitive processes* (pp. 35–70). Cambridge, MA: MIT Press.

Altmann, E.M. (2002). Functional decay of memory tasks. *Psychological Research, 66*, 287–297.

Anderson, M. C., & Neely, J. H. (1996). Interference and inhibition in memory retrieval. In E. L. Bjork & R. A. Bjork (Eds.), *Memory* (pp. 237–313). New York: Academic Press.

Atkinson, R. C., & Shiffrin, R. M. (1971). The control of short-term memory. *Scientific American, 225*, 82–90.

Bacon, W. F., & Egeth, H. E. (1997). Goal-directed guidance of attention: Evidence from conjunctive visual search. *Journal of Experimental Psychology: Human Perception and Performance, 23*, 948–961.

Baddeley, A. D. (1986). *Working memory.* New York: Oxford University Press.

Baddeley, A. D. (2000). The episodic buffer: A new component of working memory? *Trends in Cognitive Sciences, 4*, 417–423.

Baddeley, A. D. (2001). Is working memory still working? *American Psychologist, 56*, 851–864.

Baddeley, A. D., Gathercole, S., & Papagno, C. (1998). The phonological loop as a language learning device. *Psychologial Review, 105*, 158–173.

Baddeley, A. D., & Hitch, G. (1974). Working memory. In G. H. Bower (Ed.), *The psychology of learning and motivation: Advances in research and theory* (Vol. 8, pp. 47–89). New York: Academic Press.

Barrouillet, P., Bernadin, S., & Camos, V. (2004). Time constraints and resource sharing in adults' working memory spans. *Journal of Experimental Psychology: General, 133*, 83–100.

Bleckley, M. K., Durso, F. T., Crutchfield, J. M., Engle, R. W., & Khana, M. M. (2003). Individual differences in working memory capacity predict visual attention allocation. *Psychonomic Bulletin & Review, 10*, 884–889.

Bunting, M. F. (2006). Proactive interference and item similarity in working memory. *Journal of Experimental Psychology: Learning, Memory, and Cognition, 32*, 183–196.

Butler, K. M., Zacks, R. T., & Henderson, J. M. (1999). Suppression of reflexive saccades in younger and older adults: Age comparisons on an antisaccade task. *Memory & Cognition, 27*, 584–591.

Case, R., Kurland, M. D., & Goldberg, J. (1982). Operational efficiency and the growth of short-term memory span. *Journal of Experimental Child Psychology, 33*, 386–404.

Conway, A. R. A., Cowan, N., & Bunting, M. F. (2001). The cocktail party phenomenon revisited: The importance of working memory capacity. *Psychonomic Bulletin & Review, 8*, 331–335.

Conway, A. R. A., Cowan, N., Bunting, M. F., Therriault, D., & Minkoff, S. (2002). A latent variable analysis of working memory capacity, short-term memory capacity, processing speed, and general fluid intelligence. *Intelligence, 30*, 163–183.

Conway, A. R. A., & Engle, R. W. (1994). Working memory and retrieval: A resource-dependent inhibition model. *Journal of Experimental Psychology: General, 123*, 354–373.

Conway, A. R. A., & Engle, R. W. (1996). Individual differences in working memory capacity: More evidence for a general capacity theory. *Memory, 4*, 577–590.

Conway, A. R. A., Kane, M. J., & Engle, R. W. (1999). Is Spearman's g determined by speed or working memory capacity? Book review of

Jensen on Intelligence-g-Factor. *Psycoloquy, 10* (074), Article 16.

Conway, A.R.A., Kane, M.J., & Engle, R.W. (2003). Working memory capacity and its relation to general intelligence. *Trends in Cognitive Sciences, 7*, 547–552.

Cowan, N. (1995). *Attention and memory: An integrated framework.* Oxford, UK: Oxford University Press.

Cowan, N. (2001). The magical number 4 in short-term memory: A reconsideration of mental storage capacity. *Behavioral and Brain Sciences, 24*, 87–185.

Cowan, N. (2005a). Understanding intelligence: A summary and an adjustable-attention hypothesis. In O. Wilhelm & R. W. Engle (Eds.), *Handbook of understanding and measuring intelligence* (pp. 469–488). Thousand Oaks, CA: Sage.

Cowan, N. (2005b). *Working memory capacity.* New York, New York: Psychology Press.

Cronbach, L. J., (1957). The two disciplines of scientific psychology. *American Psychologist, 12*, 671–684.

Crowder, R. G. (1982). The demise of short-term memory. *Acta Psychologica, 50*, 291–323.

Daneman, M., & Carpenter, P. A. (1980). Individual differences in working memory and reading. *Journal of Verbal Learning and Verbal Behavior, 19*, 450–466.

Daneman, M., & Merikle, P. M. (1996). Working memory and language comprehension: A meta-analysis. *Psychonomic Bulletin & Review, 3*, 422–433.

De Jong, R. (2001). Adult age differences in goal activation and goal maintenance. *European Journal of Cognitive Psychology, 13*, 71–89.

Engle, R. W., Cantor, J., & Carullo, J. J. (1992). Individual differences in working memory and comprehension: A test of four hypotheses. *Journal of Experimental Psychology: Learning, Memory, and Cognition, 18*, 972–992.

Engle, R.W., & Kane, M.J. (2004). Executive attention, working memory capacity, and a two-factor theory of cognitive control. In B. Ross (Ed.) *The psychology of learning and motivation* (pp. 145–199). New York: Academic Press.

Engle, R. W., Kane, M. J., & Tuholski, S. W. (1999). Individual differences in working memory capacity and what they tell us about controlled attention, general fluid intelligence and functions of the prefrontal cortex. In A. Miyake & P. Shah (Eds.), *Models of working memory: Mechanisms of active maintenance and executive control* (pp. 102–134). New York: Cambridge University Press.

Engle, R. W., Tuholski, S. W., Laughlin, J. E., & Conway, A. R. A. (1999). Working memory, short-term memory and general fluid intelligence: A latent variable approach. *Journal of Experimental Psychology: General, 128*, 309–331.

Eriksen, C. W., & Murphy, T. D. (1987). Movement of attentional focus across the visual field: A critical look at the evidence. *Perception and Psychophysics, 42*, 299–305.

Friedman, N. P., & Miyake, A. (2004). The reading span test and its predictive power for reading comprehension ability. *Journal of Memory and Language, 51*, 136–158.

Haarmann, H. J., Davelaar, E. J., & Usher, M. (2003). Individual differences in semantic short-term memory capacity and reading comprehension. *Journal of Memory and Language, 48*, 320–345.

Hasher, L., & Johnson, M. K. (1975). Interpretive factors in forgetting. *Journal of Experimental Psychology: Human Learning and Memory, 1*, 567–575.

Hasher, L., & Zacks, R. T. (1988). Working memory, comprehension, and aging: A review and a new view. In G. H. Bower (Ed.), *The psychology of learning and motivation: Advances in research and theory* (Vol. 22, pp. 193–225). San Diego: Academic Press.

Hitch, G. J., Towse, J. N., & Hutton, U. M. Z. (2001). What limits children's working memory span? Theoretical accounts and applications for scholastic development. *Journal of Experimental Psychology: General, 130*, 184–198.

Jensen, A. R. (1998). *The g factor: The science of mental ability.* Westport, CT: Praeger.

Jonides, J., Reuter-Lorenz, P. A., Smith, E. E., Awh, E., Barnes, L. L., Drain, M., Glass, J., Lauber, E. J., Patalano, A. L., & Schumacher, E. H. (1996). Verbal and spatial working memory in humans. *Psychology of Learning and Motivation, 35*, 43–88.

Kail, R., & Salthouse, T. A. (1994). Processing speed as a mental capacity. *Acta Psychologica, 86*, 199–225.

Kane, M. J., Bleckley, M. K., Conway, A. R. A., & Engle, R. W. (2001). A controlled-attention view of working-memory capacity. *Journal of Experimental Psychology: General, 130,* 169–183.

Kane, M. J., & Engle, R. W. (2000). Working memory capacity, proactive interference, and divided attention: Limits on long-term memory retrieval. *Journal of Experimental Psychology: Learning, Memory, and Cognition, 26,* 333–358.

Kane, M. J., & Engle, R. W. (2002). The role of prefrontal cortex in working-memory capacity, executive attention, and general fluid intelligence: An individual-differences perspective. *Psychonomic Bulletin & Review, 9,* 637–671.

Kane, M. J., & Engle, R. W. (2003). Working-memory capacity and the control of attention: The contributions of goal neglect, response competition, and task set to Stroop interference. *Journal of Experimental Psychology: General, 132,* 47–70.

Kane, M. J., Hambrick, D. Z., & Conway, A. R. A. (2005). Working memory capacity and fluid intelligence are strongly related constructs: Comment on Ackerman, Beier, and Boyle (2005). *Psychological Bulletin, 131,* 66–71.

Kane, M. J., Hambrick, D. Z., Tuholski, S. W., Wilhelm, O., Payne, T. W., & Engle, R. W. (2004). The generality of working memory capacity: A latent-variable approach to verbal and visuo-spatial memory span and reasoning. *Journal of Experimental Psychology: General, 133,* 189–217.

Kane, M. J., Poole, B., Tuholski, S. W., & Engle, R. W. (2003). *Working memory capacity and executive control in search and switching.* Presented at the annual meeting of the Psychonomic Society, Vancouver, Canada.

Kane, M. J., Poole, B. J., Tuholski, S. W., & Engle, R. W. (2006). Working memory capacity and the top-down control of visual search: Exploring the boundaries of "Executive attention." *Journal of Experimental Psychology: Learning, Memory, and Cognition, 32,* 749–777.

Klein, K., & Fiss, W. H. (1999). The reliability and stability of the Turner and Engle working memory task. *Behavior Research Methods, Instruments & Computers, 31,* 429–432.

Kyllonen, P. C., & Christal, R. E. (1990). Reasoning ability is (little more than) working-memory capacity?! *Intelligence, 14,* 389–433.

Logan, G. D. & Bundesen, C. (2003). Clever homunculus: Is there an endogenous act of control in the explicit task-cuing procedure? *Journal of Experimental Psychology: Human Perception and Performance, 29,* 575–599.

Lustig, C., May, C. P., & Hasher, L. (2001). Working memory span and the role of proactive interference. *Journal of Experimental Psychology: General, 130,* 199–207.

MacDonald, A. W., III, Cohen, J. D., Stenger, V. A., & Carter, C. S. (2000). Dissociating the role of the dorsolateral prefrontal and anterior cingulate cortex in cognitive control. *Science, 288,* 1835–1838.

MacDonald, M. C., & Christiansen, M. H. (2002). Reassessing working memory: Comment on Just and Carpenter (1992) and Waters and Caplan (1996). *Psychological Review, 109,* 35–54.

McNamara, D. S., & Scott, J. L. (2001). Working memory capacity and strategy use. *Memory & Cognition, 29,* 10–17.

Melton, A. W. (1963). Implications of short-term memory for a general theory of memory. *Journal of Verbal Learning and Verbal Behavior, 2,* 1–21.

Miller, G. A. (1956). The magical number seven, plus or minus two: Some limits on our capacity for processing information. *Psychological Review, 63,* 81–97.

Miyake, A., Friedman, N. P., Rettinger, D. A., Shah, P., & Hegarty, M. (2001). How are visuospatial working memory, executive functioning, and spatial abilities related? A latent-variable analysis. *Journal of Experimental Psychology: General, 130,* 621–640.

Monsell, S., & Driver, J. (Eds.). (2001). *Attention and performance XVIII: Control of cognitive processes.* Cambridge, MA: MIT Press.

Nairne, J. S. (2002). Remembering over the short term: The case against the standard model. *Annual Review of Psychology, 53,* 53–81.

Norman, D. A., & Shallice, T. (1986). Attention to action: Willed and automatic control of behavior. In R. J. Davidson, G. E. Schwartz, & D. Shapiro (Eds.), *Consciousness and self-regulation: Advances in research and theory* (vol. 4, pp. 1–18). New York: Plenum Press.

Pearson, D. G. (2001). Imagery and the visuo-spatial sketchpad. In J. Andrade (Ed.), *Working memory in perspective* (pp. 33–59). Hove, UK: Psychology Press.

Rogers, R. D., & Monsell, S. (1995). The cost of a predictable switch between simple cognitive tasks. *Journal of Experimental Psychology: General, 124,* 207–231.

Rosen, V. M., & Engle, R. W. (1998). Working memory capacity and suppression. *Journal of Memory and Language, 39,* 418–436.

Salthouse, T. A., & Craik, F. I. M. (2001). Closing comments. In F. I. M. Craik & T. A. Salthouse (Eds.), *The handbook of aging and cognition* (2nd ed.). Mahwah, NJ: Lawrence Erlbaum Associates.

Shah, P., & Miyake, A. (1996). The separability of working memory resources for spatial thinking and language processing: An individual differences approach. *Journal of Experimental Psychology: General, 125,* 4–27.

Toth, J. P., & Hunt, R. R. (1999). Not one versus many, but zero versus any: Structure and function in the context of the multiple memory systems debate. In J. K. Foster & M. Jelicic (Eds.), *Memory: Systems, process, or function?* (pp. 233–272). Oxford, UK: Oxford University Press.

Treisman, A. M., & Gelade, G. (1980). A feature-integration theory of attention. *Cognitive Psychology, 12,* 97–136.

Tuholski, S. W., Engle, R. W., & Baylis, G. C. (2001). Individual differences in working memory capacity and enumeration. *Memory & Cognition, 29,* 484–492.

Turley-Ames, K. J., & Whitfield, M. M. (2003). Strategy training and working memory task performance. *Journal of Memory and Language, 49,* 446–468.

Turner, M. L., & Engle, R. W. (1989). Is working memory capacity task dependent? *Journal of Memory and Language, 28,* 127–154.

Underwood, B. J. (1975). Individual differences as a crucible in theory construction. *American Psychologist, 30,* 128–134.

Underwood, B. J., & Ekstrand, B. R. (1967). Studies of distributed practice XXIV: Differentiation and proactive inhibition. *Journal of Experimental Psychology, 74,* 574–580.

Unsworth, N., & Engle, R. W. (2006). Verbal working and short-term memory spans and their relation to fluid abilities: Evidence from list-length effects. *Journal of Memory and Language, 54,* 68–80.

Unsworth, N., Heitz, R. P., Schrock, J. C., & Engle, R. W. (2005). An automated version of the operation span task. *Behavioral Research Methods, 37,* 498–505.

Wolfe, J. M. (1994). Guided search 2.0: A revised model of visual search. *Psychonomic Bulletin and Review, 1,* 202–238.

Wood, N., & Cowan, N. (1995). The cocktail party phenomenon revisited: How frequent are attention shifts to one's name in an irrelevant auditory channel? *Journal of Experimental Psychology: Learning, Memory, and Cognition, 21,* 255–260.

Wundt, W. (1912/1973). *An introduction to psychology.* Originally published by G. Allen, London. Reprinted by Arno Press, New York.

3

Individual Differences in Working Memory Capacity and Reasoning Ability

KLAUS OBERAUER, HEINZ-MARTIN SÜß,
OLIVER WILHELM, and NICOLAS SANDER

A substantial number of studies have shown that working memory capacity (WMC) is the best single predictor identified so far of reasoning ability as measured by intelligence tests (Ackerman, Beier, & Boyle, 2002; Colom, Flores-Mendoza, & Rebollo, 2003; Conway, Cowan, Bunting, Therriault, & Minkoff, 2002; Engle, Tuholski, Laughlin, & Conway, 1999; Kyllonen & Christal, 1990; Oberauer, 1993; Süß, Oberauer, Wittmann, Wilhelm, & Schulze, 2002; for reviews see Ackerman, Beier, & Boyle, 2005; Oberauer, Schulze, Wilhelm, & Süß, 2005; Kane, Hambrick, & Conway, 2005). This robust finding is an important step toward understanding psychometric intelligence in terms of theories from cognitive psychology. How much we gain from such a link depends on how well we can specify WMC itself. Much of our group's research, therefore, has been devoted to capture more precisely—both on a conceptual and a measurement level—the variance of WMC that is responsible for its tight relationship to reasoning ability.

On the measurement level we feel that it is important to operationalize WMC by a variety of heterogeneous indicators (i.e., tasks). This helps to delineate the generality and boundaries of the construct and to investigate its factorial structure. When we conducted a factor-analytic study on a large sample of tasks used in the literature to assess WMC and related constructs (Oberauer, Süß, Schulze, Wilhelm, & Wittmann, 2000), we were surprised by the large commonality among many of these tasks. This is matched by the high generality of the reasoning factor in structural models of intelligence. Our analyses show that the relationship between measures of WMC and of reasoning is highest on a high level of aggregation. This implies that the common variance among a broad set of different working memory tasks, not the specific variance of one task or task family, is related to reasoning ability, where reasoning ability also stands for the common variance of a diverse set of reasoning tasks.

On a conceptual level, we are looking for a theoretically meaningful characterization of WMC as a limiting factor for reasoning ability. It should capture the requirements shared by reasoning tasks and those tasks in the working memory literature that are good predictors of reasoning, while at the same time excluding tasks only weakly related to reasoning ability. Our current working hypothesis is this: *working memory capacity* reflects the ability to keep several chunks of information simultaneously available for direct access. The critical underlying mechanism for this ability is the flexible, temporary binding of chunks to positions in a common cognitive coordinate system. The binding to a position provides a cue, or "address," by which the chunk can be accessed as input for a cognitive operation. The common coordinate system provides the basis for the construction of new relations between the chunks. We believe that the construction of new structures out of representational elements is the common requirement of all reasoning tasks that sets them apart from other tasks not loading highly on the reasoning factor. Working memory capacity is a general limiting factor for the generation of new structural representations; therefore, it is a critical source of variance for all reasoning tasks.

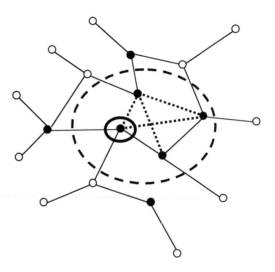

Figure 3.1. The concentric model of working memory. Nodes connected by continuous lines represent the network of associated representations in long-term memory; activated representations are highlighted in black. The large, broken circle delineates the region of direct access, in which a few elements are bound to positions in a cognitive coordinate system. In addition to the pre-existing associations, new relations (dotted lines) can be established between them. The small, continuous circle represents the focus of attention that selects one element as the object of a cognitive operation.

THEORETICAL FRAMEWORK

Our theoretical model of working memory is mainly inspired by the work of Cowan (1988; 1995) and of Halford and colleagues (Halford, Wilson, & Phillips, 1998). We think of working memory as a system responsible for making representations in long-term memory (LTM) available for intentional (i.e., goal-directed) processing. As such, working memory is not a memory system in itself, but a system for attention to memory, an idea shared by several other authors (Baddeley, 1993; Engle, Kane, & Tuholski, 1999; Moscovitch, 1992). A schematic illustration of the model is given in Figure 3.1.

Memory representations are selected for processing on three levels (Oberauer, 2002). On the first level, representations in LTM are activated above baseline. Activation has its source in perceptual input and in representations currently held in the central parts of working memory, and it spreads along associations in LTM. The degree of activation can be regarded as a quick on-line "estimate" of the expected relevance of each representation for the current goal (Anderson & Lebiere, 1998). There is no inherent limit to the amount of activation allocated to memory representations, but activating too many representations (including irrelevant ones) can impair performance as much as activating too few.

On a second level, a subset of the activated representations is held in the region of direct access. This means that they are temporarily bound to positions in a cognitive coordinate system, which could be a literal representation of space, as when a chess player represents the position of several pieces on the board in working memory. It can also be a temporal dimension, as when a participant in a working memory experiment memorizes the temporal order of words read to her. Much evidence on the short-term recall of temporal serial order supports the assumption that elements of a series are bound to positions on a temporal context representation (Burgess & Hitch, 1999; Henson, Norris, Page, & Baddeley, 1996). Very often a quasi-spatial medium is used to represent nonspatial relations between elements, for example, when comparative relations (e.g., "Jim is taller than John") are represented as spatial arrays of tokens, as was first suggested by De Soto, London, and Handel (1965). The idea that people use representations of space in a metaphorical way to capture nonspatial relations has been elaborated on and supported by numerous examples in cognitive linguistics (Lakoff & Johnson, 1980; Langacker, 1986). Not all relations between objects, events, and persons, however, can be mapped onto spatial relations, and so we assume that working memory also uses schemata to organize its contents. Schemata are abstract templates for structural representations that contain placeholders for elements that can be bound to them to fill specific roles. For example, elements can be bound to the roles of agent and object in causal-force schemata (Talmy, 1988). Language processing also involves temporary binding of sentence constituents into syntactic roles in a schema. This form of binding, however, seems to draw on a specialized mechanism that is not limited by general WMC (see Chapter 11).

Currently, we have no fixed position on how this binding in working memory is accomplished (for various proposals see Halford et al., 1998; O'Reilly, Busby, & Soto, 2003; Raffone & Wolters, 2001; Usher, Haarmann, Cohen, & Horn, 2001). All current mechanisms for temporary binding suggest that there is a limit to the number of independent information elements (i.e., chunks) that can be kept separate and bound to different positions or argument slots at the same time. We see this as the source of the capacity limit of working memory. The limiting factor for reasoning tasks thus arises from the limited capacity to keep up several temporary

bindings simultaneously in the region of direct access. The idea that WMC primarily limits the complexity of new structures has been forcefully advanced by Halford et al. (1998) on the basis of a connectionist model of binding in working memory. Robin and Holyoak (1995) and Waltz et al. (1999) have argued for a link between *relational integration* and the prefrontal cortex (see also Christoff et al., 2001). We borrow their term here to refer to the ability to coordinate elements into new structures in the direct-access region of working memory.

A third component of the model is the focus of attention. Its role is to select one chunk at a time from the contents of the direct-access region as the object of a cognitive operation. For instance, when the task is to add two three-digit numbers, the role of the direct-access region is to link the six digits to their respective roles (e.g., the ones of the first number, the tens of the second number). The role of the focus is to pick out one digit, increment it by the amount indicated by the second digit, and thereby transform its value to obtain the sum (Oberauer, 2003).

Our model is similar to that of Cowan (1995, 1999) in that it distinguishes between the activated part of LTM and a more central component with limited capacity. Unlike Cowan, we differentiate the central part of working memory into the direct-access region, in which several elements can be held and related to each other, and the focus of attention, which is limited to a single element.[1] We also make more explicit assumptions about the functions of the various components of the model and their qualitative differences. Activation in LTM marks a representation as likely to be relevant, thus making it easier to retrieve it (i.e., bring it into the region of direct access). Moreover, activated representations can prime or bias cognitive operations and overt responses, for instance, by generating a feeling of familiarity in a recognition task (Oberauer, 2001). Only the contents of the direct-access region, however, provide relational representations as input to cognitive operations. For example, when a chess player's decision depends on whether the queen is to the left or in front of the king, the two figures must be encoded in the direct-access region.

The focus of attention serves to pick out the one object that is actually manipulated by a cognitive operation or an action—e.g., the player needs to decide whether to move the queen or the king, and this selection is done by taking only one figure into the focus of attention. One further point on which we differ from Cowan (2001) is that we are not committed to the "magical number 4" as a constant to describe the capacity of the direct-access region.

ANSWERS TO THE
FOUR QUESTIONS

We now provide concise answers to the four questions posed by the editors, which will be elaborated in the remainder of this chapter.

1. The theoretical framework we found useful to integrate our results is the three-layer model of working memory outlined above (Oberauer, 2002), which is an extension of the model proposed by Cowan (1995). A second important source of our work is facet theory (Canter, 1985), in particular the two-facet structure of the Berlin Intelligence Structure (BIS) model (Jäger, Süß, & Beauducel, 1997). Facet theory can be regarded as the equivalent of an experimental design in correlational research: it is assumed that the variance of any manifest (i.e., measured) variable is affected by the variance of several latent (i.e., hypothetical) variables that are levels of orthogonal factors (called *facets*). Our factor model of working memory assumes two facets, one related to content and the other to cognitive functions. On the content facet, we distinguish between two sources of variance, one related to verbal-numerical content and the other to visuospatial content. On the functional facet, we differentiate storage and processing, relational integration, and executive functions. The latent variables can be represented as factors in structural equation models. Each manifest variable is assumed to reflect variance

from (at least) one content factor and one functional factor. A facet model provides a matrix for classifying existing manifest variables and rules for guiding the construction of new variables (i.e., test tasks) for specific cells of the matrix (for instance, the construction of a verbal storage-and-processing task). Test tasks can be constructed by varying their features according to the facets, just as experimental conditions are varied according to a design factor (e.g., changing the content to be memorized from digits to spatial matrices corresponds to a variation in the content facet). Whether manipulations of tests according to facet have an effect can be investigated by testing whether the manipulation changes a task's correlation with other tasks. For instance, a storage-and-processing task with verbal content should load on a verbal factor, whereas one with spatial matrices as content should load on a spatial factor. For a review of facet models of intelligence see Süß and Beauducel (2005).

2. We believe that the critical source of individual differences in WMC is the ability to provide direct access to several independent information elements (chunks) at the same time. This capacity rests on a mechanism that quickly establishes and dissolves temporary bindings between these elements and positions in a cognitive coordinate system, or placeholders in a schema. Direct access to a multitude of separate elements is necessary to construct new relations between them and integrate them into new structural representations. The limited capacity for relational integration is the most important limiting factor for reasoning ability. We focus on this source of variance because it seems to be a parameter of the cognitive system that affects a large number of different tasks, thereby explaining the common variance of many experimental working memory tasks, reasoning tasks from intelligence tests, and potentially complex cognitive achievements in everyday life.

3. One other source of individual differences in cognition that has attracted much attention recently is the efficiency of executive functions. Our results (Oberauer, Süß, Wilhelm, & Wittmann, 2003) suggest that at least one prototypical executive function, switching between task sets, is not strongly related to WMC. We venture that this is not an exception. We think that the capacity of working memory cannot be reduced to the efficiency of executive functions, and currently there is no compelling evidence that executive functions contribute substantial variance to reasoning ability.

Another construct, related to executive functions but not identical to it, is the ability to inhibit irrelevant representations (Hasher, Zacks, & May, 1999, see also Chapter 9). We believe there is some evidence that this source of variance contributes to individual differences in working memory and other complex cognitive functions (e.g., reading ability). The role of the inhibition function within our model is to reduce the activation of irrelevant representations in LTM, thereby reducing the amount of intrusion into the more central parts of working memory (Oberauer, 2001). Inhibition efficiency, however, cannot account for the common variance of all working memory tasks.

4. Factor-analytic studies of individual differences can help us to figure out which cognitive functions belong closely together and which are relatively independent of each other; this is an important contribution to the shaping and sharpening of concepts such as working memory. Our research thus far has yielded two important insights. First, working memory has a limited capacity that constrains cognitive performance in a wide variety of tasks. Their common feature is probably that they all require simultaneous access to several independent elements of information. Second, WMC cannot be reduced to the efficiency of executive functions. Therefore, we argue that working memory and executive functions be treated as separate constructs.

THE FACTOR STRUCTURE OF WORKING MEMORY

The factor-analytic approach to individual differences provides a tool to simultaneously identify associations and dissociations between indicators of cognitive functions. These indicators can be raw performance scores in tasks designed to tap a particular function, or derived measures (e.g., task-switching costs or interference effects) used to assess specific functions. Our approach is to model the correlational structure of large sets of indicators by theoretically specified structural equation models. We regard this as an important complement to experimental and neuropsychological research, which usually focuses on dissociations of cognitive functions. Through factor analysis one can test the assumptions of generalizability, which is implicit in all experimental work that uses a specific paradigm. By investigating which indicators of cognitive functions are highly correlated and which are not, we can assess whether a phenomenon observed in an experimental paradigm is in fact representative of the construct it is meant to operationalize.

In two large factor-analytic studies (Oberauer et al., 2000; Oberauer et al., 2003) we tested a facet model of the structure of working memory. The basic framework was borrowed from the Berlin Intelligence Structure (BIS) model (Jäger et al., 1997). It specifies two dimensions by which cognitive performances, or the indicators used to measure them, can be classified. One distinguishes content (verbal, numerical, and spatial-figural materials), the other, cognitive functions. In the BIS, cognitive functions are described as *processing capacity* (i.e., reasoning), *creativity* (i.e., fluency of ideas), *memory* (i.e., remembering supra-span sets of items for brief periods), and *processing speed*. In the working memory model, we distinguished between three functions: *simultaneous storage and processing*, *coordination* (i.e., relational integration), and *supervision* (i.e., executive functions).

In the first study (Oberauer et al., 2000) we used a large pool of tasks sampled from the literature (up to 1995) in an attempt to cover the whole range of measures proposed by scholars to capture working memory and executive functions. Among the tasks were classics such as reading span (Daneman & Carpenter, 1980) and random generation (Baddeley, 1986), tasks used in research on cognitive aging such as memory updating (Salthouse, Babcock, & Shaw, 1991), and tasks developed to measure relational integration (i.e., "coordination"; Oberauer, 1993), together with indicators of executive functions such as task-set switching (Allport, Styles, & Hsieh, 1994).

Since most of these tasks were complex mixtures of various cognitive functions, we attempted a more analytical approach in the second study (Oberauer et al., 2003). We constructed new tasks designed to reflect specifically the three functions proposed in our model: simultaneous storage and processing, relational integration, and supervision of cognitive processes. We do not claim that we succeeded in constructing pure indicators of the constructs we intended to measure, but our new tasks arguably reflected the cognitive functions we targeted more than other functions.

First, we chose to reduce the measures of "simultaneous storage and processing" to the essence of what this construct description requires, that is, processing some information while concurrently memorizing a briefly presented list of items. We constructed dual-task combinations of memory for serial order and choice reaction-time (RT) tasks. First, the memory lists were presented, then participants worked through several trials of a two-choice RT task for 5 s, and finally they reproduced the memory list. This task schema was realized with verbal, numerical, and spatial materials.

We attempted to construct tasks that require relational integration but no storage, in that no information had to be kept available when it was no longer present in the environment. In these so-called structure-monitoring tasks, participants observed a set of objects on the computer screen, which changed independently

from time to time. The task was to detect the emergence of specific relations between the objects. In the finding squares task, for example, participants saw 10 dots randomly placed in fields of a 10×10 matrix. Every 1.5 s two dots jumped to a new position. Participants had to indicate by a key press when four of the dots formed a square somewhere in the matrix (see Fig. 3.2, left panel). This task required representing the ever-changing relations between the dots and integrating them into larger structures to detect patterns that form a square (or a partial square, such that attention can be directed to the critical positions in which the appearance of a dot would complete a square). We constructed structure-monitoring tasks with verbal, numerical, and spatial content. For each task there was one version without need to memorize any information, and a complementary version in which some information was erased from the screen briefly after presentation so that it had to be memorized.

As a measure of executive function we used four versions of the task-set switching paradigm introduced by Rogers and Monsell (1995). This paradigm is used to compare pure blocks, in which a single task is repeated, with mixed blocks, in which two tasks alternate every second trial. We derived two indicators for the efficiency of executive function. Specific switch costs were defined as the RT difference between trials following a switch and trials following no switch within the mixed blocks. General switch costs were defined as the RT difference between no-switch trials in the mixed blocks and trials in the pure blocks.

The major results of the two studies were the following:

1. The factor representing storage and processing and the relational-integration factor were highly correlated and in one case (Oberauer et al., 2000) indistinguishable. Most of their variance was shared, and we regard this shared variance as the core of working memory capacity.
2. The factors representing indicators of supervision or executive functions were only weakly correlated with the other two working memory factors.

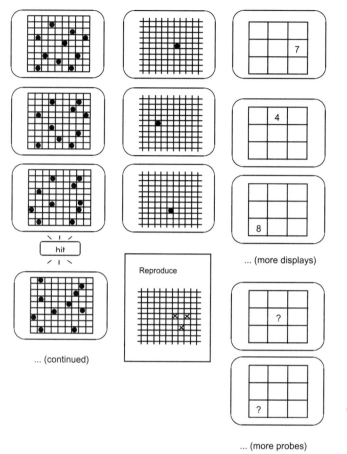

Figure 3.2. Schematic example trials from working memory tasks. *Left column*: Finding squares task (Oberauer et al., 2003). *Middle column*: Spatial short-term memory task (Oberauer, 1993). Note that a correct response requires only reproduction of the relations between dots, not their absolute locations in the matrix. *Right column*: Memory updating (numerical) task, STM version (modified from Salthouse et al., 1991).

3. Verbal and numerical working memory loaded on the same factor. The factors for verbal-numerical and for spatial working memory were highly correlated, but a small proportion of their variance seems to be specific for each domain.

4. As in other studies (Ackerman et al., 2002; Kyllonen & Christal, 1990; Kyllonen, 1994, but see Conway et al., 2002), WMC was highly correlated with factors reflecting processing speed. Nonetheless, speed variables always formed a distinct separate factor.

One representative model is displayed in Figure 3.3 (for factor loadings see Table 3.1). This model is based on the data from Oberauer et al. (2003), integrating two models reported in that article into one. The model had a satisfactory fit, with $\chi^2 (141) = 198.7$, CFI = .966, and RMSEA = .056, despite the lack of content-specific factors, which did little to improve the fit. The right part of the model represents the choice RT variables from the pure and the mixed blocks. A general speed factor captures the variance common to all choice RT measures. A more specific factor captures the residual variance shared by all variables taken from the mixed blocks; it thereby represents the common variance of general switch costs. A third, even more specific factor represents the variance shared by only the switch RTs, thus reflecting the common variance associated with specific switch costs. The two factors reflecting general and specific switch costs have substantial loadings from most of their variables, supporting the hypothesis that these switch costs have something in common beyond particular tasks and even across content domains.

The left part of the model represents the two working memory factors. The storage and processing factor represents memory performance from the dual tasks, and the relational integration factor represents accuracy in the structure-monitoring tasks. The model could not be improved significantly by adding correlations between both working memory factors and both switching factors (i.e., general and specific switch costs); the improvement in χ^2 was only 4.0 (df $= 4$). In other words, WMC is related to the basic speed of choice reactions, but not to the additional variance captured by general switch costs and by specific switch costs.

THE BASIC MECHANISM: BINDING AND RELATIONAL INTEGRATION

What is the common variance of tasks measuring simultaneous storage and processing and tasks measuring relational integration? As outlined above, our current hypothesis is that WMC reflects the limited ability to bind several elements simultaneously to different positions in a cognitive coordinate system, or argument placeholders in schemata.

Relational Integration Tasks

Relational integration obviously depends on a binding mechanism. For example, building a new temporal relation such as "A happened before B" can be accomplished by binding the elements A and B to argument slots in a propositional schema BEFORE(x,y) (c.f., Halford et al., 1998). Alternatively, it can be accomplished by binding A and B to two positions on a temporal dimension in a cognitive coordinate system, thereby generating a mental model of the two elements' temporal order (c.f. Schaeken, Johnson-Laird, & d'Ydewalle, 1996).

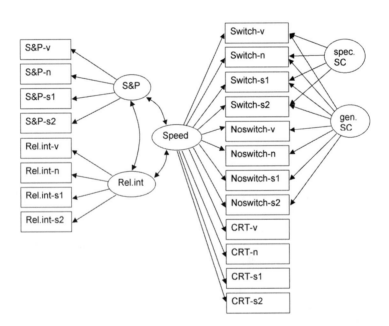

Figure 3.3. Structural equation model of data from Oberauer et al. (2003), N = 131. S&P = memory performance from dual-task combinations of storage and concurrent processing; Rel.-int = structure-monitoring tasks used to measure relational integration; CRT = choice reaction times from pure blocks; Noswitch = choice reaction times from no-switch trials in mixed blocks; Switch = choice reaction times from switch trials in mixed blocks. All reaction times were log transformed and multiplied by −1. Suffixes: n = numerical; v = verbal; s1 and s2 refer to two versions of spatial material. Error terms (omitted here for clarity) between reaction time tasks with the same material (e.g., CRT-n, Noswitch-n, and Switch-n) were correlated freely.

TABLE 3.1. Factor Loadings of Variables in the Model in Figure 3.3

Variable	Speed	gen. SC	spec. SC	S&P	Rel.Int
Switch-v	.72	.18	.29		
Switch-n	.65	.34	.53		
Switch-s1	.66	.18	.42		
Switch-s2	.69	.17	.31		
Noswitch-v	.76	.34			
Noswitch-n	.69	.57			
Noswitch-s1	.68	.27			
Noswitch-s2	.73	.10			
CRT-v	.78				
CRT-n	.76				
CRT-s1	.77				
CRT-s2	.71				
S&P-v				.47	
S&P-n				.50	
S&P-s1				.76	
S&P-s2				.64	
Rel.Int-v					.60
Rel.Int-n					.69
Rel.Int-s1					.61
Rel.Int-s2					.60

All loadings were significant with $p < .05$, except the loading of switch-s1 on the general switch cost factor ($p = .052$). $N = 131$, $\chi^2 = 198.7$, df = 141. Errors were uncorrelated except S&P-v with S&P-n (.38) and Rel.Int-v with Rel.Int-n (.41). Switch = choice reaction times from switch trials in mixed blocks; v = verbal; n = numerical; s1, s2 = two versions of spatial material; Noswitch = choice reaction times from no-switch trials in mixed blocks; CRT = choice reaction times from pure blocks; S&P = memory performance from dual-task combinations of storage and concurrent processing; Rel.Int = structure-monitoring tasks used to measure relational integration.

The tasks we used to measure relational integration mostly required establishing a structure within a spatial coordinate system. For example, two tasks developed by Oberauer (1993), called *spatial short-term memory* (STM) and *spatial coordination*, display a sequence of dots in different cells of a 10×10 matrix (see Fig. 3.2, middle panel). The dots are displayed one by one, and the participants are asked to imagine how they would look if they appeared simultaneously and reproduce the resulting pattern in an empty matrix. This can be done either by an absolute coding of each dot's position, based on bindings between each dot and its position in a representation of the matrix, or by a relative coding, based on binding dots to argument slots in schemata such as TWO-

CELLS-LEFT-OF(x,y). Both approaches work, because reproduction of an absolute position is not asked for in the instructions. Both approaches require quickly establishing temporary bindings.

In the verbal monitoring task designed by Oberauer et al. (2003), participants see a 3×3 matrix with one word displayed in each cell. Every 2 s, one of the words is replaced by a new one. Participants have to signal with a key press whenever three words in a horizontal, vertical, or diagonal row rhyme with each other. To detect this structure, one has to bind the words to their spatial positions in the matrix. It is not sufficient to activate the representations of all currently presented words and to detect that some of them rhyme. It is also necessary to be aware of the rhyming words' (relative or absolute) positions. Once again, accurate performance depends on binding elements to positions in a cognitive coordinate system, and efficient performance requires that subjects build up and resolve bindings quickly.

Storage and Processing Tasks

Performance on tasks measuring storage and processing is usually assessed by the accuracy of recall of a list in serial order. This requires memory not only for the particular items in the list but also for their ordinal position in the list. One way to accomplish this is to bind list elements temporarily to positions in a mental coordinate system in which one dimension represents temporal order. Several computational models of serial recall use a mechanism that links list elements to a context representation changing over time (Brown, Preece, & Hulme, 2000; Burgess & Hitch, 1999; Henson, 1998). The efficiency of a mechanism that establishes temporary bindings can therefore be expected to be critical for the accuracy of serial recall.

This account raises one question: there is ample evidence that serial recall tasks combined with a concurrent processing task (so-called complex spans) are better predictors of reasoning and other complex tasks than serial recall alone (so-called simple spans) (Ackerman et al., 2005; Daneman & Merikle, 1996; Engle, Tuholski et al., 1999; Kane et al., 2005; Kane et al., 2004;

Oberauer, 1993; Oberauer et al., 2005), at least in the verbal domain. (with spatial material the available data are more ambiguous—Miyake, Friedman, Rettinger, Shah, & Hegarty, 2001, could not differentiate simple and complex spatial span tasks; Kane et al., 2004, could separate them, but spatial simple span tasks contributed unique variance to explaining fluid intelligence over and above a domain-general complex-span factor). Why should this be the case? One plausible explanation is that there is a specialized mechanism for recall in forward serial order, which is disrupted by concurrent processing, so that the system can rely on it for simple span tasks, but has to fall back onto the more general mechanism of temporary binding for complex span tasks.

One such specialized mechanism could be a primacy gradient, as proposed by two further computational models of serial recall (Farrell & Lewandowsky, 2002; Page & Norris, 1998). In these models, activation or encoding strength of each successive list item gradually decreases as the list progresses, and the resulting gradient is used to reconstruct the order of encoding. Such a mechanism requires no binding. Its limitation, however, is that every event intervening between two list items or occurring after list presentation could easily leave behind a representation with its own activation (or strength) level. The activation of representations decreases only slowly once they become irrelevant (Oberauer, 2001), therefore, their activation is likely to distort the primacy gradient at recall. Hence, at recall, keeping the relevant list items from the now irrelevant material separate from the intervening processing task requires the binding mechanism after all, at least to bind list items to one context and representations from the processing task to another.

A variant of this explanation is to assume a specialized system for keeping the serial order only of phonemes—a "phonological loop" in the model of Baddeley (1986). The processing task, introducing additional phonological material (e.g., reading sentences aloud in reading span), would interfere with this system, leaving recall of the memory list at the mercy of the general binding mechanism (Oberauer, Lange, & Engle,

2004). This variant would be specific to verbal material, consistent with Miyake et al.'s (2001) findings, who did not obtain a distinction between simple and complex spans with spatial material.

Our theory predicts that the addition of a concurrent processing component is just one way to turn a simple span task into a working memory task (i.e., a powerful predictor of complex cognitive performance), and it might not even be the best way. Another way to disrupt the specialized mechanism for forward recall would be to require recall of a list in random order. This is what we did in an adaptation of the (numerical) memory updating task designed by Salthouse et al. (1991). In what we called the "STM version" of this task, participants saw a number of digits, each in a separate frame on the screen. Later a subset of the frames was probed for recall in random order (see Fig. 3.2, right panel). No processing had to be done in the meantime. What makes this task different from ordinary serial recall is the allocation of the list elements to spatial positions and the probing of recall in an order that differed from presentation order. This task had very high loading on a working memory factor and a first-order correlation with the BIS reasoning scale of $r = .40$ (Oberauer et al., 2000), not much less than tasks combining storage and processing (e.g., reading span: $r = .56$).

Although this result is certainly preliminary and in need of replication, it gains additional support by the fact that several spatial tasks requiring only storage but no processing also did very well as predictors of reasoning. For example, the spatial STM task (Fig. 3.2, middle panel) was one of the best single predictors of the BIS reasoning factor in three studies (Oberauer, 1993, Süß et al., 2000, 2002), with first-order correlations ranging from .54 to .59. Likewise, Miyake et al. (2001) found that one spatial task measuring short-term retention without additional processing, the dot memory task, was as highly correlated with two spatial reasoning tasks (termed "spatial visualization") as were the complex span tasks combining storage and processing ($r \approx .40$). In both the spatial STM and dot memory tasks, participants have to memorize the locations of several dots in a matrix, presented either sequentially or simultaneously. Arguably, this taps directly into the ability to integrate spatial relations between the dots within a common coordinate system. Future research will have to disentangle whether it is the spatial nature of these tasks or the fact that they require relational integration that makes them good predictors of reasoning ability.

WORKING MEMORY CAPACITY AND EXECUTIVE FUNCTIONS

Several authors believe there is a very strong link between WMC and the efficiency of executive functions. Within the framework of Baddeley's (1986) theory, the capacity of the central executive is the most natural candidate to account for the relationship between WMC and reasoning ability (Bayliss, Jarrold, Gunn, & Baddeley, 2003). A strong association between WMC, reasoning ability (or fluid intelligence, which is almost the same in practice), and the executive functions of the prefrontal cortex has been postulated by several authors (see Chapters 2 and 10).

The term *executive function* is often used in a loose and very encompassing way, sometimes including all cognitive operations performed on some stimuli or memory contents. Here we use the term for the set of cognitive processes that serve to keep cognition and action in line with the current primary goal. Thus, we distinguish between primary cognitive operations, which work on the representation currently held in the focus of attention according to a set of parameters (called a *task set*), and executive processes that ensure that the primary operations function properly in the service of the person's overarching goal (cf. Chapter 7). For the present purpose, we distinguish between two kinds of executive processes: (1) cognitive processes that control and manipulate the task sets, and (2) processes that inhibit irrelevant, potentially distracting representations. Briefly stated, the former ensure that the right task is executed, and the latter make sure that it is executed with the right information. The two

categories can, of course, overlap, for instance, when inhibition is applied to task sets themselves (Mayr & Keele, 2000). A third category of processes that is often subsumed under executive functions is the updating of working memory (Miyake et al., 2001). The tasks used to measure this process combine storage and processing in working memory (in fact, they are virtually identical to the "memory updating" tasks used in our studies), so we regard performance on these tasks as reflecting WMC and not executive functions.

Control of Task Sets

Task-set switching (Allport et al., 1994; Rogers & Monsell, 1995) is clearly a prototypical case of the first category of executive functions, the manipulation of task representations. Currently there are two major theoretical interpretations of the time costs of switching between two tasks (i.e., specific switch costs). One, advanced by Rogers and Monsell (1995), is that these costs reflect the time needed for a process of task-set reconfiguration. Thus, specific switch costs directly reflect the speed of one executive process. The other view, first proposed by Allport et al. (1994), sees these costs as a reflection of proactive interference from the old task set when it has to be replaced by a new one. Specific switch costs can then be interpreted as the efficiency with which the cognitive system overcomes this proactive interference. Overcoming proactive interference from no-longer relevant task sets can be accomplished by inhibiting the old task set, boosting activation of the new task set, or a mixture of both (for a computational model of task-set switching using these mechanisms see Gilbert & Shallice, 2002). This reads like a perfect job description for the "supervisory attentional system" (Norman & Shallice, 1980; Shallice & Burgess, 1991), which Baddeley (1986) used as the blueprint for his "central executive."

Therefore, we regard specific task-set switching costs as one of the least disputable means of measuring executive functions available today. Moreover, general switch costs can best be interpreted as reflecting the need to coordinate two task sets held available at the same time, which would appear to be a typical assignment for the central executive. The finding that neither specific nor general switching costs correlate substantially with WMC factors is therefore a serious challenge for theories assuming a strong link between executive functions and working memory.

One might dismiss this finding as being exceptional. First, it could be argued that the specific way in which we implemented task-set switching was responsible for our low correlations. This seems not to be the case. Other authors who investigated individual or age differences in switching costs, using different variants of the paradigm, also reported weak to non-existent correlations of switching costs with working memory tasks such as operation span (Miyake et al., 2000), backward digit span (Cepeda, Kramer, & Gonzalez de Sather, 2001), or a composite of three complex span tasks (Kray & Lindenberger, 2000). Recently, Friedman et al. (2006) have shown that task-set switching ("shifting" in their terminology) is not significantly related to fluid intelligence, further strengthening the case that WMC and task-set switching measure different constructs.

Second, it could be argued that switching is an atypical representative of the concept of executive functions, and other indicators of this construct correlate better with WMC measures. There is indeed an impressive number of studies showing that complex span tasks are related to indicators of executive functions such as speed and errors in the antisaccade task (Kane, Bleckley, Conway, & Engle, 2001; Unsworth, Schrock, & Engle, 2004), Stroop interference in blocks with few conflict trials (Kane & Engle, 2003), and verbal fluency tasks (Rosen & Engle, 1997). Establishing a strong link between WMC and executive functions, however, requires much more. First, one would have to show that different measures of executive function correlate high enough to warrant conceptualizing them through a single overarching construct (Salthouse, Atkinson, & Berish, 2003). The studies by Miyake et al. (2000) and Salthouse et al. (2003) have provided some preliminary evidence in that direction, but others have failed to find substantial associations between indicators

of executive function (Duncan, Johnson, Swales, & Freer, 1997; Kramer, Humphrey, Larish, Logan, & Strayer, 1994; Shilling, Chetwynd, & Rabbitt, 2002; Ward, Roberts, & Phillips, 2001). Second, one would have to demonstrate that a factor representing this construct is correlated with a WMC factor to a degree that goes beyond the moderate positive correlation to be expected from the "positive manifold," that is, the tendency toward positive correlations among all cognitive tasks. The case for such a strong connection between WMC and a general executive factor has not been made so far, and we doubt that it can be made.

Inhibition of Irrelevant Information

One potential source of individual differences in complex cognition is the efficiency with which irrelevant or no-longer relevant information is inhibited. The inhibition hypothesis was first advanced by Hasher and Zacks (1988) in the context of cognitive aging, but was soon applied to individual differences within one age group as well (e.g., Conway & Engle, 1994). There is now considerable evidence consistent with the assumption that the efficiency of inhibiting irrelevant information is related to measures of WMC (Conway, Cowan, & Bunting, 2001; Gray, Chabris, & Braver, 2003; Lustig, May, & Hasher, 2001; May, Hasher, & Kane, 1999). Moreover, De Beni and colleagues (De Beni, Palladino, Pazzaglia, & Cornoldi, 1998; De Beni & Palladino, 2000) linked inhibition of irrelevant words in a working memory task to performance in text comprehension (see also Meiran, 1996). There has been some progress toward establishing an inhibition factor that captures the common variance of several measures of cognitive inhibition (Friedman & Miyake, 2004), but it has not yet been established that this factor is substantially related to a factor reflecting WMC. In the study of Friedman et al. (2006), a latent factor measuring inhibition was not correlated with fluid intelligence, a finding that should dampen our expectations of finding a strong relationship with WMC.

One scenario that deserves serious consideration is that correlational links between measures of WMC and indicators of inhibition exist on a relatively low level of generality. For instance, it is theoretically plausible that the ability to inhibit irrelevant memory representations is helpful in a task such as reading span, where one must recall the sentence-final words but not words from the remainder of the sentence (De Beni et al., 1998). But the same ability might be much less important in a task such as our spatial STM task (Oberauer, 1993), in which all information presented on each trial has to be recalled. On the other hand, the ability to inhibit an already initiated action (Logan & Cowan, 1984) might contribute to variance in the structure-monitoring tasks of Oberauer et al. (2003) by helping to reduce false alarms (i.e., pressing the key when the required structure is absent), but be unrelated to complex span tasks that require no suppression of action. This highlights the importance of distinguishing levels of generality when it comes to relating constructs (Wittmann, 1988), which we will return to again in the section on working memory and reasoning.

INTERLUDE: WORKING MEMORY CAPACITY AND SPEED

In many studies, WMC was found to be strongly related to measures of processing speed (Ackerman et al., 2002; Kyllonen & Christal, 1990; Kyllonen, 1994; Salthouse, 1991, 1994, see also Chapter 8), and this is also apparent in Figure 3.3. One obvious potential explanation is that many working memory tasks are complex span tasks that involve a processing component themselves, and the speed of performing this component is one source of variance in complex span tasks (see Chapters 5 and 6). However, this cannot be the whole story, because not all WMC tasks are complex span tasks, and speed measures are also correlated to working memory tasks lacking a processing component. A clear example of this is the study by Conway et al. (2002), who found a substantial correlation of speed with a factor that extracted the common variance of short-term and working memory tasks, but none with a second factor capturing the specific variance of working memory. This is the opposite of what one would

expect if speed is related to complex span through the processing component of the latter. One might even speculate on the basis of Conway et al.'s findings that the WMC–speed relationship is due to the STM component in complex span tasks. A high correlation with speed indicators, however, was also obtained with relational integration tasks (see Fig. 3.3), part of which have no STM component. Taken together, these findings suggest that the link between speed and WMC cannot be reduced to shared components between tasks used to measure the two constructs. We should look for an explanation for this relationship on a higher level of generality.

We believe that the binding account of WMC advanced here can offer such an explanation, although at present it is largely speculative. Speed tasks require the fast execution of a rule mapping categories of stimuli onto categories of responses. Often, these rules must be implemented ad hoc according to the instructions (e.g., when a left key press is to be made in response to the letter A and a right key press in response to a B). Several attention theorists have argued that these tasks are executed as a "prepared reflex" (Logan, 1978) once a task set or action plan incorporating the rule has been set up. The task set specifies all parameters for the action to be executed in advance, except those that depend on the stimulus, and then the stimulus can immediately trigger the action by "direct parameter specification" (Neumann & Klotz, 1994).

The task set or action plan implements the stimulus–response (S-R) mapping in a way that makes it immediately executable in reaction to an appropriate stimulus. Thus, the task set differs from a representation of the rule one acquires, for instance, from reading the instructions. Knowledge of a rule does not in itself make an organism prepared to react to a stimulus according to the rule. Once a task set is established, however, an appropriate stimulus activates the response mapped to it automatically (Logan & Schulkind, 2000), although this activation might not be sufficient for execution (Lien & Proctor, 2002). For a fast and accurate response to a stimulus it is therefore critical that the task set be firmly established, such that an incoming stimulus can "pass through" without requiring extra cognitive work.

A task set is a temporary binding between representations of the relevant stimulus categories and representations of the corresponding responses (c.f. Hommel, 1998), which is probably held in working memory. The bindings must be temporary because they can overcome established long-term associations (e.g., one can respond to the letter A by saying "B" and the other way round), without having to unlearn these associations (i.e., after executing the A-B mapping a thousand times, the letter A is still associated more with saying "A" than with saying "B"). The ability to set up temporary bindings between arbitrary representations, which we argue underlies WMC, should therefore also be highly relevant for efficient execution of speeded responses to stimuli according to S-R-mapping rules. A high correlation between WMC measures and speed in such tasks is therefore to be expected.

This argument suggests one important prediction: the correlation between WMC tasks and speed tasks should depend on the degree of S-R compatibility in the speed task. According to Kornblum, Hasbroucq, and Osman (1990), S-R compatibility is high when (a) there is a high degree of dimensional overlap between stimuli and responses, and (b) stimuli are mapped to those responses that correspond to them on the dimensions they share. For instance, when the task is to press a button in response to one of four lights arranged in a horizontal line, an arrangement of the four response keys in a horizontal line would be one with high dimensional overlap. Given this overlap, a mapping in which the left–right order of the lights corresponds to the left–right order of the keys to be pressed is one with a maximum of S-R compatibility. A random mapping would be an example of low S-R compatibility, although the dimensional overlap is still high. Another way to have low S-R compatibility is to eliminate dimensional overlap, for example, by having participants call out one of four arbitrarily chosen female names in response to each light.

Kornblum et al. (1990) assume two processing paths from a stimulus representation to a response. One is mediated by pre-existing associations between stimulus and response representations (e.g., between the printed letter A and saying "A") and enables a stimulus to automatically activate its corresponding response. This path is operative only in cases with dimensional overlap between stimulus and response. The second path is mediated by a representation of the task rule, and can implement any arbitrary S-R mapping. The second path is always operative and determines which response is correct. When the S-R mapping is compatible, this is just a quick verification of the already activated response; when it is incompatible, the activated response must be suppressed and replaced by the correct one. In case of no dimensional overlap, the second path does all the S-R translation on its own. In our interpretation, the second path is mediated through a task set implemented by temporary bindings. Tasks with low S-R compatibility will have to rely heavily on this task set, whereas tasks with high S-R compatibility will be less dependent on a well-established task set, because it is needed just to confirm the already activated response. This line of reasoning leads to the hypothesis that tasks with high S-R compatibility will correlate less (although not necessarily zero) with a measure of WMC than tasks with low S-R compatibility.

Two of us have recently tested this hypothesis (Wilhelm & Oberauer, 2006). In a study involving four-choice RT tasks with compatible and with arbitrary S-R mapping we identified two latent factors, one general RT factor capturing the common variance of all RT tasks, and an arbitrary-mapping factor capturing the residual variance shared by all tasks with arbitrary S-R mapping. The general RT factor was correlated substantially with a latent factor reflecting WMC, but the specific arbitrary-mapping factor had an even higher correlation with WMC.

The only other study we are aware of that contrasts high and low S-R compatibility within the same task is the study by Kane et al. (2001), who compared groups of people with high and low WMC on the speed and accuracy of executing prosaccades (i.e., eye movements toward a suddenly appearing cue in the periphery) and antisaccades (i.e., eye movements away from the cue). Obviously, the prosaccade task has high S-R compatibility, whereas the antisaccade has lower compatibility. Kane et al. (2001) found that the two capacity groups differed in performance on the antisaccade task but not on the prosaccade task.

Unfortunately, there is an alternative explanation, the one advanced by Kane et al. (2001): the better performance of high-capacity people on the antisaccade task could reflect their greater ability to suppress the saccade toward the cue, which is a strongly prepotent response. One way to decide between the inhibition interpretation and an interpretation in terms of S-R bindings would be to compare high- and low-capacity groups on the speed and accuracy of saccades in response to arbitrary cues presented centrally (e.g., when the fixation point turns into a square, move the eyes to the left; if it turns into a circle, move the eyes to the right). An account based on inhibition of prepotent responses would not predict a correlation of this task with WMC, because there is no prepotent action to be inhibited. Our binding account, in contrast, predicts that this arbitrary saccade task correlates as strongly with WMC as the antisaccade task.

WORKING MEMORY CAPACITY AND REASONING

What it is about working memory capacity that makes it such an important prerequisite for successful reasoning? Reasoning tasks found in intelligence tests tend to load on a single factor, even though they share hardly any cognitive operations apart from those common to virtually all tasks. For example, the analyses of component processes of inductive- and deductive-reasoning tasks performed by Sternberg (1985) reveal hardly any common processes beyond "encoding" and "response selection." Nonetheless, Wilhelm (2005) was unable to obtain separate factors for inductive and deductive reasoning. The most important limiting factor for these tasks must be one they have in common, independent of the diverse cognitive operations used to perform each of them.

We think that what is common to all reasoning tasks is the fact that their solutions require the construction of new structural representations. This means that given elements must be combined by new relations. The complexity of the new structures is limited by the capacity of working memory. The capacity of the direct-access region sets a limit on the number of elements that can be placed simultaneously within a common cognitive coordinate system, and thereby be integrated into a new structure. We will demonstrate this for a few prototypical examples in the following section.

Reasoning and Relational Integration

Three categories of reasoning tasks are commonly found in intelligence tests as well as in experimental studies of human reasoning. The first, *deductive reasoning*, can be defined as drawing inferences from premises with logical necessity. The premises are given as verbal statements (as in syllogisms) or in mathematical form (as in equations to be solved), but spatial-figural formats can also be designed (c.f., Wilhelm, 2000). *Inductive reasoning* is defined as drawing a plausible, but not necessary, inference from given information. In psychological tests and experiments this involves inferring a rule or category from particular instances (e.g., categorization or series completion) or transferring information from one instance to another (e.g., analogical reasoning). *Transformations* can be defined as tasks in which an initial state of some object or situation must be mentally transformed into a final state by the application of given operators. Problem solving can be seen as a subset of this category because it is usually defined as transforming an initial state into a goal state by means of a set of operators (Newell & Simon, 1972). Problem-solving tasks loading high on reasoning factors are typically from the well-defined variety for which the states and operators are given, and one has to look for an optimal combination of operators to attain the desired transformation.

Currently the most successful theory of deductive reasoning is the theory of mental models (Johnson-Laird & Byrne, 1991; Johnson-Laird, 2001). According to this theory, deductive inferences are drawn from mental models representing the truth conditions of the premises. This means that representations of the objects or events referred to in the premises are arranged according to the relations expressed in the premises. For example, in reasoning about temporal relations (Schaeken et al., 1996), tokens representing individual events must be arranged into an array corresponding to their temporal order. In syllogistic reasoning (Johnson-Laird & Bara, 1984), tokens representing individual members of the categories must be arranged such that the category relations stated in the premises are true. Mental models make use of geometrical constraints even when they represent nonspatial relations. Consider, for example, the mental model of the syllogism "All A are B. No B is C" (each line represents one individual with its features A, B, C, or any combination of them):

$$A = B$$
$$A = B$$
$$B$$
$$C$$

Constructing the model according to the premises results in a spatial arrangement of the tokens, which represent the individuals. The new relationship between the "end terms" A and C emerges through the geometric constraints of the medium: no C token can lie on the same line as an A token, and therefore the model supports the conclusion "No A is C." Thus, the deductive inference relies on binding the tokens to places in a quasi-spatial mental coordinate system and making use of the emerging relations not explicitly mentioned in the premises.

Typical inductive reasoning tasks are series completion, matrices, and analogies. All of these tasks depend on detecting relations between relations, that is, mapping relations onto each other. This has been spelled out most elaborately for analogical reasoning (e.g., Gentner, 1989). Gentner defined an *analogy* as a mapping of the structure of a base domain onto a target domain. Analogical reasoning thus requires identifying relations in the base domain

and at least in part also in the target domain, then identifying mappings (i.e., relations of identity or similarity) between these relations. A good analogy is characterized by systematicity, that is, preferentially mapping coherent systems of relations. Finding the most systematic mapping between two domains requires representing complex structures in both the base and the target domains simultaneously. It should be obvious that this requires extensive binding of elements into the argument placeholders of the relations in question. A computational model of analogies demonstrating the central role of bindings was developed by Hummel and Holyoak (1997).

Matrices and series completions can be analyzed as special cases of analogical mapping. In series-completion tasks, the rule generating the series is repeated after n items. In order to detect the rule, together with the value of n, one must try to map the first n elements of the series onto the next n elements (for varying values of n). In matrices (such as Raven's) the relations between elements in a row must be mapped across columns, and the relationships between elements in a column must be mapped across rows. According to this analysis, the limiting factor for Raven's matrices is not memorizing several hypotheses or rules, as Carpenter, Just, and Shell (1990) assumed, but simply representing three structures, each one linking three elements, at the same time to figure out their mapping. Partly supporting this contention, Unsworth and Engle (2005) found that the correlation between a WMC task (operation span) and Raven items did not increase with the number of rules to be applied for solving the Raven item.

A prototypical problem-solving task investigated in numerous studies is the Tower of Hanoi (e.g., Carpenter et al., 1990; Kotovsky, Hayes, & Simon, 1985). Several discs are stacked on one of three rods, ordered by size. The tower has to be moved to another rod, with the constraints that only one disc can be moved at a time, and a larger disc must never be placed on top of a smaller one. Problem-solving tasks usually require the construction of a sequence of operations (e.g., movements of individual discs) that transform the given state into the goal state. If the task is not to be solved by blind trial and error, at least part of the sequence must be planned in advance. This means building a mental structure to bring individual steps into a temporal order. Often the plan is also hierarchical because of the goal–subgoal structure, extensively analyzed for the Tower of Hanoi problem (e.g., Karat, 1982).

Other transformation tasks used in intelligence tests such as the BIS test involve the mental rotation, translation, or folding of objects or their parts in space (e.g., paper-folding tasks, puzzle-assembly tasks) or the recombination of symbols (e.g., anagram tasks). These tasks highlight a second aspect of relational integration in mental transformations: the states are often structures of objects, object parts, or symbols, and the operations are rearrangements of the structure's elements (e.g., the discs of the Tower of Hanoi, the sides of a cube to be folded from a two-dimensional cut-out, the letters in an anagram tasks). To keep track of the current state in planning, one has to continuously update the structure of the state one transforms. This again requires the flexible, temporary binding of representations of the independent objects or parts (e.g., the discs) to their places in a cognitive coordinate system (e.g., the rod positions).

This analysis shows that many reasoning tasks share the requirement of constructing new relational representations, often with considerable complexity, and updating them quickly and efficiently. Constructing new structural representations requires a mechanism that flexibly sets up and dissolves temporary bindings of elements into argument slots of a schema or positions in a mental coordinate system. According to our model, a schema or coordinate system is made available by the direct-access region of working memory, such that new elements can be bound to it. Updating structural representations often involves picking out selectively one element in the structure to manipulate it by a cognitive operation (e.g., moving one disc while leaving the others on their rod). This is the role of the focus of attention in working memory. An important feature of structural

representations is that individual elements can be changed without affecting the other elements. This is accomplished by the division of labor between the direct-access region and the focus of attention, thus enabling the system to attend to several elements concurrently. A structural representation is thus formed, and at the same time one element is selected exclusively as the object of a cognitive operation (Oberauer, 2002).

The above analysis of reasoning tasks should also explain why some tasks used to measure executive functions have been observed to correlate highly with measures of WMC and spatial reasoning (Miyake et al., 2001). These tasks are characterized by a mixture of demands on cognitive functions, among which may indeed be executive functions. Importantly, they all also place heavy demands on relational integration. Miyake et al. (2001) operationalized executive function through use of the Tower of Hanoi and a random-generation task (i.e., the generation of a sequence of digits that fulfils criteria of randomness such as equal frequency of all possible digits and digit transitions). As shown above, the Tower of Hanoi is a problem-solving task that relies heavily on the construction of new structures. The random-generation task requires constant monitoring of the sequence produced thus far, with careful attention to systematic patterns, that is, relations and structures that repeat themselves inadvertently. This comes down to a series completion task performed on the memory of one's own output—again, a task that relies considerably on relational integration. It is therefore not surprising that these tasks are strongly correlated with WMC and reasoning factors, and it proves in no way the crucial role of executive functions.

Our reinterpretation of some putative executive tasks leads to the prediction that removing the executive aspect from these tasks should not diminish their correlation with indicators of WMC and reasoning. The Tower of Hanoi problem, for example, is assumed to have executive demands because problem solvers must manage goals and subgoals and plan an appropriate sequence of moves (Miyake et al., 2001). A version without this requirement could be constructed in which participants receive an initial state and a sequence of operations, and their task is to determine what the final state will look like. Random generation is assumed to require the central executive because participants must suppress prepotent schemata and switch between generation strategies repeatedly (Baddeley, Emslie, Kolodny, & Duncan, 1998). A version with much reduced executive demand could be constructed in which participants are asked to monitor a sequence of digits and detect certain deviations from randomness (e.g., the repetition of a sequence of n digits or the emergence of a constant generation rule). We predict that these versions with diminished executive demand will correlate as highly as the originals with factors reflecting WMC and reasoning ability.

Relating Reasoning to Working Memory—Levels of Generality and Symmetry

In both our factor-analytic studies mentioned above, we also asked participants to take a test for the BIS (Jäger et al., 1997). Consistent with previous studies, we found a strong correlation between a factor representing WMC and the reasoning factor extracted from the BIS test (Süß, Oberauer, Wilhelm, & Wittmann, 2000; Süß et al., 2002). Because of the facet-theoretical framework of both the BIS and our structural model of working memory, we were able to investigate the relation between WMC and intelligence on different levels of generality. This investigation provided an opportunity to apply the multivariate reliability theory developed by Wittmann (1988) to the prediction of intelligence test scores from measures of working memory (and related constructs).

The central idea of multivariate reliability theory is that each measure is a composite of wanted and unwanted variance. *Wanted variance* is the variance due to the construct one intends to measure. *Unwanted variance* consists of variance due to other psychological variables one is not interested in (e.g., content-related variance when the intention is to measure a content-independent construct, or speed variance in a speeded reasoning test), task-specific

variance (which one is usually not interested in either), and random error. Only random error can be suppressed by increasing the number of items in a test; the first two components of unwanted variance are systematic and therefore don't drop out through longer testing with items of the same type. So in order to obtain a relatively pure estimate of the intended construct (i.e., the wanted variance), it is necessary to aggregate over several indicators of this construct. These indicators should not be clones of each other, distinguished only by trivial variations; heterogeneity is important to suppress systematic unwanted variance in the composite.

This requirement raises the question of the right amount of heterogeneity, or, in other words, the right level of generality. For an ability construct such as WMC, a minimum requirement is that its indicators are positively correlated, such that their shared variance can be interpreted as manifestation of the ability. Thus, one obvious means to assess what level of generality is adequate for an ability construct—that is, what set of indicators has an adequate level of heterogeneity—is to investigate the correlations in a large set of potential indicators, as we did above for WMC and related constructs. A second, complementary approach is to investigate the relationship to external criteria on different levels of generality. The rationale is given by the principles of *symmetry* in the Brunswik lens model (Tucker, 1964), illustrated in Figure 3.4 (after Wittmann, 1988). The figure shows a predictor and a criterion construct, each measured on three levels of generality (illustrated as the manifest variables and two levels of latent variables in a structural equation model). Assuming that the constructs share most (or even all) of their true variance, the highest correlations will be measured when symmetrical measures are related to each other. Symmetrical measures are measures on the same level of aggregation that reflect corresponding constructs with the same scope, represented by the thick, continuous lines in the figure. Asymmetrical relations (broken lines) lead to smaller correlations, because either the predictor or the criterion measure contains variance that has no counterpart on the other side. An example for

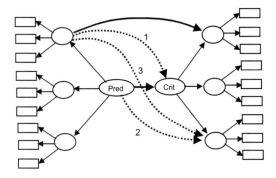

Figure 3.4. Principles of symmetry in predictor–criterion relations (after Wittmann, 1988). Thin lines represent factor loadings; thick lines represent predictor–criterion paths. Solid paths are symmetrical, broken paths are asymmetrical. Three kinds of asymmetry are illustrated: (1) the predictor variable is too specific relative to the criterion variable; (2) the criterion variable is too specific relative to the predictor variable; (3) predictor and criterion variables measure different subsets of the variance shared between predictor construct and criterion construct.

an asymmetric relationship would be to predict general intelligence (a highly general criterion) from a single measure of WMC such as reading span (path 1 in Fig. 3.4). An example of the converse asymmetry would be to use a battery of working memory tests to predict success in solving the Tower of Hanoi problem (path 2 in Fig. 3.4).

On the basis of this logic, we can use the correlations between WMC (and related constructs) and intelligence test measures on different levels of aggregation to search empirically for the most symmetric level for their relationship. Here we illustrate this approach with a reanalysis of data from our two studies (Oberauer et al., 2003; Süß et al., 2002).

The first level of generality is to correlate individual working memory tasks with the reasoning scale from the BIS. Table 3.2 shows three examples using classical WMC tasks. The correlations on this level are already substantial but leave enough room for doubting that WMC and reasoning ability are actually identical psychometric constructs (e.g., Ackerman et al., 2005). Many studies in the literature report relationships between single measures of WMC and some criterion variable, and the correlations are rarely larger than $r = .50$.

For a second level of generality we averaged the z scores of all tasks measuring predominantly storage and processing and all tasks measuring predominantly relational integration, separately

TABLE 3.2. Correlations between Working Memory Measures and Reasoning Ability and General Intelligence, on Four Levels of Generality

	Reasoning*	General Intelligence*	Reasoning[†]	General Intelligence[†]
Reading span	.57	.64	.47	.51
Computation span	.54	.52	.24	.29
Spatial STM	.59	.55	.58	.44
S&P-vn (7,5)	.69	.66	.53 (5)	.52
S&P-spat (3,2)	.68	.59	.58 (2)	.50
Rel.Int-vn (3,4)	.61	.61	.67 (4)	.64
Rel.Int-spat (5,7)	.65	.64	.67 (7)	.57
WMC (18, 18)	.77	.75	.76 (18)	.69
Speed/Exec (6, 16)	.59	.71	.55	.54
WMC + Speed/Exec (24, 34)	.76	.82	.77	.72

*Data from Süß et al. (2002), $N = 129$.
[†]Data from Süß et al. (2000), for task descriptions see Oberauer et al. (2003); $N = 133$. Numbers in parentheses behind composites represent the number of individual tasks entering into the respective composite (first entry = study 1, second entry = study 2). The Speed/Exec composite of Süß et al. (2002) consists of the tasks loading on the speed/executive functions factor in Oberauer et al. (2000); the Speed/Exec composite of Süß et al. (2000) consists of the choice response time tasks in single blocks and task-set switching blocks (i.e., the 16 manifest variables on the right side of Figure 3.3). STM = short-term memory; WMC = working memory capacity. For other abbreviations see Table 3.1.

for verbal-numerical and for spatial contents. The composite WMC scores correlate somewhat higher with reasoning ability. This is the level of generality attained by a number of studies using a latent-variable approach to measuring WMC and intelligence constructs. Most of these studies operationalized WMC by composites of complex span tasks with verbal or numerical content (e.g., reading span, operation span, counting span). This corresponds to the variable storage and processing with verbal or numerical material (S&P-vn) in Table 3.2.

On the third level of generality, we averaged the four composite variables to form a single indicator of WMC. The correlations with reasoning ability were higher still. When we move to an even higher level of generality on the predictor side, including variables reflecting processing speed and executive functions (e.g., reaction times from task-set switching paradigms), the correlations with reasoning level off. This suggests that the gain in reliability obtained through the larger number of test items is now offset by a reduction in symmetry.

Table 3.2 also contains correlations of all the WMC variables with a general intelligence score, obtained from the BIS test by aggregating the four functional scales (reasoning, creativity, memory, and speed). This illustrates a move to a higher level of generality on the criterion side. Relative to the correlations obtained with the reasoning scale, this move doesn't increase the correlations with the predictor variables, with one exception: the combination of WMC with speed and executive function was related more to general intelligence than to reasoning in the study of Süß et al. (2002).

Taken together, these data suggest that the most symmetric relationships are between the most comprehensive composite of WMC and reasoning ability, and, on a higher level of generality, between the even more encompassing composite of WMC, speed, and executive functions and general intelligence. The more elaborate analyses reported in Süß et al. (2002) show that the relationship on the highest level of generality can be summarized as (1) a strong association between WMC and reasoning, as shown above, and (2) a strong association between speed and

executive functions with the processing speed and memory factors of the BIS test.

A third kind of asymmetry (path 3 in Fig. 3.4) is obtained when two measures on the same level of generality are correlated that reflect different portions of the variance shared between the two constructs. An example from cognitive abilities is relating measures from different content domains. Although we and others found that content-specific WMC factors tend to be highly correlated, a separation of verbal-numerical from figural-spatial working memory factors is often warranted (Kyllonen, 1994; Oberauer et al., 2000; see Chapters 6 and 8), and at least in one study their correlation turned out to be quite low (Shah & Miyake, 1996). Therefore, correlating WMC measures consisting exclusively (Conway et al., 2002) or mostly (Ackerman et al., 2002) of verbal-numerical tasks with measures of fluid intelligence or reasoning based only on spatial-figural material (such as the Raven matrices or Cattell's Culture Fair Test) will result in an underestimation of the true relationship between WMC and fluid intelligence and reasoning.[2]

A structural equation model reported in Süß et al. (2002) illustrates this. In that model (Figure 10 in Süß et al., 2002), we used separate factors for spatial-figural WMC and for verbal-numerical WMC to predict the three content scales from the BIS test (verbal, numerical, and spatial-figural). The spatial-figural WMC factor predicted the spatial-figural factor of the BIS with a path coefficient of .70, whereas the path coefficients to the numerical factor (.35) and the verbal factor (−.26) were low. Conversely, the verbal-numerical WMC factor predicted verbal abilities in the BIS (.87) and numerical abilities (.52), but not spatial-figural abilities (.12).

To conclude, many correlations obtained in published studies on the relationship between WMC and reasoning or fluid intelligence, though impressively high, might actually underestimate the true amount of shared variance between the two constructs. Still, we do not believe that the two can be identified. Evidence that fluid intelligence cannot be completely reduced to WMC comes again from the content dimension. Whereas verbal and numerical content could never be factorially separated in sets of WMC tasks (Kyllonen & Christal, 1990; Oberauer et al., 2000, 2003), they are clearly different on the side of intelligence in general (Carroll, 1993) and reasoning ability in particular (Jäger et al., 1997). Reasoning is, after all, a little bit more than working memory.

CONCLUSIONS

We see converging evidence that WMC is a highly general parameter of the cognitive system, one that acts as an important limiting factor for a wide variety of complex cognitive tasks. In this chapter we argued that the common denominator of all cognitive functions limited by WMC is the temporary binding of representations. The more a performance on any task relies on the establishment of multiple temporary bindings maintained simultaneously and consistently, the more we expect it to load on a general WMC factor. First direct support for this prediction comes from a study showing that short-term recognition tasks (such as the Sternberg task and the *n*-back task) correlate with WMC only if they involve a high demand on bindings (Oberauer, 2005a).

Working memory capacity, in turn, is the best single predictor of reasoning ability, explaining at least half of the systematic variance in tests of reasoning or fluid intelligence. This relationship seems to exist on a high level of generality. It is not due to associations between particular WMC tasks and particular reasoning tasks, but rather is a manifestation of a highly general limiting factor that affects both working memory and reasoning. We hypothesize that this factor is the limited ability of our nervous system to establish multiple temporary bindings at the same time, thereby enabling the construction of new relational representations. The construction of new relational representations is a requirement shared by most tasks commonly used in established reasoning tests and in experiments on reasoning.

Temporary bindings are also needed to establish task sets implementing arbitrary links between stimulus and response categories. Although speculative at the moment, this paradigm can offer an explanation for the strong association between WMC measures and many speed tasks, a relationship largely ignored in the working memory literature so far. At the same time, WMC cannot be reduced to mental speed; factors representing WMC and factors representing speed have always been separable in comprehensive studies.

Finally, our view differs in one respect from the majority opinion in the field, in that we don't assume a special link between WMC and executive function. The evidence available thus far suggests that different executive function measures have little variance in common. Some of them are related to WMC, but we think this is not because they reflect executive functions but because of some other feature. For example, choice RTs obtained in task-set switching paradigms correlate with WMC factors, but no more than do RTs in the same tasks without switching. Planning tasks such as Tower of Hanoi correlate with WMC because of their demand on relational integration, not because of their demand on executive functions to select individual moves.

The challenge to theories that link working memory and executive functions is perhaps the most significant contribution of our studies to theories of working memory. It is just one example of the general potential inherent in individual-difference studies. They can serve to validate, and invalidate, experimental tasks and variables as indicators of theoretical constructs, and they can test theories about associations, as well as dissociations, between constructs (cf. Oberauer, 2005b). Factor analyses of large samples of tasks have, for example, helped to establish working memory as an important theoretical concept in cognitive psychology. Factor-analytic research, however, raises serious doubts about the usefulness of a unitary construct subsuming all executive functions. Experimental research helps us to understand the cognitive processes going on when a person is confronted with a specific situation or task. Individual-differences research tells us whether these processes are in fact representative of the theoretical concepts the experimentalist assumes them to represent.

BOX 3.1. SUMMARY ANSWERS TO BOOK QUESTIONS

1. THE OVERARCHING THEORY OF WORKING MEMORY

We think of working memory as a system that provides access to memory representations for goal-directed processing on three successive levels: (1) activation in LTM, (2) temporary binding of content representations to positions in a cognitive coordinate system or placeholders in a schema in the region of direct access, and (3) selection as the object of manipulation by the focus of attention. Further, we use facet theory to organize the sources of variance among individuals that affect performance on particular tasks.

2. CRITICAL SOURCES OF WORKING MEMORY VARIATION

The capacity limit of working memory is a limit on the simultaneous binding of several independent chunks in a common coordinate system or schema in the region of direct access. This limit constrains how many independent chunks can be accessed simultaneously, and thereby constrains the ability to construct new

relational representations between them, and the ability to take existing relations into account in cognitive operations. People with low working memory capacity are assumed to have a specific problem with establishing and maintaining robust bindings.

3. OTHER SOURCES OF WORKING MEMORY VARIATION

We consider two other sources of variability: the efficiency of executive function and the efficiency of inhibition. We believe that both these functions can be dissociated from working memory capacity.

4. CONTRIBUTIONS TO GENERAL WORKING MEMORY THEORY

Our research shows that the limited capacity of working memory affects a wide variety of tasks, its scope reaching beyond the classical characterization as subserving simultaneous storage and processing. Working memory, however, cannot be equated with executive function.

Notes

1. For this reason, we renamed "focus of attention" in the model of Cowan (1995) as "region of direct access" in our model.
2. In light of this, it is impressive how high the relationships obtained in these two studies were, as Conway et al. (2002) pointed out.

Acknowledgments

The research reported in this chapter was supported by Deutsche Forschungsgemeinschaft (DFG, grants WI 1390/1, KL 955/4, and OB 121/3).

References

Ackerman, P. L., Beier, M. E., & Boyle, M. O. (2002). Individual differences in working memory within a nomological network of cognitive and perceptual speed abilities. *Journal of Experimental Psychology: General, 131*, 567–589.

Ackerman, P. L., Beier, M. E., & Boyle, M. O. (2005). Working memory and intelligence: The same or different constructs? *Psychological Bulletin, 131*, 30–60.

Allport, A., Styles, E. A., & Hsieh, S. (1994). Shifting intentional set: Exploring the dynamic control of tasks. In C. Umiltá & M. Moscovitch (Eds.), *Attention and Performance* (Vol. XV, pp. 421–452). Cambridge, MA: MIT Press.

Anderson, J. R., & Lebiere, C. (1998). *The atomic components of thought*. Mahwah, NJ: Erlbaum.

Baddeley, A. D. (1986). *Working memory*. Oxford: Clarendon Press.

Baddeley, A. D. (1993). Working memory or working attention? In A. Baddeley & L. Weiskrantz (Eds.), *Attention: Selection, awareness, and control* (pp. 152–170). Oxford: Clarendon Press.

Baddeley, A. D., Emslie, H., Kolodny, J., & Duncan, J. (1998). Random generation and the executive control of working memory. *Quarterly Journal of Experimental Psychology, 51A*, 819–852.

Bayliss, D. M., Jarrold, C., Gunn, D. M., & Baddeley, A. D. (2003). The complexities of complex span: Explaining individual differences in working memory in children and adults. *Journal of Experimental Psychology: General, 132*, 71–92.

Brown, G. D. A., Preece, T., & Hulme, C. (2000). Oscillator-based memory for serial order. *Psychological Review, 107*, 127–181.

Burgess, N., & Hitch, G. J. (1999). Memory for serial order: A network model of the phonological loop and its timing. *Psychological Review, 106*, 551–581.

Canter, D. (1985). *Facet theory.* Berlin: Springer.

Carpenter, P., Just, M. A., & Shell, P. (1990). What one intelligence test measures: A theoretical account of the processing in the Raven Progressive Matrices Test. *Psychological Review, 97*, 404–431.

Carroll, J. B. (1993). *Human cognitive abilities: a survey of factor-analytic studies.* New York: Cambridge University Press.

Cepeda, N. J., Kramer, A., & Gonzalez de Sather, J. C. M. (2001). Changes in executive control across the life span: Examination of task-switching performance. *Developmental Psychology, 37*, 715–730.

Christoff, K., Prabhakaran, V., Dorfman, J., Zhao, Z., Kroger, J. K., Holyoak, K. J., et al. (2001). Rostrolateral prefrontal cortex involvement in relational integration during reasoning. *NeuroImage, 14*, 1136–1149.

Colom, R., Flores-Mendoza, C., & Rebollo, I. (2003). Working memory and intelligence. *Personality and individual Differences, 34*, 33–39.

Conway, A. R. A., Cowan, N., & Bunting, M. F. (2001). The cocktail party phenomenon revisited: The importance of working memory capacity. *Psychonomic Bulletin & Review, 8*, 331–335.

Conway, A. R. A., Cowan, N., Bunting, M. F., Therriault, D. J., & Minkoff, S. R. B. (2002). A latent variable analysis of working memory capacity, short-term memory capacity, processing speed, and general fluid intelligence. *Intelligence, 30*, 163–183.

Conway, A. R. A., & Engle, R. W. (1994). Working memory and retrieval: A resource-dependent inhibition model. *Journal of Experimental Psychology: General, 123*, 354–373.

Cowan, N. (1988). Evolving conceptions of memory storage, selective attention, and their mutual constraints within the human information-processing system. *Psychological Bulletin, 104*, 163–191.

Cowan, N. (1995). *Attention and memory: An integrated framework.* New York: Oxford University Press.

Cowan, N. (1999). An embedded-process model of working memory. In A. Miyake & P. Shah (Eds.), *Models of working memory. Mechanisms of active maintenance and executive control* (pp. 62–101). New York: Cambridge University Press.

Cowan, N. (2001). The magical number 4 in short-term memory: A reconsideration of mental storage capacity. *Behavioral and Brain Sciences, 24*, 87–185.

Daneman, M., & Carpenter, P. A. (1980). Individual differences in working memory and reading. *Journal of Verbal Learning and Verbal Behavior, 19*, 450–466.

Daneman, M., & Merikle, P. M. (1996). Working memory and language comprehension: a meta-analysis. *Psychonomic Bulletin & Review, 3*, 422–433.

De Beni, R., & Palladino, P. (2000). Intrusion errors in working memory tasks. Are they related to reading comprehension ability? *Learning and Individual Differences, 12*, 131–143.

De Beni, R., Palladino, P., Pazzaglia, P., & Cornoldi, C. (1998). Increases in intrusion errors and working memory deficit of poor comprehenders. *Quarterly Journal of Experimental Psychology, 51A*, 305–320.

DeSoto, C., London, M., & Handel, S. (1965). Social reasoning and spatial paralogic. *Journal of Personality and Social Psychology, 2*, 513–521.

Duncan, J., Johnson, R., Swales, M., & Freer, C. (1997). Frontal lobe deficits after head injury: Unity and diversity of function. *Cognitive Neuropsychology, 14*, 713–741.

Engle, R. W., Kane, M. J., & Tuholski, S. W. (1999). Individual differences in working memory capacity and what they tell us about controlled attention, general fluid intelligence, and functions of the prefrontal cortex. In A. Miyake & P. Shah (Eds.), *Models of working memory. Mechanisms of active maintenance and executive control* (pp. 102–134). New York: Cambridge University Press.

Engle, R. W., Tuholski, S. W., Laughlin, J. E., & Conway, A. R. A. (1999). Working memory, short term memory and general fluid intelligence: A latent variable approach. *Journal of Experimental Psychology: General, 128,* 309–331.

Farrell, S., & Lewandowsky, S. (2002). An endogenous distributed model of ordering in serial recall. *Psychonomic Bulletin & Review, 9,* 59–79.

Friedman, N. P., & Miyake, A. (2004). The relations among inhibition and interference control functions: a latent variable analysis. *Journal of Experimental Psychology: General, 133,* 101–131.

Friedman, N. P., Miyake, A., Corley, R. P., Young, S. E., DeFries, J. C., & Hewitt, J. K. (2006). Not all executive functions are related to intelligence. *Psychological Science, 17,* 172–179.

Gentner, D. (1989). The mechanisms of analogical learning. In S. Vosniadou & A. Ortony (Eds.), *Similarity and analogical reasoning* (pp. 199–241). Cambridge: Cambridge University Press.

Gilbert, S. J., & Shallice, T. (2002). Task switching: A PDP model. *Cognitive Psychology, 44,* 297–337.

Gray, J. R., Chabris, C. F., & Braver, T. S. (2003). Neural mechanisms of general fluid intelligence. *Nature Neuroscience, 6,* 316–322.

Halford, G. S., Wilson, W. H., & Phillips, S. (1998). Processing capacity defined by relational complexity: Implications for comparative, developmental, and cognitive psychology. *Behavioral and Brain Sciences, 21,* 803–864.

Hasher, L., & Zacks, R. T. (1988). Working memory, comprehension, and aging: A review and a new view. In G. H. Bower (Ed.), *The psychology of learning and motivation* (Vol. 22, pp. 193–225). New York: Academic Press.

Hasher, L., Zacks, R. T., & May, C. P. (1999). Inhibitory control, circadian arousal, and age. In D. Gopher & A. Koriat (Eds.), *Attention and performance* (pp. 653–675). Cambridge, MA: MIT Press.

Henson, R. N. A. (1998). Short-term memory for serial order: The Start-End Model. *Cognitive Psychology, 36,* 73–137.

Henson, R. N. A., Norris, D. G., Page, M. P. A., & Baddeley, A. D. (1996). Unchained memory: Error patterns rule out chaining models of immediate serial recall. *Quarterly Journal of Experimental Psychology, 49A,* 80–115.

Hommel, B. (1998). Event files: Evidence for automatic integration of stimulus-response episodes. *Visual Cognition, 5,* 183–216.

Hummel, J. E., & Holyoak, K. J. (1997). Distributed representations of structure: A theory of analogical access and mapping. *Psychological Review, 104,* 427–466.

Jäger, A. O., Süß, H.-M., & Beauducel, A. (1997). *Test für das Berliner Intelligenzstrukturmodell (BIS).* Göttingen: Hogrefe.

Johnson-Laird, P. N. (2001). Mental models and deduction. *Trends in Cognitive Sciences, 5,* 434–442.

Johnson-Laird, P. N., & Bara, B. G. (1984). Syllogistic inference. *Cognition, 16,* 1–61.

Johnson-Laird, P. N., & Byrne, R. M. J. (1991). *Deduction.* Hillsdale, NJ: Erlbaum.

Kane, M. J., Bleckley, M. K., Conway, A. R. A., & Engle, R. W. (2001). A controlled-attention view of working-memory capacity. *Journal of Experimental Psychology: General, 130,* 169–183.

Kane, M. J., & Engle, R. W. (2003). Working-memory capacity and the control of attention: The contributions of goal neglect, response competition, and task set to Stroop interference. *Journal of Experimental Psychology: General, 132*(47–70).

Kane, M. J., Hambrick, D. Z., & Conway, A. R. A. (2005). Working memory capacity and fluid intelligence are strongly related constructs: comment on Ackerman, Beier, and Boyle (2004). *Psychological Bulletin, 131,* 66–71.

Kane, M. J., Hambrick, D. Z., Tuholski, S. W., Wilhelm, O., Payne, T. W., & Engle, R. W. (2004). The generality of working-memory capacity: A latent-variable approach to verbal and visuospatial memory span and reasoning. *Journal of Experimental Psychology: General, 133,* 189–217.

Karat, J. (1982). A model of problem solving with incomplete constraint knowledge. *Cognitive Psychology, 14,* 538–559.

Kornblum, S., Hasbroucq, T., & Osman, A. M. (1990). Dimensional overlap: Cognitive basis for stimulus-response-compatibility—a model and taxonomy. *Psychological Review, 97,* 253–270.

Kotovsky, K., Hayes, J. R., & Simon, H. A. (1985). Why are some problems hard? Evidence from Tower of Hanoi. *Cognitive Psychology, 17,* 248–294.

Kramer, A. F., Humphrey, D. G., Larish, J. F., Logan, G. D., & Strayer, D. L. (1994). Aging and inhibition: Beyond a unitary view of inhibitory processing in attention. *Psychology & Aging, 9,* 491–512.

Kray, J., & Lindenberger, U. (2000). Adult age differences in task switching. *Psychology and Aging, 15,* 126–147.

Kyllonen, P. C. (1994). Aptitude testing inspired by information processing: A test of the four-sources model. *Journal of General Psychology, 120,* 375–405.

Kyllonen, P. C., & Christal, R. E. (1990). Reasoning ability is (little more than) working-memory capacity?! *Intelligence, 14,* 389–433.

Lakoff, G., & Johnson, M. (1980). *Metaphors we live by.* Chicago: University of Chicago Press.

Langacker, R. W. (1986). An introduction to cognitive grammar. *Cognitive Science, 10,* 1–40.

Lien, M.-C., & Proctor, R. W. (2002). Stimulus-response compatibility and psychological refractory period effects: Implications for response selection. *Psychonomic Bulletin & Review, 9,* 212–238.

Logan, G. D. (1978). Attention in character-classification tasks: Evidence for the automaticity of component stages. *Journal of Experimental Psychology: General, 107,* 32–63.

Logan, G. D., & Cowan, W. B. (1984). On the ability to inhibit thought and action: A theory of an act of control. *Psychological Review, 91,* 295–327.

Logan, G. D., & Schulkind, M. D. (2000). Parallel memory retrieval in dual-task situations: I. Semantic memory. *Journal of Experimental Psychology: Human Perception and Performance, 26,* 1072–1090.

Lustig, C., May, C. P., & Hasher, L. (2001). Working memory span and the role of proactive interference. *Journal of Experimental Psychology: General, 130,* 199–207.

May, C. P., Hasher, L., & Kane, M. J. (1999). The role of interference in memory span. *Memory & Cognition, 27,* 759–767.

Mayr, U., & Keele, S. W. (2000). Changing internal constraints on action: The role of backward inhibition. *Journal of Experimental Psychology: General, 129,* 4–26.

Meiran, N. (1996). Is reading ability related to activation dumping speed? Evidence from immediate repetition priming. *Memory & Cognition, 24,* 41–59.

Miyake, A., Friedman, N. P., Emerson, M. J., Witzki, A. H., Howerter, A., & Wager, T. D. (2000). The unity and diversity of executive functions and their contributions to complex "frontal lobe" tasks: A latent variable analysis. *Cognitive Psychology, 41,* 49–100.

Miyake, A., Friedman, N. P., Rettinger, D. A., Shah, P., & Hegarty, M. (2001). How are visuospatial working memory, executive functioning, and spatial abilities related: A latent-variable analysis. *Journal of Experimental Psychology: General, 130,* 621–640.

Moscovitch, M. (1992). Memory and working-with-memory: A component process model based on modules and central systems. *Journal of Cognitive Neuroscience, 4,* 257–267.

Neumann, O., & Klotz, W. (1994). Motor responses to nonreportable, masked stimuli: Where is the limit of direct parameter specification? In C. Umiltá & M. Moscovitch (Eds.), *Attention and Performance* (Vol. XV, pp. 124–150). Cambridge: MIT Press.

Newell, A., & Simon, H. A. (1972). *Human problem solving.* Englewood Cliffs, N.J.: Prentice Hall.

Norman, D. A., & Shallice, T. (1980). *Attention to action. Willed and automatic control of behavior* (CHIP Report No. 99): University of California San Diego.

O'Reilly, R., Busby, R. S., & Soto, R. (2003). Three forms of binding and their neural substrates: Alternatives to temporal synchrony. In A. Cleeremans (Ed.), *The unity of consciousness: binding, integration, and dissociation* (pp. 168–192). Oxford, UK: Oxford University Press.

Oberauer, K. (1993). Die Koordination kognitiver Operationen. Eine Studie zum Zusammenhang von "working memory" und Intelligenz. *Zeitschrift für Psychologie, 201,* 57–81.

Oberauer, K. (2001). Removing irrelevant information from working memory. A cognitive aging study with the modified Sternberg task. *Journal of Experimental Psychology: Learning, Memory, and Cognition, 27,* 948–957.

Oberauer, K. (2002). Access to information in working memory: Exploring the focus of attention. *Journal of Experimental Psychology: Learning, Memory, and Cognition, 28,* 411–421.

Oberauer, K. (2003). Selective attention to elements in working memory. *Experimental Psychology, 50,* 257–269.

Oberauer, K. (2005a). Binding and inhibition in working memory individual and age differences in short-term recognition. *Journal of Experimental Psychology: General, 134,* 368–387.

Oberauer, K. (2005b). The measurement of working memory capacity. In O. Wilhelm & R. W. Engle (Eds.), *Handbook of understanding and measuring intelligence* (pp. 393–408). Thousand Oaks: Sage.

Oberauer, K., Lange, E., & Engle, R. W. (2004). Working memory capacity and resistance to interference. *Journal of Memory and Language, 51,* 80–96.

Oberauer, K., Schulze, R., Wilhelm, O., & Süß, H.-M. (2005). Working memory and intelligence—their correlation and their relation: A commend on Ackerman, Beier, and Boyle (2005). *Psychological Bulletin, 131,* 61–65.

Oberauer, K., Süß, H.-M., Schulze, R., Wilhelm, O., & Wittmann, W. W. (2000). Working memory capacity—facets of a cognitive ability construct. *Personality and Individual Differences, 29,* 1017–1045.

Oberauer, K., Süß, H.-M., Wilhelm, O., & Wittmann, W. W. (2003). The multiple faces of working memory—storage, processing, supervision, and coordination. *Intelligence, 31,* 167–193.

Page, M. P. A., & Norris, D. (1998). The primacy model: A new model of immediate serial recall. *Psychological Review, 105,* 761–781.

Raffone, A., & Wolters, G. (2001). A cortical mechanism for binding in visual working memory. *Journal of Cognitive Neuroscience, 13,* 766–785.

Robin, N., & Holyoak, K. J. (1995). Relational complexity and the functions of prefrontal cortex. In M. S. Gazzaniga (Ed.), *The cognitive neurosciences* (pp. 987–997). Cambridge, MA: MIT Press.

Rogers, R. D., & Monsell, S. (1995). Costs of a predictable switch between simple cognitive tasks. *Journal of Experimental Psychology: General, 124,* 207–231.

Rosen, V. M., & Engle, R. W. (1997). The role of working memory capacity in retrieval. *Journal of Experimental Psychology: General, 126,* 211–227.

Salthouse, T. A. (1991). Mediation of adult age differences in cognition by reductions in working memory and speed of processing. *Psychological Science, 2,* 179–183.

Salthouse, T. A. (1994). The aging of working memory. *Neuropsychology, 8,* 535–543.

Salthouse, T. A., Atkinson, T. M., & Berish, D. E. (2003). Executive functioning as a potential mediator of age-related cognitive decline in normal adults. *Journal of Experimental Psychology: General, 132,* 566–594.

Salthouse, T. A., Babcock, R. L., & Shaw, R. J. (1991). Effects of adult age on structural and operational capacities in working memory. *Psychology and Aging, 6,* 118–127.

Schaeken, W., Johnson-Laird, P. N., & d'Ydewalle, G. (1996). Mental models and temporal reasoning. *Cognition, 60,* 205–234.

Shah, P., & Miyake, A. (1996). The separability of working memory resources for spatial thinking and language processing: An individual differences approach. *Journal of Experimental Psychology: General, 125,* 4–27.

Shallice, T., & Burgess, P. (1991). Higher-order cognitive impairments and frontal lobe lesions in man. In H. S. Levin, H. M. Eisenberg & A. L. Benton (Eds.), *Frontal lobe function and dysfunction* (pp. 125–138). New York: Oxford University Press.

Shilling, V. M., Chetwynd, A., & Rabbitt, P. M. A. (2002). Individual inconsistency across measures of inhibition: an investigation of the construct validity of inhibition in older adults. *Neuropsychologia, 40,* 605–619.

Sternberg, R. J. (1985). *Beyond IQ.* New York: Cambridge University Press.

Süß, H.-M., & Beauducel, A. (2005). Faceted models of intelligence. In O. Wilhelm & R. W. Engle (Eds.), *Handbook of understanding and measuring intelligence* (pp. 313–332). Thousand Oaks, CA: Sage.

Süß, H.-M., Oberauer, K., Wilhelm, O., & Wittmann, W. W. (2000). *Can working memory capacity explain reasoning ability?* Paper presented at the XXVII International Congress of Psychology, Stockholm, Sweden.

Süß, H.-M., Oberauer, K., Wittmann, W. W., Wilhelm, O., & Schulze, R. (2002). Working memory capacity explains reasoning ability and a little bit more. *Intelligence, 30,* 261–288.

Talmy, L. (1988). Force dynamics in language and cognition. *Cognitive Science, 12,* 49–100.

Tucker, L. R. (1964). A suggested alternative formulation in the developments by Hursch, Hammond and Hursch, and by Hammond, Hursch and Todd. *Psychological Review, 77,* 528–530.

Unsworth, N., & Engle, R. W. (2005). Working memory capacity and fluid abilities: Examining the correlation between operation span and Raven. *Intelligence, 33,* 67–81.

Unsworth, N., Schrock, J. C., & Engle, R. W. (2004). Working memory capacity and the antisaccade task: Individual differences in voluntary saccade control. *Journal of Experimental Psychology: Learning, Memory, and Cognition, 30,* 1302–1321.

Usher, M., Haarmann, H. J., Cohen, J. D., & Horn, D. (2001). Neural mechanism for the magical number 4: Competitive interactions and nonlinear oscillation. *Behavioral & Brain Sciences, 24,* 151–152.

Waltz, J. A., Knowlton, B. J., Holyoak, K. J., Boone, K. B., Mishkin, F. S., de Menezes Santos, M., et al. (1999). A system for relational reasoning in human prefrontal cortex. *Psychological Science, 10,* 119–125.

Ward, G., Roberts, M. J., & Phillips, L. H. (2001). Task-switching costs, Stroop-costs, and executive control: A correlational study. *Quarterly Journal of Experimental Psychology, 54A,* 491–511.

Wilhelm, O. (2005). Measuring reasoning ability. In O. Wilhelm & R. W. Engle (Eds.), *Handbook of understanding and measuring intelligence* (pp. 373–392). Thousand Oaks: Sage.

Wilhelm, O., & Oberauer, K. (2006). Why are reasoning ability and working memory capacity related to mental speed? An investigation of stimulus-response compatibility in choice-reaction-time tasks. *European Journal of Cognitive Psychology, 18,* 18–50.

Wittmann, W. W. (1988). Multivariate reliability theory. Principles of symmetry and successful validation strategies. In J. R. Nesselroade & R. B. Cattell (Eds.), *Handbook of multivariate experimental psychology* (pp. 505–560). New York: Plenum.

4

Explaining the Many Varieties of Working Memory Variation: Dual Mechanisms of Cognitive Control

TODD S. BRAVER, JEREMY R. GRAY,
and GREGORY C. BURGESS

Virtually all working memory (WM) theorists agree that control processes are a critical component of WM function. Some set of internal mechanisms must be responsible for (1) selecting information for active maintenance in WM; (2) ensuring that it can be stored for an appropriate length of time; (3) protecting it against sources of interference; (4) updating it at appropriate junctures; and (5) using it to influence other cognitive systems (i.e., perception, attention, memory and action). Yet, equally clear to most theorists is the observation that the ability to exert control over WM varies substantially, both within individuals (across time and task situations) and across individuals. In some sense, this observation poses perhaps the core paradox regarding cognitive control: why is cognitive control so important, yet simultaneously so fragile and vulnerable to disruption? Why does it appear that our ability to exert control is so strong in some cases but so weak in others? If exerting cognitive control seems to be the optimal response in many situations, why does it seem as if behavior is suboptimally controlled much of the time in many individuals, and at least some of the time in all individuals?

In this chapter, we put forth a theory of cognitive control in WM that attempts to explain this variability. Our central hypothesis is that cognitive control operates via two distinct operating modes: *proactive control* and *reactive control*. We will present arguments suggesting that these two modes are dissociable on a number of dimensions, such as computational properties, neural substrates, temporal dynamics, and consequences for information processing. We will suggest that although most formulations of cognitive control in WM only consider proactive control, reactive control mechanisms may be more dominant. We will further suggest that by distinguishing between these two modes we will be able to (1) resolve some of the apparent inconsistencies in the existing WM literature; (2) understand how and why the impact of cognitive control processes in WM can vary so strongly within individuals across time and task situations; (3) gain insight into the nature of cognitive control impairments found in healthy aging (and possibly in other populations suffering from neuropsychiatric disorders); (4) understand some of the critical underlying mechanisms related to individual differences in WM function; and (5) account for potentially surprising data indicating that putatively "noncognitive" variables such as mood states and personality traits (e.g., extraversion, neuroticism) may also influence WM function.

The general theoretical framework that we advance here for understanding the sources of variation that affect WM and cognitive control is termed the *dual mechanisms of control*, or DMC account. It is worth noting that, although we have been developing this framework for several years now, this chapter marks the first comprehensive treatment of the theory and its empirical support. As such, we combine discussion of both published and not-yet-published experimental data in the sections below, to better make the case for how the DMC theory provides a fully integrated account of a variety of cognitive-control phenomena. Moreover, before turning to experimental findings, we first provide important theoretical background that motivated the development of this new theory.

A GENERAL THEORETICAL MODEL OF WORKING MEMORY

In this section, we describe the overarching theoretical framework that guides our work (i.e., Question #1). Our theoretical model attempts to specify critical WM components in terms of underlying neurobiologically based computational mechanisms (Botvinick, Braver, Barch, Carter, & Cohen, 2001; Braver & Cohen, 2000; O'Reilly, Braver, & Cohen, 1999) (see Fig. 4.1 for schematic of model). The central hypothesis is that the core of WM is controlled processing: the ability to flexibly adapt behavior to particular task demands, favoring the processing of task-relevant information over competing sources of information and emphasizing goal-compatible behavior over habitual or otherwise dominant responses. This definition is fairly

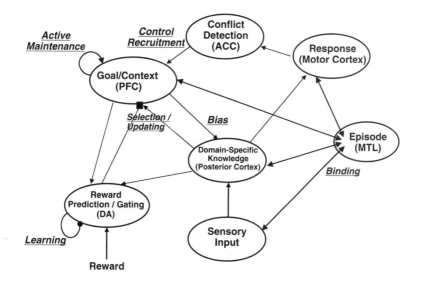

Figure 4.1. Schematic diagram of theoretical framework of working memory. Lines with single arrowheads reflect excitatory interconnection; bold lines with double arrowheads reflect encoding and retrieval of traces via episodic memory. The excitatory connection from prefrontal cortex (PFC) back to itself represents recurrent connectivity in PFC that mediates active maintenance. The line ending in a square reflects the ability of dopaminergic (DA) projections to modulate or gate inputs into PFC. The line with a circle reflects gradual learning and plasticity involved in reward prediction. ACC = anterior cingulate cortex; MTL = medial temporal lobe.

similar to others that have been put forth in the literature (e.g., Duncan, Emslie, Williams, Johnson, & Freer, 1996; Norman & Shallice, 1986) and in this volume (e.g., Chapters 2 and 7). We suggest that controlled processing is an emergent phenomenon, arising from dynamic interactions between specialized processing subsystems in the brain. Considering each subsystem in isolation cannot fully account for any of the mechanistic properties of WM functionality. Nevertheless, we argue that a number of core brain systems play critical roles in WM function because of their specialized computational properties. A central feature of our theoretical framework is that these specializations arise in neural tissue as a means of optimizing a fundamental computational trade-off. The interaction between these specialized systems enables a kind of global constraint satisfaction process to occur, whereby maximal flexibility is ensured across the entire range of information-processing situations.

In particular, we suggest that the prefrontal cortex (PFC) is an especially influential structure in WM because of its extensive connectivity with other brain regions and specialized processing capabilities. As discussed in much greater detail below, the PFC is hypothesized to play a central role in the *active maintenance* of internally represented context information, allowing it to *bias* processing in other neural systems in accordance with this maintained information (e.g., goals, instructions, intermediate products of mental computation). The PFC is aided in this function by its interactive connectivity with the hippocampus–medial temporal lobe complex (MTL), the midbrain dopamine (DA) system, and the anterior cingulate cortex (ACC). The MTL complex augments PFC functions through rapid, associative *binding* of active representations throughout the brain, which can then serve as an auxiliary form of storage in WM tasks (O'Reilly et al., 1999; a similar type of mechanism is described in Chapter 3). The DA system is postulated to regulate the contents of PFC via a *dynamic updating* mechanism sensitive to reinforcement contingencies (Braver & Cohen, 2000). The ACC is postulated to modulate the general

responsiveness of PFC through a *performance-monitoring* mechanism that continuously indexes the need for top-down control via a computation of ongoing processing conflict (Botvinick et al., 2001). The PFC also interacts extensively with posterior brain systems, which store domain-specific content knowledge. The content-specific computational specializations within posterior cortex may contribute to domain-specific components of WM, such as the storage of sequential-order information associated with verbal WM, and the storage of configural and/or movement-based representations associated with visuospatial WM.

THE PREFRONTAL CORTEX AND PROACTIVE COGNITIVE CONTROL

Our research has primarily focused on understanding the role of the PFC in cognitive control and WM. There is general agreement that PFC plays a critical role in control functions, but much less agreement concerning the particular computational and neural mechanisms that enable it to play such a role. A great deal of data on PFC function has come from single-cell recording studies in nonhuman primates during simple WM tasks, such as the delayed-response paradigm. In these studies, a highly reliable finding is that PFC neurons (particularly in dorsolateral regions of PFC) show elevated and sustained activity during the retention interval (Fuster, 1997). This pattern of activity, along with related results, has been taken as evidence that PFC subserves storage functions in WM. Human neuroimaging data have provided some support for this notion, showing sustained lateral PFC responses during WM maintenance periods (e.g., Cohen et al., 1997). However, a growing trend within the neuroimaging literature has been to emphasize PFC involvement in cognitive control rather than WM per se (Smith & Jonides, 1999). Indeed, a number of imaging studies have suggested that WM tasks involving simple storage may not engage PFC at all, or at least not the dorsolateral regions targeted in primate neurophysiology studies (e.g., Postle, Berger, & D'Esposito, 1999).

Yet, at the same time, there is no clear consensus as to what the specific control functions are that engage PFC.

Our own work has been guided by the hypothesis that PFC is central to cognitive control and WM because it is specialized to enable the representation and active maintenance of *context* information. *Context* is defined as task-relevant information that is internally represented in such a form that it can bias processing in the pathways responsible for task performance. Representations of context are similar to the goal representations of other theoretical formulations (e.g., Norman & Shallice, 1986), but are flexible enough to influence not only action systems but also perception, attention, memory, and emotion. Likewise, some context representations should be considered micro-goals, in that they operate over short timescales or act to bias a narrow range of target representations.

Representations of context are particularly important in situations where there is strong competition for response selection. These situations may arise when the appropriate response is relatively infrequent (such as the color name in the Stroop task). Because context representations are maintained on-line, in an active state, they are continually available to influence processing. Consequently, context can be thought of as one component of WM. Specifically, context can be viewed as the subset of representations within WM that govern how other representations are used. In this manner, context representations simultaneously subserve both mnemonic and control functions. This aspect of the model differentiates it from classical models of WM (e.g., Baddeley, 1986), which postulate a strict separation of representations for storage vs. control (but for an updated view, see Baddeley, 2003).

An important component of our account of PFC function concerns the interaction between PFC and the DA neurotransmitter system, which projects strongly to this region of the brain. We suggest that active maintenance of context within PFC occurs via local recurrent connectivity, resulting in a stable, self-sustaining pattern of neural activity (i.e., an attractor, in computational terms). The DA system is postu-lated to regulate active maintenance within PFC, by gating the entrance of information into PFC, such that only task-relevant context will be actively maintained. We claim that this regulatory action occurs in response to phasic bursts of DA release within PFC, which produce a neuromodulatory effect on PFC neurons, enabling them to update and actively maintain afferent inputs arriving from other brain regions (Braver & Cohen, 2000). Without such a synchronous burst of DA activity at the time of external inputs, they will only be transiently represented within PFC, decaying shortly after the external input stops. For this reason, actively maintained representations of task-relevant context in PFC will be relatively robust to interference from task-irrelevant inputs.

Importantly, the DA system is postulated to also play a critical role in learning based on predictions of expected reward (i.e., reinforcement-based learning; Schultz, Dayan, & Montague, 1997). Because of this learning role, the DA system can self-organize to develop the appropriate timing of gating signals to enable the appropriate updating and maintenance of relevant context. As such, the system is not a "homunculus," in that it uses simple principles of learning to dynamically configure and adaptively regulate its own behavior. Moreover, our hypotheses regarding the functional roles of PFC and DA and their interaction have been studied within implemented computational models (e.g., Braver & Cohen, 2000).

For example, we have developed a model of PFC function in a simple delayed-response paradigm known as the AX-CPT, in which contextual cues must be actively maintained over a retention interval to bias processing to a subsequent probe item. A key aspect of the task is that in some trial conditions (termed *BX*), the contextual information must be used to inhibit a dominant response tendency, whereas in other trials (termed *AY*) context serves an attentional biasing function. In our computational model of the AX-CPT, the representation and maintenance of the context provided by the cue is postulated to occur within PFC. The DA system regulates the access of this context information to PFC, such that context can be appropriately updated on a trial-by-trial basis and sustained over the delay without interference. In a systematic series of simulation and empirical studies (Braver, Cohen, & Barch, 2002), we demonstrated that the model can account for a wide range of behavioral and brain imaging data in both healthy young adults and different WM-impaired populations (older adults and schizophrenia patients). Thus, the model appears to provide a good description of the control and WM mechanisms that might underlie AX-CPT performance, their relationship to PFC and DA function, and the consequences of their breakdown.

The simulation studies with the AX-CPT suggest some of the specific mechanistic properties of cognitive control. In particular, the simulations suggest that successful WM performance is achieved via a proactive strategy of actively maintaining contextual information provided by the cue within PFC regions, such that this information can appropriately prepare the system to respond most effectively to subsequent events. Thus, context maintenance can drive attentional expectancies for perceptual inputs and prime predicted responses. More generally, our model has implications for how control can be effectively achieved in many cognitive tasks—by actively maintaining representations in PFC that can serve as a source of top-down bias on pathways that are directly involved in task performance. We suggest that this bias influences a number of dimensions of information processing: enhancing perceptual fluency, orienting attention, configuring response selection parameters, structuring action-sequencing systems, and coordinating the operation of domain-specific storage buffers. Critically, in situations where the upcoming need for cognitive control is signaled by a pre-occurring contextual cue, the suggestion is that this contextual information must be successfully encoded into PFC, and actively sustained over the intervening delay for control to be achieved. Based on our model of DA-PFC interactions, we further hypothesize that such encoding and sustained maintenance depends on a specific pattern of DA system activity. Specifically, at the time of cue presentation there must be a strong phasic burst of DA activity to enable this information to appropriately engage PFC. In contrast, during the delay interval, tonic

DA activity levels must be neither too low nor too high, to ensure that this information is appropriately sustained without interference or decay.

THE DUAL MECHANISMS OF CONTROL ACCOUNT

Our previous theory and modeling work focused exclusively on how proactive cognitive control might be implemented, and the benefits accrued by such a control mechanism. Our current account of cognitive control substantially refines this earlier view, by suggesting a dual-process framework that we term the *DMC account*. Specifically, the DMC account suggests that cognitive control may be achieved not only by proactive mechanisms but also through *reactive* mechanisms. Importantly, we believe that the DMC account provides important new insight into WM and cognitive control by elucidating the intrinsic variability at the core of this domain. In other words, the DMC account is primarily an account of why there is variation within WM and cognitive control (i.e., Question #2). Moreover, as we develop further below, the DMC account provides a coherent explanation of how different types of empirically observed sources of variation in WM function—task or situational factors, neural dysfunction, cognitive individual differences or even noncognitive (i.e., affective and personality) variables—might relate to the distinction between proactive and reactive control. In this section, we describe the DMC account in detail, focusing on how reactive control can be distinguished from proactive control and the relationship between these two mechanisms. The critical distinctions between proactive and reactive control are summarized in Table 4.1.

What is reactive control? As the name suggests, reactive control is engaged after, rather than before, the occurrence of some imperative event. Prior to this event, the system remains relatively unbiased, and so is more influenced by bottom-up inputs. Furthermore, reactive control mechanisms are engaged only as needed, on a "just-in-time" basis rather than consistently, and in advance of critical events. Finally, when

TABLE 4.1. Distinctions between Proactive and Reactive Control

	Proactive Control	Reactive Control
Computational properties	Future-oriented, early selection, preparatory attention	Past-oriented, late correction, interference resolution
Information processing	Strong goal-relevant focus, global control effects	Increased goal-irrelevant processing, item-specific control
Temporal dynamics	Sustained, activation prior to imperative stimulus	Transient, activation after imperative stimulus
Neural substrates	Lateral PFC, midbrain DA (phasic activity)	ACC, lateral PFC (transient response), MTL, others

ACC = anterior cingulate cortex; DA = dopamine; MTL = medial temporal lobe; PFC = prefrontal cortex.

control depends upon the use of context information, the activation of such information by reactive mechanisms occurs transiently rather than in a sustained fashion, and thus decays away quickly. As a consequence, in situations when the same context must be repeatedly accessed, this must occur through full reactivation of the information each time it is needed.

The distinction between proactive and reactive control can be thought of as a distinction between early selection and late correction (Jacoby, Kelley, & McElree, 1999). Concrete examples can help illustrate the proactive–reactive distinction. A real-world example might be the typical prospective memory situation in which an intention is formed about a behavioral goal to be completed at some later point, such as stopping at the dry cleaners after leaving work, before they close. A proactive control strategy would require the goal information to be actively sustained from the time the intention is formed until the goal is satisfied (e.g., the end of the day). The usefulness of such a proactive strategy is that plans and behaviors can be continually adjusted to facilitate optimal completion of the goal (e.g., not scheduling a late meeting). In contrast, with a reactive control strategy the goal would only be transiently activated at the time of intention, and then need to be reactivated again by an appropriate trigger event (e.g., opening the car door). Because of this need for repeated reactivation, there is greater dependence on the trigger events themselves, since if these are insufficiently salient or discriminative they will not drive reactivation (e.g., the dry cleaning errand might only be re-

membered because of the cleaning ticket left on the car seat).

The AX-CPT task, described above, provides another example. A proactive control strategy would result in a context representation being activated by the cue stimulus, and maintained at full strength over the intervening delay prior to the probe. During this delay, cognitive control would be achieved by priming the perceptual and response systems in accordance with cue-driven attentional expectancies. In contrast, a reactive control strategy would result in context information being only transiently represented following the cue. During the delay between cue and probe, context activation and, as a result, response-related priming would be minimal. Upon presentation of the probe, context would need to be reactivated via retrieval. Once contextual representations reached full activation strength they could be used to overcome interference that had occurred in the interim, due to probe-related biases. Thus, in the AX-CPT, proactive control means control engaged by the cue, whereas reactive control means control driven by the probe.

The hypothesized distinction between proactive and reactive control extends to neural mechanisms. In particular, we have suggested above that proactive control requires that context representations be sustained over extended periods, whereas in reactive control the representation of context occurs only transiently, as needed. Our theory assumes that the representation and active maintenance of context occur in PFC, and most specifically in lateral (rather than medial) PFC regions. Thus, when proactive control is engaged, sustained activity should be found in these PFC regions during the interval between the initial presentation of context and the point at which it is used. Under proactive control conditions, PFC activity should be present reliably across events, and not just on those in which it is most needed. In contrast, under conditions of reactive control, PFC activity will be (1) transient rather than sustained; (2) present only for those events that directly require the reactivation of context to mediate appropriate performance; and (3) activated after rather than before the onset of an imperative stimulus. Additionally, the two control mechanisms should differ in terms of the involvement of the DA system. We have suggested that the ability to sustain inputs in PFC requires a phasic DA-mediated gating signal occurring at the time of context presentation. Without such a gating signal, PFC can only be transiently activated. Thus, our hypothesis is that under conditions of proactive control, presentation of contextual input is accompanied by a phasic change in DA, whereas under reactive conditions there is no DA-mediated gating signal. In the absence of DA gating, PFC can only be transiently activated, and only in situations where there is a strong enough association between the context representation and the triggering stimulus to produce spreading activation.

Under reactive conditions, we would also expect that other brain systems in addition to PFC would be more strongly involved in mediating performance. For example, if reactive control can be achieved through the activation of long-term memory traces or through retrieval of episodic information, then we would expect to see engagement of either posterior cortical regions or the hippocampal–MTL complex. Another brain system that might be critical for reactive control is the ACC. A currently influential account of ACC function postulates that this brain region indexes the demand for cognitive control by detecting the presence of response conflict or uncertainty due to either interference, weak response strength, the activation of an erroneous response, or the estimated high-likelihood of making an erroneous response (Botvinick et al.,

2001; Brown & Braver, 2005). Critically, conflict-related ACC signals are postulated to modulate activation in lateral PFC regions that can implement an increase in top-down control to resolve such conflict. Thus, the conflict signal in ACC might be used to increase the tendency to use proactive control on subsequent trials, as has been postulated by current theory (Botvinick et al., 2001). However, it might also be the case that the ACC serves as a core component of reactive control processing, by rapidly signaling the need for increased control on the current trial, to resolve interference, increase response strength, or correct an impending error. In preliminary computational modeling work, we have been exploring the hypothesis that the ACC may serve a dual role in proactive and reactive control through outputs to different PFC systems (De-Pisapia & Braver, 2006).

COSTS AND BENEFITS OF PROACTIVE AND REACTIVE CONTROL

We have just described some of the functional and neural characteristics that distinguish reactive from proactive control. Yet an obvious question is the following: why postulate such a dual-process account at all, given the virtues of parsimony and the wisdom of Occam's razor? This question can best be answered by considering that there may be both costs and benefits associated with proactive and reactive control, such that a computational trade-off exists. By using both mechanisms to varying degrees through a dual-process control architecture, the cognitive system is best able to overcome these trade-offs, and in so doing optimize behavioral performance across a wide range of environments and task demands. Indeed, this type of dual-process architecture, involving a mixture of proactive and reactive control mechanisms, is one that tends to be present in many existing computer systems. Specifically, most computer operating systems tend to operate with a standard top-down flow of control driven by a stored program (i.e., proactive control), but with a separate built-in mechanism to deal with interrupts (i.e., reactive control). Likewise, general-purpose symbolic computational cognitive architectures, like Soar (Newell, 1990), frequently operate in two distinct control modes: one in which problem spaces are traversed according to the dictates of a pre-existing goal stack (similar to proactive control), and a second mode that initiates to resolve unexpected impasses or conflicts (similar to reactive control). Thus, on purely computational grounds it is sensible to argue that a dual-process or mixture model mechanism of control is one that serves to optimize information processing. Nevertheless, it is important to consider these computational trade-offs between proactive and reactive control more explicitly, since they provide insights into the factors that should affect which control mode is dominant in specific situations and for specific individuals.

Below, we list some of the limitations and disadvantages of proactive control, followed by the negative consequences of reactive control:

Proactive control requires the presence of predictive contextual cues. Many times predictive contextual information is not present in the environment, and as such, control cannot be prepared in advance. In these circumstances, the only possible control strategy is a reactive one.

Proactive control requires predictive contextual cues to be highly reliable. In situations where predictive cues turn out to be invalid, there can be a strong cost if the cue-based contextual information is used as a basis for proactive control. Such cue invalidity costs can be seen in a range of cognitive situations (e.g., the Posner spatial cued reaction time task; Posner, Snyder, & Davidson, 1980). Thus, adoption of a proactive control strategy is only likely in situations where contextual cues serve as highly reliable predictors of upcoming events or required actions.

Proactive control is metabolically costly. According to our theoretical model, the active maintenance of goal-relevant information requires a high and sustained level of neuronal activity in lateral PFC during the entire retention interval. Such extended periods of high firing are likely to require additional metabolic resources (e.g., for glucose consumption, waste removal, neurotransmitter recycling, etc.) that may not always be available, or at the minimum, reduce the amount available for other purposes. Even without considering metabolic requirements directly, it seems clear that proactive control is capacity demanding, since only a small number of goals can be actively maintained in the focus of attention (Cowan, 2001). Thus, proactive control draws away resources from other active maintenance demands. Consequently, it is likely to only be used if sufficient capacity is available (i.e., other WM demands are low, general cognitive resources are high, and cortical arousal is optimal).

Proactive control is prohibitive with very long retention intervals. Because the sustained, active context maintenance associated with proactive control is so resource demanding, the longer the interval between the maintenance initiation and context utilization, the less feasible this strategy becomes. Thus, proactive control is unlikely with retention intervals longer than a few minutes. Certain prospective memory tasks are the best example of situations in which the interval between goal formation and goal realization can be hours or days. In such situations, actions are accomplished through reactive control—that is, by transiently reactivating the goal (via episodic retrieval) at the appearance of an appropriate trigger stimulus such that it can bias the goal-relevant behavior. This idea is consistent with the bulk of the prospective-memory literature, which has suggested that retrospective processes are the primary mechanisms guiding delayed-intention behavior (Einstein & McDaniel, 1996). Nevertheless, recent studies have begun to suggest that in certain experimental prospective-memory paradigms, preparatory control may be occurring, even across longer timescales of retention (Smith, 2003). It will be important to determine more conclusively whether, and under what constraints, active maintenance processes are being used in such paradigms.

Proactive control is less sensitive to changes in reward–punishment contingencies. Because environments are typically non-stationary, contingencies can often change without warning. The active representation of goals during proactive control modes causes the system to be biased to attend primarily to goal-relevant features of the environment, and to be predisposed to interact with these features in a goal-driven manner. This leads to a reduction in incidental encoding of goal-irrelevant or goal-incongruent features, which may, in fact, serve as cues that the environment is changing. Theorists have suggested that continuous monitoring of environmental (or internal) background information is a critical function of motivationally oriented neural systems. For example, such mechanisms can lead to optimal detection of low-probability but potential threats (Goschke, 2003). Thus, high demands or a pre-existing bias for background monitoring (such as when vigilance toward potential threats is required) will make the use of proactive control less likely.

Proactive control impedes the natural progression toward automatization. There is a fundamental tension between the exertion of cognitive control and the development of automaticity, which has been termed the "control dilemma" (Goschke, 2003). Because automatic processes are robust, fast, and efficient, it is likely that there is an inherent computational pressure or bias on the cognitive system to automatize processing wherever possible, via strengthening of internal associations and stimulus–response bindings. Proactive control processes oppose such mechanisms by providing a sustained top-down flow of information that enables contextual goals to override default processing. Indeed, it is reactive rather proactive control that allows for the best optimization of the control dilemma, by introducing a

highly transient and minimalist (i.e., only-as-needed) form of intervention, that allows habits, skills, and procedures to be learned while still enabling the system to override these forces if necessary.

Reactive control is more susceptible to proactive interference. Control mechanisms are necessary because many times the effects of past experience conflict with current goals. However, such sources of proactive interference (PI) cannot be completely counteracted by a reactive control strategy. This is because reactive control is initiated by post-stimulus processing, such that potentially interfering stimulus-based associations will already be activated by the time control mechanisms are engaged. In contrast, proactive control may lead to complete suppression of PI, via optimal attentional configuration. Thus, in conditions where PI effects are very strong and the costs of interference are high, the disadvantages of reactive control will be most apparent.

Reactive control is suboptimal when stimulus-driven processing is insufficient. Because reactive control is stimulus driven rather than preparatory, it is always a suboptimal control strategy. However, the limitations of reactive control are most prominent in conditions where perceptual information is weak, response selection parameters are underdetermined, and/or when there is a premium on optimal performance (i.e., high speed and accuracy constraints).

Reactive control does not maximize rewards. Maximizing reward often depends upon the ability to predict its occurrence and magnitude. Proactive control aids in maximizing rewards through the use of predictive contextual cues that can bias action selection. The strong link between proactive control and reward prediction can be seen in the phasic DA signals postulated to engage proactive control processes in PFC, according to the DMC account, and also appear to signal reward-related salience of predictive cues, according to influential reinforcement learning models (Schultz et al., 1997). In contrast, reactive control is not geared toward maximization of rewards but rather toward resolving interference and facilitating the transition to automaticity. Thus, in conditions where processing is oriented toward reward maximization, and where reward attainment depends on precise focusing of attention or optimal response preparation, a reactive control strategy will be highly disadvantageous.

As the above discussion indicates, there are a number of advantages and limitations associated with both reactive and proactive control, thus successful cognition may depend on some mixture of both proactive and reactive control strategies. Indeed, it may be the case that the two systems are fully independent, and thus may be both engaged simultaneously. Nevertheless, there is likely to be some bias favoring one type of control strategy over the other. It is our hypothesis that a default mode for the cognitive system is one favoring reactive control, given its greater applicability (i.e., use in more situations), lower demands on metabolic resources, and maximal compatibility with the development of automatization. However, other factors may be present that exert pressures on the system to engage in proactive control. These factors can be characteristics of the task situation, but may also be characteristics of the individual. Indeed, we believe that the DMC account provides a unifying framework for understanding both intra-individual and inter-individual variability in normal WM function in terms of shifting biases toward proactive vs. reactive control. Likewise, because of the putative dependence of proactive control on specific neural mechanisms (e.g., DA interactions in lateral PFC), the DMC framework also provides a coherent explanation as to why specific populations suffering from breakdown or dysfunction in these neural systems might also experience specific changes in WM and cognitive-control function. Finally, the DMC account suggests that there should be an important role for "noncognitive" factors in producing WM variation. This is due to the role played by constructs such as reward prediction and background-threat monitoring in altering the

balance between proactive and reactive control. These constructs are likely to be impacted by related state (e.g., mood) and trait (e.g., personality) variables.

In the sections that follow, we elaborate each of these points in turn, discussing how the DMC account makes specific predictions regarding different sources of variability on WM and cognitive-control function: (a) within-individual variation; (b) cognitive individual differences; (c) neural dysfunction; and (d) noncognitive factors. Moreover, we describe results of recent studies designed to provide empirical support for each of these components of the DMC account.

Within-Individual Variation

A central assumption of the DMC framework is that a change in situational factors will result in alteration of the weighting between proactive and reactive control strategies. These situational factors include (1) the availability and reliability of predictive information; (2) length of time provided to engage in preparation; (3) demands on speed and accuracy; (4) length of retention interval; (5) strength of habit or response biases; (6) expectation of proactive interference; (7) arousal level; (8) motivational focus (reward vs. punishment); (9) expected WM load; and (10) available capacity. Changes in any or all of these factors are thus predicted to produce a change in cognitive-control strategy. Thus, the DMC account naturally leads to the idea that there will be considerable variability in the control strategies employed by healthy individuals across different task situations. Indeed, it is possible that potentially subtle differences between otherwise similar tasks might lead to large changes in an individual's preferred cognitive-control strategy. These control-mode differences would be expected to result in shifts in both behavioral performance characteristics and brain activation profiles. In recent work, we have examined this aspect of the DMC account, by directly manipulating factors expected to influence cognitive-control strategy during the performance of WM (and other cognitive) tasks. These experiments were all conducted using a within-participants design, to determine whether we could observe intra-individual variation in cognitive-control processes.

In one such study (Speer, Jacoby, & Braver, 2003), we examined whether WM load—in terms of number of items to be simultaneously maintained over a delay—would impact the use of proactive vs. reactive control during performance of a classic WM task: Sternberg item recognition (Sternberg, 1966). The key aspect of this study was that we were interested not in the direct effect of memory load manipulations, which has well-established effects on performance (Sternberg, 1966) and brain activity (Grasby et al., 1994), but rather in the effect of *expected* memory load. Thus, we investigated whether participants' expectations of the number of items they would have to maintain influenced the control processes they used to perform the task, irrespective of the actual number of items they were to maintain on a given trial. This manipulation of expectancy was achieved by having participants perform task blocks in which memory-set size varied randomly from trial to trial. However, in one block of trials the average memory load was low (~3 items), while in another the average load was high (~8 items). Critically, however, there was a subset of trials (25%) in each block that were exactly equivalent in memory load (6 items). The analysis focused exclusively on comparing performance and brain activity dynamics (through the use of event-related fMRI) on these load-matched trials.

The reason for examining load expectancy rather than the load effect itself is that the DMC account suggests that a critical source of variation in WM tasks is not the representations used for short-term storage per se (which involve domain-specific mechanisms such as the phonological loop, and which should be affected directly by WM load), but rather the way in which such representations are used and controlled to bias response selection. Specifically, we hypothesize that proactive control in a task such as the Sternberg translates into whether, *during the delay period*, items stored in short-term memory get represented in a form that is useful for rapid target decisions—i.e., a goal-based representational code that might take something of the form, "if probe is X (or Y or Z), make target response, otherwise make non-target response." Such goal-based proactive representations are postulated to be present within lateral PFC. Conversely, reactive control processes would ensure that probe information, *once presented*, could be represented in a form that could drive a successful matching (e.g., familiarity evaluation) or retrieval operation (e.g., episodic search) with memory-set items. Importantly, such reactive control processes would also be facilitated by having memory-set items stored in a highly activated and accessible trace. Thus, the proactive–reactive distinction reflects both a distinction in the types of control processes that engage with short-term memory representations to bias response decisions and a distinction in the time course of activation for these control processes.

Our specific hypothesis was that the use of a proactive control strategy in the Sternberg task would be most likely under conditions of low WM load. With only a few items to be maintained, it should be easier to activate a goal-based representation of memory-set items during the delay period and begin to use such a representation to bias target-detection processes. Conversely, under high load conditions, this type of control strategy would be more difficult and thus less likely activated. Thus, a reactive control strategy would likely be preferred. However, our key prediction was that the preferential engagement of proactive vs. reactive control would be truly strategic, and thus tied primarily to expectations of what would be most successful, rather than directly constrained by specific task conditions. Of course, it is important to note that the term *strategic* should not be taken to imply that such processes are necessarily consciously engaged by participants, since we are not at all convinced that consciousness has anything to do with the process. Instead, we use the term *strategic* to imply that the preferential engagement of one control process or the other is somewhat optional (i.e., variable), rather than fully constrained, but is likely tied to a (potentially implicit) evaluative process that attempts to optimize performance given the expected task conditions. Thus, the DMC account predicts that load-expectancy effects will impact the engagement of control even on the six-item trials with matched load (the role of expectancy was enhanced by presenting memory items sequentially, such that the memory load for the current trial was only known at the end of the encoding period).

The results of the study were just as predicted. Probe decisions on six-item trials were both faster and more accurate in the low-load expectancy condition. This finding is consistent with the hypothesis that in the low-load condition probe decisions were based on a rapid target-detection process associated with proactive control. However, in the high-load condition, it appeared as if probes were more deeply encoded (as assessed by a surprise delayed-recognition test for non-target probes), consistent with the hypothesis that the probes were used as retrospective retrieval or matching cues to achieve reactive control. More importantly, we observed a strong double dissociation in the pattern of activity dynamics within PFC (Fig. 4.2, see color insert). First, in a number of medial and mid-lateral PFC regions, we observed that activity in the low-load condition tended to progressively increase throughout the memory-set encoding and delay period of the six-item trials. However, in the high-load con-

dition the same six-item trials, evoked an activity pattern of rapid increase at the beginning of the memory-set encoding period, but no further increase (and, in fact, a tendency toward decreased activity) during the delay. In contrast, within a more anterior PFC region (an area that has previously been associated with episodic retrieval processes; see, e.g. Lepage, Ghaffar, Nyberg, & Tulving, 2000), activation was found to increase only during the period of probe judgment, and was significantly greater for six-item trials in the high-load condition. These observed activity patterns are consistent with the hypothesis that the mid-lateral PFC regions reflect the engagement of proactive control processes that are increased in the low-load condition, while the anterior PFC is associated with a reactive control process that is preferentially engaged in the high-load condition.

The central message of the Sternberg study is that a subtle task factor, such as the expected memory load, can dramatically influence both performance and brain activation during the performance of WM tasks. Indeed, the subtlety of the manipulation demonstrates that the cognitive-control processes engaged to achieve successful performance might be highly vari-

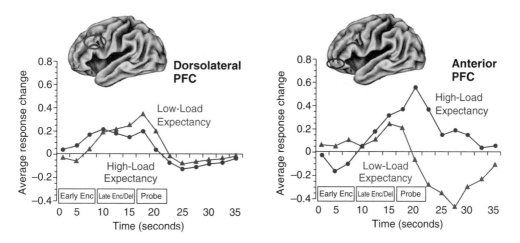

Figure 4.2. Memory strategy effects on prefrontal cortex (PFC) activity (Speer et al., 2003). *Left panel*: Left dorsolateral PFC region showing anticipatory, delay-related activation in low-load expectancy condition. *Right panel*: Left anterior PFC region showing increased probe-related activity in high-load expectancy condition. X-axis refers to the time course of activity. Y-axis refers to average percentage fMRI signal change (from baseline).

able even across very similar WM conditions. In particular, some WM conditions might be associated with a preferential engagement of proactive control, which would be reflected in sustained (or increasing) lateral PFC activity during retention periods, while other conditions might be associated with a stronger bias toward reactive control, which would be reflected in reduced retention-period activity in PFC, but potentially a greater probe-driven response in different brain regions (including other areas of PFC).

Significantly, these results have important implications for resolving some of the apparent inconsistencies and controversies in the recent neuroimaging literature investigating the role of PFC in WM task performance. The current controversy is whether PFC, and specifically dorsolateral PFC, actually subserves active maintenance functions in WM, or whether it instead performs "executive" operations (i.e., manipulation, selection) on maintained items, but does not subserve maintenance itself (e.g., D'Esposito et al., 1998). Although there is quite a bit of evidence for the active-maintenance view from both primate neurophysiologic studies (Fuster, 1997) and human neuroimaging (Cohen et al., 1997), findings from some more recent studies have directly called into question the maintenance account. The strongest evidence comes from fMRI studies using event-related designs that isolate PFC activity to different periods of a trial, in which the activation of PFC has been observed to be transient rather than sustained and most prominent during the encoding or response period rather than the maintenance interval (Rowe, Toni, Josephs, Frackowiak, & Passingham, 2000).

Our results suggest such cross-study differences in the dynamics of PFC activity might actually be due to cross-study differences in whether proactive vs. reactive control processes were preferred for task performance. Thus, the lack of sustained delay–period activity in lateral PFC might reflect the presence of tasks or subtle task factors that encourage reactive rather than proactive control strategies on the part of participants. Indeed, undetected cross-study differences in the use of proactive vs. reactive control may constitute an uncontrolled source of

variability that can confound clear interpretations of the results of WM studies.

Critically, the DMC account suggests that there are a number of task factors, in addition to expected WM load, that could lead to variability in the type of cognitive control strategy preferred across different task situations. Furthermore, we postulate that such condition-related variability in cognitive control may not only impact WM tasks but also other cognitive domains that place a high demand on control processes. Indeed, in other studies that we are currently conducting, we have observed substantial within-individual variation in proactive vs. reactive control associated with interference expectancy in the Stroop task (Braver & Hoyer, 2006), trial-by-trial fluctuations during task switching (Braver, Reynolds, & Donaldson, 2003; Reynolds et al., 2006), and motivational incentives in the AX-CPT (Locke & Braver, 2006). Such work will help to provide a better foundation on which to design and interpret WM studies by taking into account potential sources of cognitive-control variation.

Cognitive Individual Differences

An important factor that likely has an influence on the selection of control strategy is individual differences in cognitive abilities. We make this claim because many of the psychological factors that should influence cognitive control strategies are likely to vary in a stable manner across individuals. These include available cognitive resources, arousal level, and motivational orientation. In terms of the effects of cognitive resources, we have suggested that engaging in proactive control is more resource demanding than engaging in reactive control. Thus it is likely that individuals possessing greater cognitive resources will be those most willing and able to adopt a proactive mode. Indeed, there has been a great deal of research suggesting that the construct of cognitive resources may index the same underlying mechanism indexed by the constructs of WM capacity and fluid intelligence (Kane & Engle, 2002). Individual differences in these constructs have been shown to have high validity in predicting performance on tasks that place a strong demand on proactive cognitive control (Duncan et al., 1996).

It is not yet clear how to directly translate these constructs into their underlying computational and neural mechanisms. Nevertheless, there is growing evidence that these constructs are closely linked to PFC function, which provides support for the idea that they have a relationship to proactive cognitive control (Duncan et al., 1996). In particular, we are highly influenced by the work of Kane, Engle and colleagues, who have suggested that the constructs of WM capacity and general fluid intelligence (gF) jointly index the efficacy of PFC function, and in particular the ability to actively maintain goal-relevant information in the face of interference (Kane & Engle, 2002; see also Chapter 2, this volume). In our framework, individuals with high WM-span and high gF should thus show an increased tendency to use proactive control strategies, but only in the task demands that most require and benefit from such strategies.

In a first test of this hypothesis, we examined the role of gF in predicting performance and brain activity in the well-known n-back WM paradigm (Gray, Chabris, & Braver, 2003). We found that gF was positively correlated with increased activation in lateral PFC and parietal cortex regions. Moreover, we found that this relationship was selective to trial conditions having the highest levels of interference (so-called lure nontargets, in which the current item is a repeat of a recent trial, but not the critical n-back trial). Most strikingly, we found that the increased PFC and parietal activation on high-interference trials statistically explained the facilitated performance that high-gF individuals exhibited on these trials. Together these findings provide important new evidence that individual differences in gF are associated with individual differences in the ability to activate control processes in lateral PFC and parietal cortex that enable the successful management of interference. However, the Gray et al. (2003) n-back study provides only an indirect test of the DMC account. The DMC account predicts that gF-related individual differences should reside primarily in the ability to use proactive control processes. In particular, evi-

dence of increased proactive control in high-gF individuals should be reflected in increased and sustained lateral PFC activity prior to onset of a target event. It is difficult to test such a hypothesis within the context of the n-back task, since the task design involves a continuous WM load (i.e., active maintenance is continuously required across each trial and intertrial interval). Thus, there is no clear way to distinguish between pre-target maintenance and preparation vs. post-target interference resolution.

To more directly test hypotheses based on the DMC account for individual differences in gF, we recently conducted a second study using the Sternberg paradigm instead of the n-back task (Burgess & Braver, 2004). The Sternberg paradigm enjoys a conceptual advantage over the n-back design, in that it enables the temporal decomposition of cognitive effects occurring at the time of the retrieval probe from those occurring during encoding or delay periods. We were interested in examining whether high-gF individuals would show an increased tendency to use proactive control during Sternberg performance. Our specific hypothesis was that high-gF individuals would preferentially engage proactive rather than reactive control mechanisms during WM performance under high-interference conditions. To examine this hypothesis within the context of the Sternberg task, we used a version that has been popularized by Jonides and colleagues (Jonides, Badre, Curtis, Thompson-Schill, & Smith, 2002). In this "recent-negative" Sternberg task, probes on some trials were "negative," in that they were not present in the current trial memory-set, but they were also "recent," in that they were present in the memory set from the *previous* trial. These recent-negative probes produce increased interference, since their high familiarity induces a bias to make an erroneous target response. As such, recent-negative trials in the Sternberg task can be thought of as being formally similar to the high-interference lure trials in the n-back task. This is consistent with the results of a series of neuroimaging studies demonstrating that recent-negative trials are associated with increased activity in left lateral PFC (Jonides et al., 2002). Consequently, a straightforward prediction, based on the Gray et al. (2003)

results and the general framework of Kane, Engle, and colleagues (Kane & Engle, 2002), is that high-gF individuals would show an increased ability to manage recent-negative interference. Moreover, these gF effects in performance should be associated with increased activation in lateral PFC. However, a more specific prediction of the DMC account is that individual differences in gF would be selectively associated with an increased ability to use proactive control mechanisms to prevent the adverse effects of interference.

An additional critical aspect of the DMC account is that the tendency to use proactive control will emerge primarily under conditions in which interference effects are not only large and costly (in terms of performance) but also reasonably anticipated. Thus, a second prediction of the theory that we tested is that the relationship between gF and proactive control would be most apparent under conditions where interference effects are frequent and expected. To test these predictions of the DMC theory, we had participants perform two different conditions of the recent-negative Sternberg task. In the *low interference expectancy* condition, recent-negative trials occurred infrequently (20% of negative probe trials), resulting in a lower occurrence of interference. In addition, 80% of "positive" probes (i.e., probes that were present in the current trial memory-set) were also "recent" (part of the memory set during the previous trial). For positive probes, the increased familiarity due to recency of previous exposure can be used to facilitate correct responding. We expected that these two factors together would lead to an increased tendency to use reactive rather than proactive control mechanisms to manage interference. Alternatively, in the *high interference expectancy* condition, the context was changed, so that recent-negative trials occurred frequently (80% of negative probes), while recent-positive trials occurred infrequently (20% of positive probes). In this condition, the tendency for familiarity (due to recency) to be incompatible with the correct response should encourage a proactive strategy aimed at resisting the impact of recency. In both conditions, the positive and negative probes that were not "recent"

were instead "novel," in that they had not been present in any memory sets from previous trials.

We conducted both a behavioral ($N = 41$) and neuroimaging study ($N = 19$) of the recent-negative Sternberg task (memory sets in both studies were five English words, presented simultaneously on a visual display) with both high- and low-gF individuals (as measured by performance on the Ravens Advanced Progressive Matrices Test, a standard experimental test of gF). Across both studies we found that high-gF individuals showed a reduced interference effect compared to that of the low-gF individuals (in terms of accuracy and/or reaction time [RT]), but that the reduction occurred selectively on the high-interference expectancy condition (behavioral study: high-expectancy gF–RT correlation, $r(39) = -.36$, $p < .05$, low-expectancy gF–RT correlation, $r(39) = .18$, $p > .1$; neuroimaging study: Accuracy gF × Condition Interaction, $F(1,17) = 6.9$, $p < .05$). In the neuroimaging study, we were able to analyze the temporal dynamics of brain activity within PFC and other regions by means of event-related fMRI. These analyses suggested that in the left lateral PFC, significantly increased activation in high-gF individuals (relative to low-gF individuals) was observed during the memory-retention interval, but only in the high-interference expectancy condition, and not in the low-interference expectancy condition (Fig. 4.3, see color insert). Thus, we observed a significant gF × Task Condition interaction $F(1,17) = 7.2$, $p < .05$. This elevated activity for high-gF individuals was found across all task trials in the high-interference expectancy condition (i.e., recent and novel negatives, and recent and novel positives). These findings support the increased use of proactive control mechanisms by high-gF individuals in the high-expectancy condition, since this type of mechanism would be engaged across all trials in advance of the probe. In other words, the use of proactive control mechanisms should not depend on whether interference is *present* on any individual trial, but instead on whether *interference is likely* across trials.

In addition, however, we also examined activation that occurred at the time of the probe

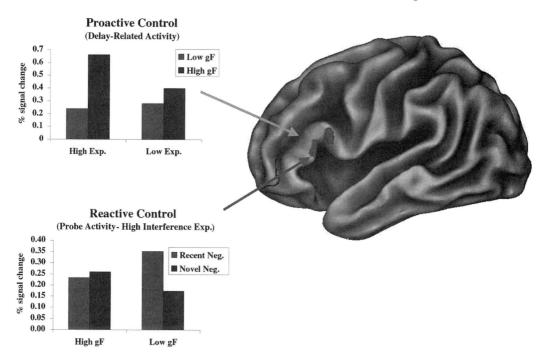

Figure 4.3. Interactions between general fluid intelligence (gF) and interference expectancy in lateral prefrontal cortex (PFC) activity (Burgess & Braver, 2004). *Top panel:* High-gF group shows that high interference expectancy leads to increased delay-related activity in left ventrolateral PFC, whereas the low gF group shows no expectancy effect. *Bottom panel:* In high-expectancy condition, low-gF group shows increased probe-related activity in a nearby left ventrolateral PFC region for recent negatives, but high-gF group does not.

and showed direct sensitivity to recent negative trials. Our motivation for examining this aspect of the data stemmed from the prior neuroimaging literature. In previous studies, Jonides and colleagues, as well as other groups, have found that left ventrolateral PFC (VLPFC) regions are selectively activated by recent-negative trials in the Sternberg task, suggesting that this region is recruited to successfully resolve interference (Jonides & Nee, 2006). Moreover, using event-related fMRI, D'Esposito and colleagues determined that the increased recent-negative activity in left VLPFC occurred at the time of probe onset (D'Esposito, Postle, Jonides, & Smith, 1999). Such an effect suggests that the left VLPFC activity indicates the presence of a reactive control process that is mobilized following the detection of interference to help resolve potential processing conflict. This is supported by the finding that older adults show increased behavioral interference on recent-

negative trials, accompanied by decreased left VLPFC activity (Jonides & Nee, 2006)

Based on the results of this literature, one might expect that it would be effective reactive control rather than proactive control that would be most strongly associated with successful interference management on recent-negative trials. However, our results did not provide strong support for that hypothesis. When collapsing across conditions and gF, we did find increased activation in left VLPFC on recent-negative trials (relative to novel negatives) at the time of the probe ($F(1,17) = 8.2$, $p < .05$). However, we did not observe the recent-negative activation to be reliably greater for high-gF individuals. In fact, in a left VLPFC region very near that observed to show control effects, recent-negative activity actually tended to be lower in high-gF individuals during the high-expectancy condition (albeit nonsignificantly; gF × Recency: $F(1,17) = 1.65$, $p > .1$; see Fig. 4.3, see color insert). At first blush, this finding is somewhat surprising, since the high-interference expectancy condition is associated with reduced interference effects in the high-gF individuals. However, the results are consistent with the DMC account, which suggests that high-gF individuals shifted from a primarily reactive to a primarily proactive control strategy in the high–interference expectancy condition. Since proactive control is thought to be a more effective strategy for preventing interference, a switch toward such mechanisms would improve performance selectively in the high gF group, while simultaneously reducing the need to engage reactive control mechanisms. Thus, the results of this study, like our other work, provide a clear and coherent interpretation of what might otherwise be counterintuitive results on the role of PFC and individual differences in mediating performance on tasks placing high demands on cognitive control processes. In future studies, it would be useful to determine whether the DMC account could also explain the effects of related individual-difference constructs on WM and cognitive control (e.g., WM span). We have recently begun to provide such evidence, by demonstrating, in a replication of the Gray et al. (2003) study, that lure interference effects in lateral PFC were associated with WM span as well as gF (Burgess et al., 2006).

Neural Dysfunction

The previous section discussed situational factors that are likely to influence control biases in healthy young adults. However, another important factor that will affect control strategy is the structural integrity of the neural systems supporting each mechanism. If one system is dysfunctional, there will be a strong bias toward adopting the other, intact control mode. Our theoretical framework suggests that the proactive control system will be most vulnerable to disruption, given its dependence on precise dynamics (i.e., sustained activation of PFC representations, strong phasic DA response to contextual cues, moderate tonic DA activity). In fact, the available evidence suggests that many neuropsychiatric disorders involving cognitive

control impairment, such as schizophrenia, Parkinson disease, and attention-deficit hyperactivity disorder (ADHD), are also associated with dysfunction in PFC and/or DA systems (Arnsten & Robbins, 2002). Consequently, our theory predicts that these populations will show primary impairments in the use of proactive strategies. Importantly, in some cases, it may be that the control impairment is completely selective, such that the reactive control system is intact. A population that likely fits this scenario is healthy older adults. The evidence is accumulating that healthy aging is associated with declines in both PFC and DA function and with impairments in cognitive control (Braver et al., 2001). However, given that healthy aging is by definition nonpathological, it is likely the case that these biological changes are relatively mild (at least in relation to clinical populations suffering dysfunction in the same systems).

From a theory-testing and validation perspective it would be ideal if there were evidence that other clinical populations showed evidence of the reverse form of impairment—intact proactive control, but impaired reactive control. However, this pure double dissociation may be unlikely given the argument that proactive control processes are the ones most vulnerable to disruption by brain dysfunction. Nevertheless, it may be the case that there are certain populations that show an overreliance on proactive control, even under conditions that should normally favor reactive strategies. Although purely speculative at this point, one population that may fit this description is patients suffering from obsessive-compulsive disorder (OCD). In particular, some theorists have suggested that OCD can be characterized as "hyper-activation" of the executive control system (Tallis, 1995). Further work will be needed to investigate this idea more directly.

In our own prior work, we have examined changes in cognitive control strategy in healthy older adults. This work has demonstrated that older adults show a reduced tendency to engage in proactive control, but still show the ability to effectively engage reactive control mechanisms. Specifically, in two studies with the AX-CPT task, older adults displayed a relative impairment on inhibitory (BX) trials, in terms of disproportionately slowed responding, yet nevertheless showed only a slight increase in error rate in this condition (Braver et al., 2001,Braver et al., 2005). The fact that older adults did not make many inhibitory errors suggests that they are able to appropriately represent context. However, the greatly increased RT interference on these trials suggests that context representation occurred in a reactive rather than a proactive fashion. That is, we hypothesize that under conditions where control is engaged reactively, context information is not represented prior to probe onset, and instead must be reactivated following the appearance of the probe. The context-activation process must happen quickly when it occurs reactively, so that it can suppress the priming effect of the probe before an error is committed. However, even in this case it is still likely that slowing of performance will occur, since during the time of context reactivation the probe has an opportunity to prime inappropriate response pathways. The low error rates but high interference in older adults indicates that they were able to achieve control, but that such control may have necessitated a more intense engagement of reactive control mechanisms on inhibitory trials (relative to the intensity needed for proactive control). In other words, it is likely that, because of their increased dependence on reactive control mechanisms, older adults had to exert compensatory effort to achieve successful inhibition.

This suggestion is consistent with recent observations from neuroimaging studies. In these studies, older adults have been found to show increases as well as decreases in brain activation during performance of difficult cognitive control tasks (Cabeza, 2001). Our hypothesis suggests that a shift from proactive to reactive control would result in both the activation of brain regions not typically activated in young adults (i.e., those subserving reactive control) and in a different pattern of activity dynamics in regions activated by young adults (i.e., greater activation in conditions most dependent on control, reduced activity in conditions with lower control demands).

In a recently completed neuroimaging study with the AX-CPT, we found evidence supporting the hypothesis that older adults showed increased neural activity in conditions low in control demands, but decreased activity in the conditions associated with proactive control (Paxton et al., 2006). In this study, 20 older (range: 66–83; mean age = 73 years) and 21 younger adults (range: 18–31; mean age = 23 years) performed the AX-CPT task under both short (1 s) and long (7.5 s) delay conditions (with total trial duration held constant across conditions at 10 s). The delay manipulation (which was blocked) enabled the isolation of brain regions involved in actively maintaining cue information, since the only variable manipulated was the proportion of the trial in which the delay occurred. In addition, task blocks alternated with control (fixation) blocks, which allowed the identification of regions generically (i.e., nonspecifically) activated by task performance. We predicted that older adults would show decreased delay-related activity in dorsolateral PFC, indicating a reduction in proactive control, while at the same time showing generalized (i.e., brain-wide) increases in task-related activation, indicating greater activation of reactive control processes.

The results confirmed the predictions (Fig. 4.4, see color insert). Younger adults showed a significant delay-related increase in dorsolateral PFC activity, in a region very similar in location to previous studies (Braver et al., 2002). In contrast, older adults actually showed a delay-related *decrease* in the activity of this region, producing a significant Age × Delay interaction $(F(1,39) = 5.6, p < .05)$. Interestingly, the interaction was of the crossover form, such that older adults showed greater activity than young adults in the short-delay condition, but less activity in the long-delay condition. Moreover, in terms of general task-related activation, older adults showed a strong trend toward greater activation in a number of brain regions, including other regions of PFC.

Taken together, these results provide initial support for the hypothesis that healthy aging produces a shift from proactive to reactive control that is observable in terms of a

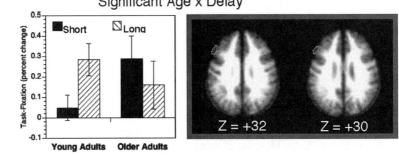

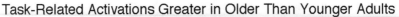

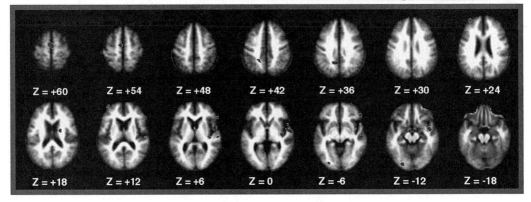

Figure 4.4. Age-related changes in prefrontal cortex (PFC) activity in the AX-CPT task (Paxton et al., 2006). *Top panel*: Right dorsolateral PFC region showing reduction in delay-related activation in older adults in long delay. *Bottom panel*: Brain regions (including PFC) showing generalized age-related increase in activation.

changing pattern of activity in PFC and other brain regions. Under conditions of high demand for proactive control (long delay), older adults showed reduced activation, while more generally showing increased activity, consistent with a greater reliance on less effective reactive control processes. Yet more direct investigation of this hypothesis is required. Specifically, these results were observed with a block-design study, which provided no information on the temporal dynamics of activity. The use of event-related fMRI would enable a test of the DMC hypothesis that older adults would show reduced activity during the cue and delay period but increased activation during the probe (specifically on inhibitory BX trials). Indeed, recent work in our lab, involving just this type of event-related design, has begun to provide more conclusive support for the DMC model (Paxton et al., 2006).

Noncognitive Factors

A unique aspect of the DMC account is that it provides a potential means for understanding how noncognitive factors might influence cognitive control. As described earlier, we believe there is a close linkage between proactive control and reward prediction. Conversely, a relationship might exist between reactive control and background threat monitoring and detection. These constructs of reward prediction and threat detection might be primarily affective in nature. Indeed, personality theorists have suggested that constructs related to reward sensitivity and threat sensitivity might represent the two fundamental affective dimensions of personality. For example, the theory of J. A. Gray (1994) has described these personality dimensions in terms of neural systems that trigger motivational and goal-directed behaviors. The behavioral approach system (BAS), which is roughly linked with extraversion, is motivated by reward-associated cues, and works to achieve appetitive outcomes. In contrast, the behavioral inhibition system (BIS), associated with neuroticism, is driven by threat cues to withdraw from potentially aversive outcomes. These trait variables are also linked to affective states, with high-BIS individuals being more susceptible to negative mood inductions and high-BAS individuals being more susceptible to positive mood inductions (Larsen & Ketelaar, 1991).

Our hypothesis is that a reward-focused motivational orientation (high BAS sensitivity) is intrinsically proactive, in that achieving complex reward goals requires anticipatory planning and attentional focusing. Conversely, a punishment-focused orientation (high BIS sensitivity) may bias a more reactive state, in which attention is diffusely vigilant and aroused, monitoring for potential threats, so that the individual can react appropriately when any threat appears. Similarly, positive moods may increase the tendency toward a reward-focused, proactive orientation, while negative moods may increase the tendency toward a punishment-focused reactive orientation. The magnitude of these effects is likely to interact with trait sensitivity (e.g., high-BIS individuals will likely have a different response to situations promoting a negative mood from that of low-BIS individuals).

The DMC theoretical framework also suggests a possible mechanistic basis on which to integrate and explain these relationships between affect or personality and cognitive control in terms of underlying neurobiology. A recent influential theoretical analysis of the neurobiology of personality has suggested that BAS/extraversion is directly related to variability in DA function (Depue & Collins, 1999) Likewise, in an extensive series of studies, Davidson and colleagues have persuasively argued that both BAS and BIS traits and positive and negative moods are associated with hemispheric shifts in lateral PFC activity (Davidson, 1995). These accounts are strikingly consistent with the reward-prediction aspects of the DMC model. As we have described above, the phasic DA response signals the reward-related salience of envi-

ronmental cues. Encoding these cues as context in PFC helps to maximize the achievement of reward. Thus, according to the DMC model, high-BAS individuals should be more able to achieve the precise neural activity dynamics required for proactive control.

The DMC account does not provide as rich a mechanistic framework for understanding the neurobiology of the BIS trait. However, if BIS/neuroticism is associated with a heightened sensitivity to threats, this should be associated with greater reactivity in a conflict-monitoring system used to detect the presence of such threats. Thus, it is noteworthy that a number of studies have reported that BIS/neuroticism is associated with increased resting-state activity within the ACC (e.g., Zald, Mattson, & Pardo, 2001), the brain region most strongly associated with conflict detection. However, these prior studies were not conducted during cognitive task performance, which makes it hard to determine whether the activity reflects increased conflict monitoring per se. Nevertheless, we speculate that high BIS may be associated with an increased bias toward reactive control strategies.

In our first preliminary studies investigating these hypotheses, we examined the role of affective states and affect-related personality traits in modulating behavioral performance and brain activity during performance of the n-back WM task (Gray & Braver, 2002b; Gray, Braver, & Raichle, 2002). Through initial behavioral studies, we found that inductions of positive and negative mood (through viewing of emotionally evocative video clips) had a striking influence on performance that selectively interacted with the n-back task condition (Gray & Braver, 2002a). Thus, when participants were induced into a positive mood, performance was facilitated when they were doing a version of the task involving verbal materials, but impaired when performing a nonverbal task variant. Conversely, when a negative mood was induced, the opposite pattern of performance modulation was observed (improved performance on the nonverbal version, impaired performance on the verbal version). This initial finding was replicated and extended in an fMRI study, where we observed that the crossover interaction effect of mood and task was expressed within lateral PFC regions (Gray et al., 2002). In particular, PFC activity was greatest in the conditions where performance was poorest (positive mood and nonverbal condition; negative mood and verbal condition). Moreover, the participants showing the greatest modulation of PFC activity by the conjunction of mood and task also showed the least modulation in behavioral performance. These patterns strongly suggest that the PFC activity served to compensate for increases in demands on cognitive control, which appear to have arisen here from the conjunction of task and affective factors. A specific explanation of the emotion–cognition interaction effect is beyond the scope of this chapter (see Gray & Braver, 2002a), but the findings are consistent with the general point of the DMC model that affective states can impact cognitive control demands and PFC activation during WM task performance.

A second set of studies examined the role of the BIS and BAS personality traits in modulating performance and brain activity during the same n-back tasks (Gray & Braver, 2002b). In a large behavioral sample, the BAS trait was found to show a weak but significant positive correlation with n-back performance $(r = .27)$ that held across both the verbal and nonverbal conditions. This finding parallels other recent results also showing BAS or extraversion associated with facilitated WM performance (Lieberman & Rosenthal, 2001). A follow-up fMRI study, using a smaller sample size $(n = 14)$, demonstrated that BAS was negatively associated with activity in caudal regions of ACC (typically associated with conflict monitoring), whereas BIS was positively associated with ACC activity. These results are consistent with the predictions of the DMC model that high-BIS individuals show an increased tendency toward reactive control (high conflict monitoring), whereas high-BAS individuals show an increased tendency toward proactive control (superior WM performance, lower conflict monitoring). Increased proactive control should be associated with a reduced demand on reactive control processes, such as conflict monitoring, since proactive control serves to anticipate and prevent conflict before it occurs. Finally, we observed that the observed personality effects

were also modulated by manipulations of affective state. Thus, the negative correlation of BAS and ACC activity was strongest following a negative mood induction, whereas the positive correlation of BIS and ACC activity was strongest following a positive mood induction. We interpret these results as suggesting that withdrawal states tend to increase task-related ACC activity by biasing a reactive control mode, but do so less for high-BAS individuals (i.e., they will be most resistant to the ACC-increasing effects of withdrawal states). Conversely, approach states will generally decrease task-related ACC activity by biasing a proactive control mode, but do so less for high-BIS individuals (i.e., they will be most resistant to the ACC-decreasing effects of approach states).

Although these preliminary studies provide an important first step in establishing the role of affect and personality factors on cognitive control processes during WM, they provide only a fairly weak test of the DMC account. In particular, the fMRI studies were conducted using a block-design approach, which does not provide a means from dissociating tonic activation from trial-specific effects. Thus, according to the DMC account, reactive control processes should be maximally engaged during high-conflict trials, and thus should exhibit trial-specific activity changes. Likewise, our original fMRI studies were conducted with a small sample size $(n = 14)$, which makes it difficult to know how consistently reliable the effects are. In recent work we have replicated our study examining personality effects in the n-back task using a much larger sample of 53 participants (Gray et al., 2005). Moreover, we used a "state-item" experimental design (Visscher et al., 2003) that enabled extraction of both trial-specific and tonic activity from the fMRI signal.

There were three sets of findings from this study that have implications for the DMC account. First, we replicated the finding that BAS was negatively correlated with caudal ACC activity $(r(51) = -.28, p < .05)$, but further observed that the correlation was found on event-related responses (i.e., was trial-specific; see Fig. 4.5, see color insert) rather than on tonic activation levels $(r(51) = .06, p > .1)$. This finding suggests more conclusively that ACC conflict-detection responses (which should occur transiently) are reduced during n-back task performance in high-BAS individuals. This is precisely what would be predicted if such individuals were more strongly biased toward a proactive control mode. Second, we also found that BAS was associated with reduced trial-specific activity in left lateral PFC ($r(51) = -.42$). Interestingly, these correlations were observed in the same lateral PFC region found to be associated with gF in our previous work (Gray et al., 2003). Yet, a multiple-regression analysis indicated that these two sources of individual-difference variation (gF, BAS) were independent predictors of lateral PFC activity. Because the gF and BAS constructs are themselves uncorrelated ($r = -.06$, $p > .1$; Gray et al., 2005), this result confirms our original intuition that both cognitive and affective dimensions of individual differences may

contribute to stable biases in cognitive control strategy, but through distinct causal pathways.

A third and final finding was that the BIS trait was observed to correlate positively with ACC activity ($r(51) = .41$, $p < .05$). However, this correlation was found in a rostral, rather than caudal, ACC region (Fig. 4.5, see color insert). Moreover, we found that the correlation was selective to tonic activity levels, rather than trial-specific responses. Although this finding is somewhat different from our earlier results (since in those results the ACC correlation with BIS was in a caudal region), they might still be consistent with the DMC framework. In particular, rostral ACC is typically deactivated during the performance of demanding cognitive tasks (Drevets & Raichle, 1998). A standard interpretation of the function of this region is that it is involved with background monitoring of negative events, particularly

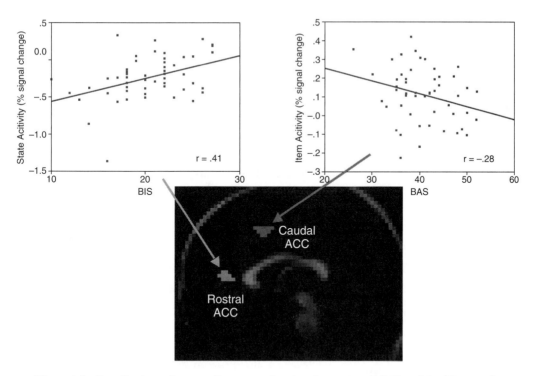

Figure 4.5. Contributions of personality to anterior cingulate cortex (ACC) activity (Gray et al., 2005). *Left panel:* Positive association between behavioral inhibition system (BIS) (punishment-sensitivity) and tonic activity in rostral ACC. *Right panel:* Negative association between behavioral approach system (BAS) (reward-sensitivity) and trial-specific activity in caudal ACC. Y-axis is percentage fMRI signal change (from baseline).

those associated with bodily states. This monitoring function is postulated to get shut off during cognitive task performance so as to free up resources for optimal performance. Thus, the failure of high-BIS individuals to deactivate rostral ACC is consistent with the idea that they continue to monitor potential threats during n-back task performance to more effectively react to such threats if they appear. However, the increased background-monitoring activity diverts resources away from proactive control processes, making them less effective.

The studies just discussed suggest an important way in which "noncognitive" factors such as personality and affect might impact cognitive control strategy. Although work in this area is just in its infancy, we strongly believe that consideration of affective influences on cognitive control is essential for a full mechanistic understanding of WM and its sources of variation. The DMC framework provides one account for synthesizing and understanding ways in which affect and personality might contribute to WM variation, by linking the more proximal constructs of reward prediction and threat detection (and their associated neural mechanisms) to proactive and reactive control modes, respectively. Nevertheless, the relationship between affect–personality and cognitive control is likely to be somewhat more complex than our original formulation, as these initial studies indicate (i.e., we had initially predicted that BIS would be associated with increased trial-specific activity in caudal ACC, but actually found an association with tonic activity in rostral ACC). Thus, further progress in this area may require more focused attention on designing WM experiments in a manner that will provide enhanced sensitivity to influences of affect and personality on cognitive control strategy, via manipulation of factors such as motivational incentives, ego threats, or emotionally evocative stimuli.

Other Sources of Variation in Working Memory

In the preceding sections we have provided evidence that many aspects of variation in WM function—within-individual effects, individual differences, effects of age and other certain types of neural dysfunction, and noncognitive influences—can all be explained by appeal to a dual-process architecture of cognitive control that we term the DMC account. In this respect, we share a common goal with the other contributors to this volume of trying to understand the common or distinct mechanisms underlying the many kinds of WM variation. In this section, we discuss how the DMC account relates to the other accounts of WM variation put forth in this volume, and more generally consider whether additional sources of variation are needed to account for the full range of empirical phenomena related to WM function (i.e., Question #4). In particular, we consider a number of outstanding issues related to variation in WM: neural and computational mechanisms, other dual-process accounts, inhibition, domain specificity vs. domain generality, development, and genetics.

Neural and Computational Mechanisms

Our view of WM variation is highly similar to the account put forward by Munakata et al. (Chapter 7), in terms of relating active maintenance and updating to the interactive function of the PFC and DA system. Likewise, we share with them a deep interest in translating WM constructs into explicit neural and computational mechanisms. The similarity of our frameworks and approach is no coincidence, as we are frequent collaborators and have developed our central theoretical ideas, for the most part, in tandem. Nevertheless, Munakata et al. place a central emphasis on the role of the basal ganglia (BG) in mediating WM updating via phasic gating signals (O'Reilly & Frank, 2006). This idea is very similar to our own ideas regarding DA and gating, but is also subtly different, focusing on how the architecture of the BG can enable hierarchical updating to occur within complex WM tasks. This is a potentially important direction for understanding WM and its potential breakdown in diseases such as Parkinson disease. It is not yet clear whether such distinctions will have any implications for the development of the DMC account.

Reuter-Lorenz and Jonides (Chapter 10) also have a neural systems-oriented view of WM variation. In their account, lateral PFC areas serve attentional-control functions in WM tasks, but they also postulate that all WM tasks require some degree of control (which explains the near ubiquity of lateral PFC activity during WM). Additionally, Reuter-Lorenz and Jonides call attention to the fact that even very subtle task manipulations can lead to substantial changes in behavioral performance and PFC activity, by altering control demands. These views are highly similar to our own, except that we further suggest that it is important to distinguish between the demands placed on proactive vs. reactive control, and to specify which mechanism is likely to be dominant in a given task context. Such distinctions in control will have important ramifications on the way in which different PFC regions are engaged in WM tasks—with either sustained or transient dynamics, and in either a cue-specific or more global manner.

Other Dual-Process Frameworks

The executive attention account described by Kane et al. (Chapter 2) is also highly compatible with our own, and has highly influenced our thinking on the role of cognitive individual differences in WM. Like our group, Kane et al. posit that variation in WM performance is primarily linked to the active maintenance of goal-relevant information rather than storage capacity per se. Kane et al. also argue that active goal maintenance, which in our terminology would refer to proactive control, is most critical when PI effects are prominent and must be overcome. Interestingly, Kane and colleagues have also begun to develop a dual-process account of executive attention, which contrasts active goal maintenance with conflict resolution. This account seems very similar to our own distinction between proactive and reactive control, since we argue that reactive control occurs precisely under conditions where high conflict is de-

tected, but not anticipated or prevented via proactive control. Kane et al. make their distinction on the basis of data from the Stroop task that indicate low-WM span individuals show heightened interference (and facilitation) effects selectively under low-interference expectancy conditions. This finding seemingly parallels our own results from the recent-negative Sternberg task (Burgess & Braver, 2004), in which low-gF individuals exhibited increased interference effects related to expectancy. However, in one way our results are exactly opposite those of Kane et al., since in our study gF differences were present selectively in the high-interference expectancy rather than low-expectancy condition. The discrepancy between these two sets of results is puzzling, but may be due to subtle cross-study differences in tasks (Stroop vs. Sternberg) and individual-difference constructs (WM span vs. gF). Nevertheless, further investigation of the issue seems warranted.

Inhibition

An important component of the DMC model is that both proactive and reactive control are often invoked in the service of interference management. This view is similar to that espoused by Hasher et al. (Chapter 9), who highlight changes in the efficacy of inhibitory control processes as a major source of both age-related and within-individual (e.g., time-of-day effects) WM variation. Like Kane et al., Hasher and colleagues have convincingly demonstrated through a series of studies that differences in WM function are unlikely to be due to storage capacity. However, Hasher et al. go further by postulating three distinct forms of inhibitory control relevant to WM: access, deletion, and restraint. Although we are sympathetic to the appeal of these types of constructs, an important distinction between the account of Hasher et al. and our own (and those of Kane et al. and Munakata et al. as well) is the causal primacy attributed to inhibitory control. In the DMC account, proactive control mechanisms serve to prevent interference, while reactive control processes can detect and suppress interference when it occurs. However, the control mechanisms themselves are not inhibitory per se, but rather achieve inhibition as an emergent consequence of active goal maintenance exerting a top-down bias on local competition within posterior brain systems. These types of emergent effects are most easily understood through the use of computational models that translate psychological constructs into specific underlying mechanisms, in often a non–one-to-one manner. Thus, we might argue that the "access" and "restraint" inhibitory functions might both relate to consequences of proactive control, but under different task contexts. Similarly, "deletion" might relate to effective DA-mediated updating in PFC. However, explicit simulations of tasks and behavioral phenomena would be required to determine whether such mappings are truly applicable.

Domain Specificity vs. Domain Generality

The DMC account can be considered a domain-general model of WM variation, since we postulate that a single source of variability, between proactive and reactive control, can account for empirical phenomena under a wide range of circumstances. There are other accounts of WM variation that are also domain-general, but which posit very distinct sources of variability. For example, a domain-general account of WM variation discussed by Hale et al. in Chapter 8 is the widely known processing-speed model. Much attention has been given to the processing-speed construct in the WM literature, especially with regard to aging, and it appears to be highly successful as a source of explanation for WM variability (Salthouse, 1994). It is our hope that the construct can be fleshed out further into mechanistic terms so that its interactions with other dimensions of information processing can be better appreciated. For example, in other recent work, Hale, Myerson, and colleagues present a mathematical model that specifies how computational speed might interact with individual differences, group differences, and task complexity to produce the diversity of speed-related behavioral phenom-

ena that have been observed in cognitive performance (Myerson, Hale, Zheng, Jenkins, & Widaman, 2003).

It is clear that any comprehensive account of WM variation will also have to deal with the obvious variation that occurs across individuals (and developmentally, within individuals) in regard to domain-specific knowledge. The brain is an organ defined by experience-dependent plasticity. Thus, individuals with different experiences are surely to have different knowledge stored in the various brain systems specialized for coding these experiences. Likewise, just as some individuals have greater perceptual acuity than others, likely as a result of domain-specific genetic variation, so might there be domain-specific differences in cognitive abilities, such as verbal and spatial reasoning, that will likely impact WM function. Indeed, these domain-specific individual differences may be as important a source of WM variation as domain-general factors. A number of chapters have provided convincing evidence supporting such a position (e.g., Chapters 6 and 8). A critical future direction for studies of WM will be to discover and explore the nature of interaction between domain-specific and domain-general sources of variability.

Development

In addition to the accounts and views of WM variation with which we hope our work intersects, we also recognize that there are likely other sources of important variation that are relevant for understanding WM function but are not within the purview of our current model. For example, developmental approaches to WM are extensively considered by a number of investigators within this volume (see Chapters 5, 6, 7, and 8). The developmental maturation of the cognitive system and the concomitant neural changes that occur with it undoubtedly serve as both important sources of variation and important tools for discovering the causal mechanisms that underlie cognitive developmental variability. We have not explored yet whether the DMC account would be useful for understanding the nature of cognitive control in young children, but this may be an important avenue of exploration. An intriguing notion is that developmental changes in WM function may be linked to the developmental trajectory of DA function in PFC (see, e.g., Diamond, 2002).

Genetics

Finally, the future of scientific investigation on WM function will likely be strongly influenced by upcoming developments in cognitive–genetic approaches. The rapid development of easily accessible genotyping methods has already provided new knowledge of how genetic variation in certain alleles may relate to phenotypic variation in cognitive and neural function among healthy individuals. For example, recent work has suggested that variations in the COMT (catechol O-methyltransferase) gene, which helps break down DA in PFC, might be strongly linked to individual-difference variation in PFC activity and behavioral performance in WM tasks such as the n-back (Mattay et al., 2003). Further studies incorporating genetically derived, independent measures of variation may provide crucial information regarding the first causal link in the pathway from biology to behavior during performance of WM tasks.

SUMMARY AND GENERAL CONTRIBUTIONS OF THE DUAL MECHANISMS OF CONTROL THEORY

In the preceding sections we have laid out what we believe is an important new direction for research into cognitive control and WM. We have argued that a comprehensive theory of cognitive control in WM requires the inclusion of at least two distinguishable and potentially independent control modes: proactive and reactive. Proactive control and reactive control can be differentiated on the basis of their information-processing characteristics, computational properties, temporal dynamics, and underlying neural systems. The existence of dual mechanisms of control is suggested because of the inherent computational trade-offs associated with

each specialized mechanism. Thus, there are both costs and benefits, advantages and limitations to the exclusive use of either proactive or reactive control strategies. Consequently, the cognitive system is likely to optimize processing by using both strategies to differing degrees, such that, in most individuals and in most task situations, a shifting mixture of both control mechanisms will be invoked.

We believe that the DMC framework contributes significantly to a general theoretical understanding of WM in a number of ways (i.e., Question #4):

- It provides clear predictions of how changes in cognitive control strategy will translate into characteristic changes in WM task performance. An example is the double dissociation in immediate vs. delayed recognition described in the Speer et al. (2003) Sternberg study.
- It clarifies the nature and temporal dynamics of lateral PFC involvement in WM tasks in terms of shifts in cognitive control mode. Examples include (1) the increased, sustained delay-related PFC activity associated with low expected WM load (i.e., proactive control) in the Speer et al. (2003) Sternberg study; and (2) the decreased transient probe-related PFC activity and reduced behavioral interference effects in high-gF individuals associated with high interference expectancy (i.e., proactive control) in the Burgess and Braver (2004) Sternberg study.
- It conceptualizes natural developmental processes, such as healthy aging, and certain types of neural dysfunction (e.g., schizophrenia) as reflecting a relatively stable shift in cognitive control strategy, with associated consequences. An example is the pattern of changes in PFC activity exhibited by older adults in the AX-CPT task, with generalized task-related activation becoming increased while specific-delay-related activity decreases (Paxton et al., 2006).
- It highlights the variety of task and individual-difference factors, many of which are either subtle in nature or not in

the traditional purview of cognitive scientists, that can influence WM task performance, by shifting which control strategy is dominant. An example is the influence of the personality traits BIS and BAS on ACC and lateral PFC activity during performance of the n-back task (Gray et al., 2005).

Probably the most important take-home message of our theoretical account to general WM theory is that of an appreciation of WM variability itself (see Box 4.1 for a summary statement of our answers to the four central chapter questions). We suggest that an understanding of the variability between proactive and reactive control is fundamental to understanding the core mechanisms of WM. The critical point of the DMC account is that variability between dual control mechanisms can be a naturally occurring part of cognition,

---

BOX 4.1.   SUMMARY ANSWERS TO BOOK QUESTIONS

1. THE OVERARCHING THEORY OF WORKING MEMORY

Our general approach is to link psychological constructs of WM to underlying neural and computational mechanisms. We suggest that WM is an emergent phenomenon arising from the interaction of multiple mechanisms (active context representation, dynamic updating, conflict detection, and binding). However, we give particular focus to the influential role of lateral PFC in mediating top-down biases over processing via actively maintained context or goal representations.

2. CRITICAL SOURCES OF WORKING MEMORY VARIATION

We suggest that the distinction between proactive and reactive cognitive control may be the core source of WM variation. Proactive control enables the optimal task preparation and prevention of interference via sustained goal maintenance in lateral PFC. Reactive control provides an as-needed, just-in-time form of interference resolution or context retrieval via transient activation of the PFC or related brain systems (e.g., MTL, ACC). Because these dual mechanisms of control each have computational advantages and disadvantages, shifts in the dominant cognitive control mode can arise from situational factors (intra-individual variation), individual differences, neural dysfunction, and noncognitive factors such as mood and personality.

3. OTHER SOURCES OF WORKING MEMORY VARIATION

Many other sources of variation should be included in a comprehensive WM theory. We consider some of the differing sources discussed by other contributors to this volume: neural mechanisms (e.g., the basal ganglia, Chapter 8), other dual-process accounts (Chapter 2), inhibition (Chapter 9), processing speed (Chapter 8), domain-specific mechanisms (Chapter 6), and development (Chapter 5). Additionally, we think that genetic variation will be an important focus of future WM research.

4. CONTRIBUTIONS TO GENERAL WORKING MEMORY THEORY

We believe that the DMC model put forward here can provide a unifying framework for understanding the many varieties of WM variation. The model (a) indicates the task and individual-difference factors that should influence WM task performance; (b) clarifies the nature and dynamics of PFC activity in WM tasks; and (c) links specific forms of neural dysfunction to stable shifts in cognitive control strategy. The conceptualization of cognitive control mechanisms in terms of computational specialization and trade-offs provides a coherent causal explanation for the occurrence of variability in complex cognitive activities, such as WM.

but can also become more prominent under various changes in internal states and external situations. Moreover, the DMC account does not posit a distinction between the types of WM variation that occur on an intra-individual basis from those that occur on an interindividual basis. In other words, regardless of the source of WM variation—task factors, state factors, cognitive individual differences, personality differences, or population differences—the proximal mechanisms of variation remain the same and have the same impact on brain activity and behavior. Thus, the DMC framework provides a unifying account that has the potential to synthesize and integrate a large body of literatures on WM function. By recognizing that there are multiple alternative routes to cognitive control, investigators may be in a better position to explore and investigate the complexity of empirical findings and thus more effectively manage the previously impossibly difficult task of defining the unifying latent WM constructs that will replicate across tasks, individuals, and cognitive domains.

References

Arnsten, A. F. T., & Robbins, T. W. (2002). Neurochemical modulation of prefrontal cortical function in humans and animals. In D. T. Stuss & R. T. Knight (Eds.), *Principles of frontal lobe function* (pp. 51–84). New York: Oxford University Press.

Baddeley, A. D. (1986). *Working memory*. New York: Oxford University Press.

Baddeley, A.D. (2003). Working memory: Looking back and looking forward. *Nature Reviews Neuroscience, 4*, 829–839.

Botvinick, M. M., Braver, T. S., Barch, D. M., Carter, C. S., & Cohen, J. C. (2001). Conflict monitoring and cognitive control. *Psychological Review, 108*, 624–652.

Braver, T. S., Barch, D. M., Keys, B. A., Carter, C. S., Cohen, J. D., Kaye, J. A., et al. (2001). Context processing in older adults: Evidence for a theory relating cognitive control to neurobiology in healthy aging. *Journal of Experimental Psychology: General, 130*, 746–763.

Braver, T. S., & Cohen, J. D. (2000). On the control of control: The role of dopamine in regulating prefrontal function and working memory. In S. Monsell & J. Driver (Eds.), *Attention and Performance XVIII* (pp. 713–738). Cambridge, MA: MIT Press.

Braver, T. S., Cohen, J. D., & Barch, D. M. (2002). The role of the prefrontal cortex in normal and disordered cognitive control: A cognitive neuroscience perspective. In D. T. Stuss & R. T. Knight (Eds.), *Principles of frontal lobe function* (pp. 428–448). New York: Oxford University Press.

Braver, T. S., Reynolds, J. R., & Donaldson, D. I. (2003). Neural mechanisms of transient and sustained cognitive control during task switching. *Neuron, 39*, 713–726.

Braver, T.S., Satpute, A.B., Rush, B.K., Racine, C.A., Barch, D.M. (2005). Context processing and context maintenance in healthy aging and early stage dementia of the Alzheimer's type. *Psychology and Aging, 20*, 33–46.

Braver, T. S., & Hoyer, C. M. (2006). *Neural mechanisms of proactive and reactive cognitive control*. Submitted manuscript.

Brown, J.W., and Braver, T.S. (2005). Learned predictions of error likelihood in the anterior cingulate cortex. *Science, 307*, 1118–1121.

Burgess, G. C., & Braver, T. S. (2004). *Dual mechanisms of cognitive control over interference*. Presented at the Cognitive Neuroscience Society, Eleventh Annual Meeting, San Francisco, CA.

Burgess, G.C., Braver, T.S., and Gray, J.R. (2006). Exactly how are fluid intelligence, working memory, and executive function related? Cognitive neuroscience approaches to investigating the mechanisms of fluid cognition. *Behavioral and Brain Sciences, 29*, 128–129.

Cabeza, R. (2001). Functional neuroimaging of cognitive aging. In R. Cabeza & A. Kingstone (Eds.), *Handbook of functional neuroimaging of cognition*. Cambridge, MA: MIT Press.

Cohen, J. D., Perstein, W. M., Braver, T. S., Nystrom, L. E., Noll, D. C., Jonides, J., et al. (1997). Temporal dynamics of brain activation during a working memory task. *Nature, 386*, 604–608.

Cowan, N. (2001). The magical number 4 in short-term memory: A reconsideration of mental storage capacity. *Behavioral and Brain Sciences, 24*, 87–185.

Davidson, R. J. (1995). Cerebral asymmetry, emotion, and affective style. In R. J. Davidson &

K. Hugdahl (Eds.), *Brain asymmetry* (pp. 361–387). Cambridge, MA: MIT Press.

DePisapia, N., & Braver, T. S. (2006). A model of dual control mechanisms through anterior cingulate and prefrontal cortex interactions. *Neurocomputing, 69*, 1322–1326.

Depue, R. A., & Collins, P. F. (1999). Neurobiology of the structure of personality: Dopamine, facilitation of incentive motivation, and extraversion. *Behavioral and Brain Sciences, 22*, 491–569.

D'Esposito, M., Aguirre, G. K., Zarahn, E., Ballard, D., Shin, R. K., & Lease, J. (1998). Functional MRI studies of spatial and nonspatial working memory. *Cognitive Brain Research, 7*, 1–13.

D'Esposito, M., Postle, B. R., Jonides, J., & Smith, E. E. (1999). The neural substrate and temporal dynamics of interference effects in working memory as revealed by event-related functional MRI. *Proceedings of the National Academy of Sciences USA, 96*, 7514–7519.

Diamond, A. (2002). Normal development of prefrontal cortex from birth to young adulthood: Cognitive functions, anatomy, and biochemistry. In D. T. Stuss & R. T. Knight (Eds.), *Principles of frontal lobe function* (pp. 466–503). New York: Oxford University Press.

Drevets, W. C., & Raichle, M. E. (1998). Reciprocal suppression of regional cerebral blood flow during emotional versus higher cognitive processes: Implications for interactions between emotion and cognition. *Cognition and Emotion, 12*, 353–385.

Duncan, J., Emslie, H., Williams, P., Johnson, R., & Freer, C. (1996). Intelligence and the frontal lobe: The organization of goal-directed behavior. *Cognitive Psychology, 30*, 257–303.

Einstein, G. O., & McDaniel, M. A. (1996). Retrieval processes in prospective memory: Theoretical approaches and some new empirical findings. In M. Brandimonte, G. O. Einstein, & M. A. McDaniel (Eds.), *Prospective memory: Theory and applications* (pp. 115–142). Mahwah, NJ: Lawrence Erlbaum Associates.

Fuster, J. (1997). *The prefrontal cortex* (3rd ed.). New York: Lippincott-Raven.

Goschke, T. (2003). Voluntary action and cognitive control from a cognitive neuroscience perspective. In S. Maasen, W. Prinz, & G. Roth (Eds.), *Voluntary action: An issue at the interface of nature and culture* (pp. 49–85). Oxford, UK: Oxford University Press.

Grasby, P. M., Frith, C. D., Friston, K. J., Simpson, J., Fletcher, P. C., Frackowiak, R. S. J., et al. (1994). A graded task approach to the functional mapping of brain areas implicated in auditory-verbal memory. *Brain, 117*, 1271–1282.

Gray, J. A. (1994). Personality dimensions and emotion systems. In P. Ekman & R. J. Davidson (Eds.), *The nature of emotion* (pp. 329–331). New York: Oxford University Press.

Gray, J. R., & Braver, T. S. (2002a). Integration of emotion and cognitive control: A neurocomputational hypothesis of dynamic goal regulation. In S. C. Moore & M. R. Oaksford (Eds.), *Emotional cognition* (pp. 289–316). Amsterdam: John Benjamins.

Gray, J. R., & Braver, T. S. (2002b). Personality predicts working memory related activation in the caudal anterior cingulate cortex. *Cognitive, Affective, & Behavioral Neuroscience, 2*, 64–75.

Gray, J. R., Braver, T. S., & Raichle, M. E. (2002). Integration of emotion and cognition in the lateral prefrontal cortex. *Proceedings of the National Academy of Sciences USA, 99*, 4115–4120.

Gray, J. R., Burgess, G. C., Schaefer, A., Yarkoni, T., Larsen, R. L., & Braver, T. S. (2005). Affective personality differences in neural processing efficiency confirmed using fMRI. *Cognitive, Affective, & Behavioral Neuroscience, 5*, 182–190.

Gray, J. R., Chabris, C. F., & Braver, T. S. (2003). Neural mechanisms of general fluid intelligence. *Nature Neuroscience, 6*, 316–322.

Jacoby, L. L., Kelley, C. M., & McElree, B. D. (1999). The role of cognitive control: Early selection versus late correction. In S. Chaiken & E. Trope (Eds.), *Dual process theories in social psychology* (pp. 383–400). New York: Guilford Press.

Jonides, J., Badre, D., Curtis, C., Thompson-Schill, S. L., & Smith, E. E. (2002). Mechanisms of conflict resolution in prefrontal cortex. In D. T. Stuss & R. T. Knight (Eds.), *Principles of frontal lobe function* (pp. 233–245). New York: Oxford University Press.

Jonides, J. & Nee, D.E. (2006). Brain mechanisms of proactive interference in working memory. *Neuroscience, 139,* 181–193.

Kane, M. J., & Engle, R. W. (2002). The role of prefrontal cortex in working-memory capacity, executive attention and general fluid intelligence: An individual-differences perspective. *Psychonomic Bulletin & Review, 9,* 637–671.

Larsen, R. J., & Ketelaar, E. (1991). Personality and susceptibility to positive and negative emotional states. *Journal of Personality and Social Psychology, 61,* 132–140.

Lepage, M., Ghaffar, O., Nyberg, L., & Tulving, E. (2000). Prefrontal cortex and episodic memory retrieval mode. *Proceedings of the National Academy of Sciences USA, 97,* 506–511.

Lieberman, M. D., & Rosenthal, R. (2001). Why introverts can't always tell who likes them: Multitasking and nonverbal decoding. *Journal of Personality and Social Psychology, 80,* 294–310.

Locke, H. S., & Braver, T. S. (2006). *Motivational influences on cognitive control: Behavior, brain activity, and individual differences.* Submitted manuscript.

Mattay, V. S., Goldberg, T. E., Fera, F., Hariri, A. R., Tessitore, A., Egan, M. F., et al. (2003). COMT genotype and individual variation in the brain response to amphetamine. *Proceedings of the National Academy of Sciences USA, 100,* 6186–6191.

Myerson, J., Hale, S., Zheng, Y., Jenkins, L., & Widaman, K. F. (2003). The difference engine: A model of diversity in speeded cognition. *Psychonomic Bulletin & Review, 10,* 262–288.

Newell, A. (1990). *Unified theories of cogntion.* New York: Cambridge University Press.

Norman, D. A., & Shallice, T. (1986). Attention to action: Willed and automatic control of behavior. In R. J. Davidson, G. E. Schwartz, & D. Shapiro (Eds.), *Consciousness and self-regulation* (Vol. 4, pp. 1–18). New York: Plenum Press.

O'Reilly, R. C., Braver, T. S., & Cohen, J. D. (1999). A biologically based computational model of working memory. In A. Miyake & P. Shah (Eds.), *Models of working memory: Mechanisms of active maintenance and executive control* (pp. 375–411). New York: Cambridge University Press.

O'Reilly, R.C. & Frank, M.J. (2006). Making working memory work: A computational model of learning in the frontal cortex and basal ganglia. *Neural Computation, 18,* 283–328.

Paxton, J.L., Barch, D. M., Racine, C. A., & Braver, T. S. (2006). *Prefrontal function in healthy aging: Context processing and proactive versus reactive cognitive control.* Submitted manuscript.

Posner, M. I., Snyder, C. R. R., & Davidson, B. J. (1980). Attention and the detection of signals. *Journal of Experimental Psychology: General, 109,* 160–174.

Postle, B. R., Berger, J. S., & D'Esposito, M. (1999). Functional neuroanatomical double dissociation of mnemonic and executive control processes contributing to working memory performance. *Proceedings of the National Academy of Sciences USA, 96,* 12959–12964.

Reynolds, J.R., Braver, T.S., Brown, J.W., Van der Stigchel, S. (2006). Computational and neural mechanisms of task-switching. *Neurocomputing, 69,* 1332–1336.

Rowe, J. B., Toni, I., Josephs, O., Frackowiak, R. S. J., & Passingham, R. E. (2000). The prefrontal cortex: Response selection or maintenance within working memory? *Science, 288,* 1656–1660.

Salthouse, T. A. (1994). The aging of working memory. *Neuropsychology, 8,* 535–543.

Schultz, W., Dayan, P., & Montague, P. R. (1997). A neural substrate of prediction and reward. *Science, 275,* 1593–1599.

Smith, E. E., & Jonides, J. (1999). Storage and executive processes in the frontal lobes. *Science, 283,* 1657–1661.

Smith, R. E. (2003). The cost of remembering to remember in event-based prospective memory: Investigating the capacity demands of delayed intention performance. *Journal of Experimental Psychology: Learning, Memory, and Cognition, 29,* 347–361.

Speer, N. K., Jacoby, L. L., & Braver, T. S. (2003). Strategy-dependent changes in memory: Effects on brain activity and behavior. *Cognitive, Affective, & Behavioral Neuroscience, 3,* 155–167.

Sternberg, S. (1966). High-speed scanning in human memory. *Science, 153,* 652–654.

Tallis, F. (1995). *Obsessive compulsive disorder: A cognitive and neuropsychological perspective.* Chichester, UK: John Wiley & Sons.

Visscher, K. M., Miezin, F. M., Kelly, J. E., Buckner, R. L., Donaldson, D. I., McAvoy, M. P., et al. (2003). Mixed block/event-related designs separate transient and sustained activity in fMRI. *NeuroImage, 19,* 1694–1708.

Zald, D., Mattson, D., & Pardo, J. (2001). Brain activity in ventromedial prefrontal cortex predicts negative temperament. *NeuroImage, 13*(6), S490.

II

Working Memory Variation
Due to Normal and
Atypical Development

5

Variation in Working Memory Due to Normal Development

JOHN N. TOWSE and GRAHAM J. HITCH

Our starting point is a popular model of working memory outlined by Baddeley and Hitch (1974) and elaborated by Baddeley (1986). We discuss this model's architecture, together with a number of conceptual issues and alternative theoretical approaches. We then consider how a family of experimental tasks designed to measure the capacity of working memory (e.g., counting span, reading span, operation span) have been used both to support the working memory model and to suggest changes to it. This leads us to discuss a research program investigating the limits of working memory span, using data from both children and adults. Our interpretation of the data seeks to provide a synthesis between individual-difference and experimental approaches, and issues concerning each approach and their relationship are raised. We provide evidence for the importance of making a careful analysis of the temporal dynamics of working memory tasks, and against the assumption that span is a straightforward measure of the resources available to working memory. We go on to suggest that some circumstances may encourage at least an integrated relationship between the processing and memory aspects of working memory, functions that are usually seen as being in direct competition with one another.

We have structured our chapter around the four questions that all contributors have been invited to address. Indeed, we interleave the answers to the four questions with the unfolding of the theoretical and empirical story, rather than attempt to keep our answers to the very end. These answers serve to summarize our position in a useful and integrative way, and therefore they work better within rather than appended to the main text. We begin with a statement of our overarching theory of working memory. This is followed by a discussion of the conceptual exploration of our own ideas that also follows in broad terms a chronological sequence. Our answers to the remaining three common questions punctuate this discussion at appropriate points. We end the chapter with short summaries of our answers to each of the four questions.

QUESTION 1: OVERARCHING THEORY OF WORKING MEMORY

What is the theory or definition of working memory that guides your research on working memory variation? Our research initially stemmed from the general framework for working memory outlined by Baddeley and Hitch (1974) and the more specific model proposed by Baddeley (1986). Furthermore, we acknowledge the relevance of working memory for understanding phenomena among children (for example, see Halliday & Hitch, 1988; Hitch & Halliday, 1983). Accordingly, we take the position that working memory is a multicomponent, limited-capacity system responsible for retaining as well as transforming fragile representations. The components of working memory are assumed to comprise a central executive, a phonological loop, and a visuospatial sketchpad. The central executive is the hub of these components, controlling and orchestrating the operation of dedicated, modality-specific memory systems. More recently Baddeley (2000) has proposed a fourth component, a multimodal episodic buffer that is closely connected to the central executive. Although the episodic buffer has not been a direct stimulus for our research, we suggest that it is quite compatible with several conclusions that come from it.

In addition to making assumptions about the architecture of working memory, and therefore the ways in which temporary information is represented, our theoretical approach stresses the importance of processing operations. In particular, we take the view that the interaction between memory and processing lies at the heart of understanding the limitations of working memory.

Our program of research has focused on working memory span. This task was first developed within a slightly different theoretical framework in which working memory is conceived as an undifferentiated general resource (Daneman & Carpenter, 1980). According to this approach, working memory span measures the ability to commit mental resources to memory as well as concurrent processing events. In terms of the multicomponent working memory model we have just articulated, working memory span is regarded as involving the central executive. However, like some others, we suspect that complex working memory tasks only partially overlap with central executive functioning. One issue is that these complex tasks likely incorporate some characteristics of slave system functioning. An additional concern is that central executive functioning is not just about servicing the requirements of these span tasks, but has independent responsibilities too.

With this in mind, we argue that variation in working memory performance can lie on several distinct dimensions. Performance on tasks involving working memory will vary as a result of which components of its architecture are accessed, for example, the degree to which verbal rehearsal contributes to the memory representation. Performance can also vary as a result of differences in the use of these components—for example, articulation speed affects the efficiency of rehearsal. Critically for us, the interplay between the processing and memory demands of complex working memory tests contributes to performance. These demands go beyond the constraints of the individual slave systems, and in this sense our theoretical account is an attempt to develop the account of working memory limitations provided by the multicomponent model.

THE THEORETICAL VISION OF WORKING MEMORY

Baddeley and Hitch's (1974) initial study on working memory represents something of a back-to-the-drawing-board approach in terms of the conceptualization of short-term memory processes. Rather than take on and attempt to develop a specific and well-worn paradigm, or adapt a theoretical model prevalent at the time, Baddeley and Hitch described a varied series of experiments into the functional characteristics of short-term memory. These were used to provide a perspective on short-term memory as a limited-capacity working memory, the "workbench of cognition" (Klatzky, 1980) or "the interface between memory and cognition" (Baddeley, 1994). Thus, it was recognized that short-term memory is not just a system for the retention of information. Instead, immediate memory processes are an integral part of cognitive activities, shaping and constraining how thought processes take place. This idea forms a cornerstone of what Baddeley (1986) subsequently referred to as *working memory—general* (WMG), the general framework within which working memory could be understood.

Baddeley and Hitch (1974) also proposed that working memory involved the combination of specialized, modality-based memory traces and more generic, flexible memory processes (part of what Baddeley, 1986, referred to as *WMS*, or working memory—specific). In particular, they focused on the idea that working memory incorporated a verbally based system that allowed individuals to remember a few items for a short period of time, supported by rehearsal of those items. They also hinted at the idea that a specialized visual memory system might also contribute to working memory. These proposals have been influential in leading to the study of the characteristics of these specialized memory systems (referred to as *slave systems*), often through the use of dual-task interference paradigms. These paradigms include articulatory suppression (repeating an irrelevant phrase during a memory trial; see Baddeley, Lewis, & Vallar, 1984), concurrent spatial tracking (Baddeley & Lieberman, 1980), and dynamic visual noise (Quinn & McConnell, 1996), where a changing visual display is watched while trying to remember a sequence of items. Different tasks cause different patterns of interference and these effects can be interpreted in terms of selective disruption of different components of working memory. There has been a steady accumulation of knowledge about these slave memory systems, and they form part of the specific model or implementation of working memory outlined by Baddeley (1986).

In the present chapter we consider the applicability of the multicomponent model to the development of working memory in children. We focus on working memory span, as this is widely used as a measure of individual differences in children and adults, and yet our understanding of this task is incomplete.

WORKING MEMORY AND COGNITIVE DEVELOPMENT

Although the multicomponent model of working memory was proposed as a theoretical account of adult memory performance, it has been fruitfully applied to a range of developmental issues. In several cases, research has shown that changes in memory among primary-school children can be attributed to variations in the strategies that children use. Verbal recoding of visually presented material (whether images or words) is not ubiquitous (see Halliday & Hitch, 1988). At around the age of 8 years, children become increasingly consistent in their sensitivity to phenomena such as word length effects and phonological similarity effects even when material is presented in a nonverbal form. Convergent with these results, children below about 7 years of age are sensitive to visual similarity effects when remembering pictorial stimuli (Hitch, Woodin, & Baker, 1989). They show confusions between items with visually overlapping features, which has been taken to suggest that their memory may be based on relatively untransformed visual representations of the initial stimuli. Exploring this last idea in more detail, Walker, Hitch, Dewhurst, Whiteley, and Brandimonte (1997) have shown that visual memory does not maintain a veridical copy of visual stimuli but rather is object based, storing both surface descriptions of objects and more abstract structural descriptions.

The multicomponent model of working memory has not just been employed to account for qualitative developmental shifts. Quantitative changes have also been explored. For example, studies of the word length effect in immediate recall in adults have demonstrated the importance of pronunciation time as a determinant of performance (Baddeley, Thomson, & Buchanan, 1975). Similarly, developmental changes in articulation speed may form one component of improved memory (Hitch, Halliday, & Littler, 1989; Hulme, Thomson, Muir, & Lawrence, 1984). Pronunciation speed is a strong predictor of short-term memory span, especially at the group level (that is, the extent to which memory ability for different age groups is predicted by their pronunciation speed). Thus, there are proportionate changes in memory performance that accompany changes to the pronunciation speed of words, and this can be understood within the notion that the phonological loop is constrained by rehearsal time.

CHILDREN'S WORKING MEMORY AS DUAL-TASK PERFORMANCE

From the perspective that working memory involves an interaction between memory and cognition, it is not surprising that there has been interest in whether working memory services the ability to carry out two tasks at the same time, and whether the development of working memory in childhood at least partly reflects the development of skills in combining separable cognitive activities; see comments in Chapter 7 that working memory span reflects a dual-task situation. We consider three aspects of this perspective.

The first aspect concerns working memory span, sometimes known as complex span. Working memory span was devised as a single task that embodied dual-task characteristics (Daneman & Carpenter, 1980). Participants are asked to carry out a processing task and retain some information associated with each processing episode. Their span is a measure of the upper limit on how much information they can retain while continuing to carry out the processing task. In these terms, working memory span involves processing and memory. In the most widely held theoretical account these two functions compete against each other. Case (1985) articulated this perspective lucidly. He argued that all children are endowed with an *executive processing space*, the capacity of which is largely invariant across age. While capacity per se remained constant, the use of this capacity underwent substantial developmental change. In particular, cognitive development was thought to involve large increases in the efficiency with which processing operations were accomplished. As the resource demands of processing dropped, a progressively increasing proportion of the EPS capacity could be allocated to other

activities, such as immediate memory. As Case notes, this model implies "one capacity that can be flexibly allocated to either of two functions" (Case, 1985, p. 120). Working memory in these terms reflects the balance between two competing activities, each of which requires access to a common pool of resources. We refer to this account as the *resource-sharing hypothesis*.

Although the present discussion focuses on children, it is important to note that, contemporaneously, Daneman and Carpenter (1980) proposed a similar theoretical view, based on an influential study of individual differences in college students. They found that working memory span was a good predictor of Scholastic Aptitude Test (SAT) scores and also that digit span, the standard measure of short-term memory, was a much poorer predictor. These findings were taken as support for the idea that working memory serves the function of combining processing and storage in cognition, whereas short-term memory is concerned merely with storage in isolation. They led to a surge of interest in identifying more precisely what limits working memory span.

The second aspect of dual-task capabilities stems from work by Towse and Houston-Price (2001), who suggested that one contributory factor to the predictive success of working memory tasks over short-term memory tasks could be the requirement to combine different task elements. To explore this idea, they developed a memory task that involved two separate components (a digit span task and Corsi span task, the latter requiring a sequence of spatial locations to be remembered). By examining individual differences in the elemental skills as well as the task in which these are brought together (a so-called combination span task, in which numbers were remembered at specific spatial locations), they tried to assay whether the combined task was more than the sum of its parts (see also Emerson, Miyake, & Rettinger, 1999; Yee, Hunt, & Pellegrino, 1991). Indeed, Towse and Houston-Price (2001) found that the combination span task was related to children's cognitive ability (as measured by their word-reading and number skills) once the relevance of both the digit and Corsi span had been statistically accounted for. This allows us to conclude the children are sensitive to complex memory tasks because of the memory requirements (here, dealing with multiple representations that cross domains) and not just because working memory tasks often incorporate processing requirements too.

For the third aspect, extending the conceptual approach outlined above, Bayliss, Jarrold, Gunn, and Baddeley (2003; Bayliss, Jarrold, Baddeley, Gunn & Leigh, 2005; see also Chapter 6, this volume) developed a novel paradigm that separated out the processing and retention components of complex span, in order to identify the emergent properties of its dual-task aspect. Instead of considering the combination of different storage tasks, Bayliss et al. (2003) focused on the combination of memory with different types of processing operations. They asked their participants to engage in a processing task that was designed to involve either visual–attention or verbal–semantic associations. They also asked participants to remember either visuospatial or verbal information in the wake of each processing event. Their working memory task thus comprised memory and processing in different combinations, and each component could be tested separately. In this skillful design, one can separate out the different elements of the task as well as consider the emergent features of the combined task. In essence, Bayliss et al. (2003) found evidence for both domain-specific and domain-general contributions to the predictive characteristics of their working memory task.

In overview, several attempts have been made to explore working memory functioning in terms of complex performance with multiple operations, in particular the need to control and orchestrate two separate mental tasks. These studies are important, particularly insofar as they show that there may be emergent properties from task "coordination" (Bayliss et al., 2003; Towse & Houston-Price, 2001). Nonetheless, the greatest concentration of research effort has been focused on working memory span, and for various reasons that will emerge later in the chapter, this paradigm may not simply represent a dual-task environment. It is impor-

tant then to understand this paradigm in its own right.

DEVELOPMENT OF PERFORMANCE ON WORKING MEMORY SPAN TASKS

An early study by Case, Kurland, and Goldberg (1982) offers an important experimental and developmental perspective on working memory span. Case et al. (1982) used a counting span task, in which children sought to find the number of target objects in an array, and then remembered this total while they counted up subsequent arrays. Six- to twelve-year-old children were assessed on the longest set of arrays that could be counted and followed by successful recall of the set of totals. An index of children's processing efficiency for counting was estimated separately by measuring their speed when counting arrays as quickly as possible. As can be seen in Figure 5.1, Case et al. found a strong linear relationship between counting span and counting efficiency. Older children, who could count arrays more quickly than younger children, also remembered more

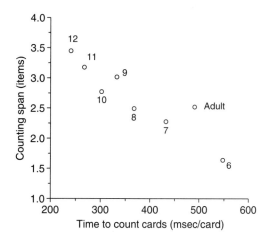

Figure 5.1. Function relating counting span to the rate of counting arrays in a separate task, replotted from data reported in Case et al. (1982). Plot labels identify the mean age of the group of children. "Adults" tested with novel number names. See text for details.

information in the counting span test, and did so in a highly lawful manner. With counting rate taken as an index of the difficulty of counting, so that younger children are regarded as slower to count because it is harder for them, the results are really quite striking. They suggest that as processing efficiency improves during development, resources are freed up for other operations, and this is reflected in improved counting-span performance across development. Thus, the data support the theoretical account outlined earlier, whereby memory and processing functions trade off against each other and the balance of this trade-off changes through development.

It is worth pointing out that in separate experiments, Case et al. (1982) investigated short-term memory span and obtained a similar linear developmental relationship against the time taken to perceptually identify the memory items, adding to the weight of argument that a general system is being tapped. Case et al. also provided an experimental test of the trade-off hypotheses. A group of adults completed a modified counting span test, counting with a sequence of non-words instead of numbers, to increase processing difficulty. Unsurprisingly, adults counted slowly with this novel sequence. More importantly, as Figure 5.1 shows, counting span was observed at a level that was in proportion to their reduced processing ability. That is, adult performance fell along the developmental function that related span and counting speed. Thus, both measures of their span and efficiency matched those of 7-year-olds and fell within the confidence interval for the regression line.[1] It should be apparent that this result is just what would be predicted by the resource-sharing hypothesis articulated above: by changing the number words and increasing adults' processing demands, their memory ability had been compromised. The critical conclusion, then, is that the change in task demands produced not only a drop in memory but also a drop in performance that provided a quantitative fit with the developmental function. In passing it is worth noting that Case et al. (1982) appear to have successfully harnessed both a correlational and an experimental approach. With respect to the former, individual differences indicated a close link between counting efficiency and counting span, and Case et al. suggested that age differences in span could be explained by corresponding differences in task-processing efficiency. With respect to the latter, Case et al. manipulated task difficulty experimentally, to buttress the argument that there is a direct relationship between memory and task difficulty.

For some time, much of the subsequent research into working memory tasks among children focused on individual differences, and examined the predictive strength of working memory span tasks for other cognitive skills. For example, Daneman and Blennerhassett (1984) administered a listening-span test to 4-year-old children in two related experiments. In the listening-span test, children listened to and attempted to comprehend sentences. They were also asked to remember the sentences (with this age group, individual words may not have been salient and therefore remembering individual words might not be straightforward). Children were also administered a more usual word span test and standardized assessment of listening comprehension (which involved matching pictures to auditorily presented sentences). A key finding was that working memory span was a strong predictor of comprehension ability, significantly more so than word span. Daneman and Blennerhassett (1984) argued on the basis of the differential sensitivity of word and listening span tests that working memory is intimately involved in those cognitive processes requiring integration and resource sharing.

Leather and Henry (1994) studied the relative contributions to early reading skills of short-term memory (word span, or "simple span"), working memory (listening span and counting span, or "complex span") and phonological-awareness tasks (e.g., tasks that required children to strip the initial consonant from words, and make sound blends). A group of 7-year-old children were recruited and reading ability was assessed in terms of reading accuracy and comprehension. An important finding was that working memory measures were able to account for significant variance in reading over and above the contribution from the word span task. Phonological-awareness tasks shared considerable variance with the complex span tasks, though they were also distinguishable. Leather and Henry (1994) speculated that the overlap might arise because both variables reflected simultaneous processing and retention demands (moreover, phonological-awareness tasks might have memory demands built into them, in having to remember and compare different stimuli). In any case, the results support the idea that working memory (that is, the retention and transformation of information) is important for developmental skills such as reading, and that complex span tasks, which they assumed tap the central executive, are better measures of working memory than simple span tasks. As was the case for Daneman and Blennerhassett, the question of interest is in the unique properties of working memory span (over short-term memory span) as an index of a developmentally sensitive cognitive ability.

The data from Leather and Henry (1994) focus on individual differences among a normal sample. Siegel and Ryan (1989) had also argued that reading and mathematical skills involved the maintenance and transformation of information, characteristics attributed to working memory span tasks. Siegel and Ryan considered whether children with learning difficulties exhibited problems on working memory span tasks. They presented working memory tests in the form of both listening span and counting span, permitting an evaluation of the generality of any deficits. Their sample comprised children with reading difficulties (RD), arithmetic difficulties (AD), and attentional difficulties (ADD).

The results for the listening span test showed that RD children were impaired relative to control children. Children with AD were not significantly different from controls, although their scores were depressed. On the counting span test, RD children again showed deficits relative to normally achieving controls, and on this task AD children showed significant span deficits as well. Children with ADD did not show significant impairments on either the listening- or the counting-span test. From these results, Siegel and Ryan (1989) argued that not all children with learning difficulties are alike; they exhibited different patterns of deficits on working memory tasks. In the present context, these results add to the evidence that working

memory span is not a domain-free measure of ability.

Theoretical Accounts of Children's Working Memory Span

One point of emphasis in the work reported above is that working memory span tests are different from short-term memory tasks in terms of their psychometric characteristics (Daneman & Blennerhassett, 1984; Daneman & Carpenter, 1980; Leather & Henry, 1984). Working memory span tests are able to account for variance in abilities such as, but not limited to, reading and arithmetic, which short-term memory tasks do not do (see Alloway, Gathercole, Willis & Adams, 2004). A second point of emphasis is that variation in working memory span arises from the way that a system such as the central executive allocates resources to the processing and memory components of the task. Changes in one can influence the other. Thus children with learning disabilities may find the processing requirements particularly taxing, and this can compromise their memory performance. However, whether this trade-off arises from a domain-specific system, or a domain-general system at the core of working memory, has been a contested question. In this section, we consider the arguments relevant to theories of children's working memory, and in particular discuss the role of experimental and correlational research in this process.

While we have described working memory span so far in terms of resource sharing, the direct evidence for a relationship between processing demands and memory ability is sparse. The data from Case et al. (1982) seem the most compelling, in that there was a linear relationship in several age groups between the efficiency of array counting and span level, as well as a child-like level of memory performance among adults when processing demands were high. Nonetheless, both these findings rely on the assumption that resource demand can be measured accurately by asking participants to count arrays as quickly as possible. Yet, the efficiency of counting also delivers an indication of how long counting span trials last. If the counting trials last a long time, the totals of each count—the information held in memory—must be retained longer. This raises the question of whether counting span varies as a function of processing resource demand (resource sharing) or just the processing duration. One reason that the duration of processing may be important is that representations in working memory are subject to rapid forgetting. For example, Hitch (1978) found that errors in mental arithmetic could be predicted from a knowledge of the sequence of processing operations and its implications for the times over which temporary information (such as partial results) had to be maintained. The idea that working memory span is limited because representations in working memory undergo rapid forgetting during the time spent processing has been termed the *task-switching account* (Towse, Hitch, & Hutton, 1998).

According to the task-switching view, the developmental function for working memory span would occur because younger children, being slower to count, have more opportunity to forget information up to the point of recall. Asking adults to count with non-words would also put them at a disadvantage because the slower counting would increase the time period over which non-words could be forgotten. Likewise, this task-switching approach could explain the pattern of data from learning-disabled children (Hitch & McAuley, 1991; Siegel & Ryan, 1989), since their processing deficits would place them at a disadvantage on working memory span trials.

Since both resource-sharing and task-switching hypotheses are able to account for much the same set of data, Towse and Hitch (1995) attempted to develop an experimental situation where the two approaches made different predictions for performance. Counting span is useful in this regard because processing is determined by the difficulty of executing the counting operation (the visual identification of targets and the articulation of an appropriate verbal label) and is also affected by the number of iterations required, that is, the number of objects to count. These factors make it possible to develop counting span materials that vary independently along the dimensions of task complexity and task duration.

Two counting span conditions labeled here *easy* (*short*) and *difficult* (*long*) differed in processing difficulty (the ease with which items could be isolated and identified for enumeration), and the time taken to complete counting. A third *easy* (*long*) condition was constructed, by increasing the array sizes and therefore the completion time requirements of the *easy* (*short*) condition so as to match that of the *difficult* (*long*) condition. Both resource-sharing and task-switching hypotheses suggest that counting span will be larger in the *easy* (*short*) condition than in the *difficult* (*long*) condition. However, the resource-sharing account also predicts higher span in the *easy* (*long*) condition than the *difficult* (*long*) condition, because of the difference in the difficulty of processing operations. In contrast, the task-switching hypothesis predicts equivalent performance in these two conditions because of the experimentally equated duration of the processing operations.

Towse and Hitch (1995) found that the prediction derived from the task-switching account was borne out in each of four different age groups of children (ranging between just under 5 and a half years of age to over 11 years of age). Counting span with *easy* (*short*) materials was significantly higher than with *difficult* (*long*) materials, but there was no discernible span difference between the *difficult* (*long*) and the *easy* (*long*) condition. There was a reliable difference in the rate of counting errors between the latter two conditions, confirming that processing resource demands were indeed greater in the *difficult* (*long*) condition.

Individual differences were also examined in this study. Counting span was found to correlate with counting speed, a result anticipated by both accounts—by resource sharing because speed is an index of processing demand, and therefore residual memory ability, and by task switching because fast counters can reach the recall cue more swiftly and therefore limit their retention interval. Partialing out the effect of age left the correlation nonsignificant. However, there are reasons to believe that there was variability in the speed measure and subsequent studies show that speed can predict span even after age is partialed out (see below).

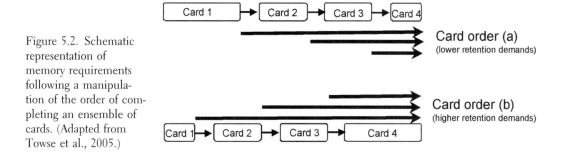

Figure 5.2. Schematic representation of memory requirements following a manipulation of the order of completing an ensemble of cards. (Adapted from Towse et al., 2005.)

Following up this result, Towse et al. (1998) presented children with working memory span tasks in which the trials involved one of two sequences of processing requirements, as shown in the schematic time line of Figure 5.2. Each card in the figure refers to a problem requiring a solution, and all solutions had to be recalled at the end of the trial. Both of the sequences, (a) and (b), contain the same problems. What differentiates them is the completion order for the problems. In set (a) there is a lengthy problem at the beginning of the trial but a short problem at the end, while the reverse occurs in set (b), where there is a short problem at the beginning of the trial and a lengthy problem at the end. As a result of this ordering, the two arrangements involve the same processing work on each trial (because the same total set of operations is involved) but differing retention times (because in set (a) the retention requirements, resulting from the completion of each problem, commence at a later point in the trial).

Towse et al. (1998) also examined the efficiency of processing operations throughout each trial. They noted that on the first card, the subject performs the task with no memory load—it is only the completion of the card that generates the first memory item. On the second card, the processing occurs with a concurrent load of one item. On the third card, if there is one, processing is accompanied by a memory load of two items, and so on. Thus as the trial progresses, the memory load increases. From a resource-sharing perspective, then, processing efficiency should decline throughout the trial. A task-switching account gives no reason to suppose that this fade in efficiency will occur.

To summarize, the paradigm offers two lines of evidence to discriminate between theoretical accounts of working memory. The manipulation of temporal order of cards should affect span according to task switching but should not affect span according to resource sharing. Card-processing efficiency within a trial should not vary according to task switching but should decline according to resource sharing.

Towse et al. (1998) reported three experiments, overall using children between 6 and 11 years of age, in which the above paradigm was used with counting span, operation span (sums were presented and the answers formed the memoranda), and reading span (children read incomplete sentences and generated a suitable end word, which formed the memoranda). They found that in each experiment, span scores were reliably affected by the order in which the ensemble of cards appeared. Where the overall retention time was smaller because memory requirements started late, spans were larger. As explained above, this fits with the prediction made by the task-switching model (for additional convergent findings with a longitudinal component, see Ransdell & Hecht, 2003). There was also no consistent evidence that participants were slower to count cards at the end of the trial rather than at the beginning; some analyses found no effects, others found a reliable speeding up, and still others, a reliable slowing down but only with some test administration orders. Overall, within-trial analyses give the impression that processing times arise from a number of flexible strategies.

Individual differences in memory were stronger in these experiments, with respect to age—older children reached higher span levels—and processing ability—span scores correlated with the speed at which the processing was accomplished. The correlation between span and processing speed persisted after partialing out the effect of age. Among children, then, memory performance is affected by the rate at which the processing operations are completed. Working memory span scores reflect the influence of processing speed in addition to any influence from immediate memory skills. In turn, this provides a basis for explaining why working memory span might involve a combination of domain-specific and domain-general abilities. Thus, if there are multiple skills that contribute to performance, some of these might be idiosyncratic to a paradigm, one that is domain specific, whereas others reflect abiding traits relevant to many related tasks.

From the final experiment in which children were tested on both operation span and reading span, there was also evidence that these two tasks were correlated, albeit modestly. Independent measures of processing speed had also been administered (from the Kit of Factor-referenced Tests; Ekstrom, French, Harman, & Dermen, 1976); consequently, it was possible to consider whether the relationship between working memory speed and span related to the task-specific processes or more global processing parameters. Reading span was predicted by reading speed but was not uniquely predicted by general speed, while operation span was predicted by general speed. The data further underline the view that working memory variation in children comprises both general and specific skills.

Hitch, Towse, and Hutton (2001) were able to reassess children from the final study of Towse et al. (1998) on operation span and reading span 1 year after their initial assessment, and collect additional measures of scholastic ability. This permits replication of the previous work on the same sample of children and introduces several new dimensions to the research. In particular it allows assessment of relationships between working memory span, reading attainment, and numerical competence as well as longitudinal analysis of performance across a 12-month interval.

Hitch et al. (2001) replicated their previous finding that span scores were reliably affected by the order in which the ensemble of cards appeared. Once again, spans were larger when the results of processing operations had to be main-tained over shorter intervals, consistent with the prediction from task switching. However, analysis of changes in the time taken to perform processing operations within a trial gave a different result from before. When data were combined across the two studies for greater power, a significant increase in processing time from the start to the end of a trial was evident in both span tasks. Such an increase is consistent with the prediction from resource sharing (although Hitch et al., 2001, suggest other explanations might be offered too; see also Saito & Miyake, 2004) and is not predicted by task switching. Thus, while it is clear that task switching has robust effects on working memory span, it is equally clear that task switching does not provide a full account. This is something we return to later.

The data collected by Hitch et al. (2001) also allowed a test of the generality of the developmental relationship between working memory span and processing speed plotted by Case et al. (1982). To recapitulate, Case and colleagues observed a linear relationship between mean counting span and the mean time to perform counting operations across age groups, such that older children's superior spans were predictable from their faster processing speed (see Fig. 5.1). In our study three age groups were tested on two separate occasions, generating six points on the graph for each span task. Figure 5.3 shows reading span plotted against reading time and operation span plotted against the time to perform arithmetic operations. Two observations are immediately clear. One is that, to a first approximation, developmental changes in each type of span are linearly related to changes in the speed of the relevant processing operations, as for counting span. Thus, a range of very different tasks reflects in general a common developmental relationship between working memory span and processing speed.

A second observation is that the slopes and intercepts of the best-fitting linear functions for each span task are different. This is further evidence for differences between working memory span tasks. Once again, observations that are common to different span tasks suggest domain-general aspects of working memory whereas differences between tasks suggest the role of domain-specific factors. As regards theoretical interpretation of the relationship between span and speed, we have already noted that it can be explained in terms of either resource sharing, as Case et al (1982) originally proposed, or task switching (Towse et al., 1998). However, Hitch et al. (2001) pointed out that task switching gives a more parsimonious account of the different functions for different tasks shown in Figure 5.3, because it does not require additional assumptions in the crossover of linear functions.

Hitch et al. (2001) also analyzed individual differences in reading span and operation span in relation to children's performance on standardized tests of number skills and word reading (as assessed by a single-word reading task). There was substantial overlap in the variance attributable to reading span and operation span with respect to each of these two measures of scholastic attainment. However, there was also evidence to distinguish reading span from operation span, because each of these tasks explained significant, unique variance in single-word reading ability. It would be simple and elegant to claim that working memory span tasks can be thought of as entirely domain specific or completely domain general. However, once again, the data do not support such an inter-

pretation. Instead, it seems necessary to conclude that there are both domain-specific and domain-general aspects to performance in working memory span tasks. The analysis of individual differences also included various measures of processing speed, taken either on-line in each span task or off-line from the Kit of Factor-referenced Tests (Ekstrom et al., 1976). As expected, there was substantial overlap between speed and span for both measures of scholastic attainment. However, in each case there was variance unique to span that was not attributable to speed. So once again, we have evidence that span is indeed complex.

Longitudinal analysis in Hitch et al.'s (2001) study showed that a combined score for reading span and operation span explained significant unique variance in both number skills and word reading some 12 months later. This was so even after taking out variance attributable to combined span scores at the time of the scholastic assessment. This result is consistent with Daneman and Carpenter's (1980) claim that working memory span is related to cognitive ability. However, it goes further in demonstrating a longitudinal relationship that is additional to any concurrent relationship. One would expect to see a longitudinal relationship if working memory is a factor in children's acquisition of reading and arithmetical skills.

One interesting aspect of our research on children has been the absence of qualitative developmental changes. Our initial view was that task switching might characterize younger children's performance, perhaps because they lacked sufficient capacity to share resources between processing operations and retention in working memory, or had yet to acquire such a strategy (Towse & Hitch, 1995). With this view, one would expect increasing evidence for resource sharing among older children. However, this was not found. To check whether we might have missed a crucial stage of development by not testing children above the age of about 11, we investigated adult performance (Towse, Hitch, & Hutton, 2000).

Results once again showed significant effects of card completion order in reading span and operation span. Thus, for both tasks, spans were larger when the card order was such that

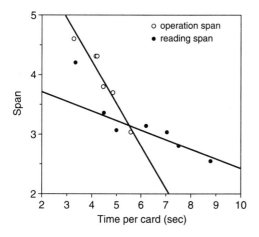

Figure 5.3. Reading span plotted against reading time and operation span plotted against the time to perform arithmetic operations. Each data point represents data on span and speed for a different age group of children at one of the two waves of testing run 1 year apart. (From Hitch et al., 2001.)

memory requirements started later rather than earlier within a trial (as in Towse et al., 1998). Furthermore, there were no discernible within-trial changes in the time taken to complete processing operations in either task. Thus, there was no evidence that processing became less efficient as the memory load increased from the start to the end of a trial. The one major contrast between adults and children was related to patterns of individual differences. Among adults, unlike children, there were no significant correlations between the speed of processing operations (whether measured on line or off-line) and span.

We interpret the adult data as showing that there is no clearly marked developmental transition from task switching to resource sharing in working memory. It seems that task switching is not an immature strategy but one that persists into adulthood. Given that task switching also provides a good account of adults' errors in doing mental arithmetic (Hitch, 1978), it seems that this conclusion generalizes beyond laboratory tasks. The qualitative developmental change was founded on the relative unimportance of individual differences in processing speed in relation to working memory span in adults compared to that of children (see Chapter 6 for similar indications of a shift away from the contribution of processing efficiency for span when moving from children to adults). However, it is not entirely clear what this means; it might reflect the greater importance of rehearsal in children's working memory (but see Hutton & Towse, 2001) or signal a difference in the balance of factors determining span, due, for example, to range effects. Thus, whereas span in children includes a component that is independent of speed as well as one that is correlated with speed, the first of these components may sweep up a much greater proportion of the variance in adults.

QUESTION 2: CRITICAL SOURCES OF WORKING MEMORY VARIATION

What is your view on the critical source(s) of working memory variability within your target population(s) of study? Why do you focus on the specific source(s) of variability in your research? Working memory span trials involve asking participants repeatedly to engage in some nontrivial processing task and remember pieces of information connected (semantically or temporally) to the processing. Span measures the maximum number of pieces of information that can be retained under these circumstances. We argue against the simple view that span is a measure of the resources available to working memory and nothing more. We argue instead that the temporal dynamics of trials are important, because children differ in the rate at which processing can be executed. This in turn affects the extent to which they are exposed to the effects of forgetting transient information, and so influences their ability to complete the task successfully.

We also suggest that there may be individual differences in the degree to which participants can sustain information in accessible form while engaged in a separate processing task. That is, overlaying the differences in the rate at which processing can be completed are differences in how destructive particular delays may be for memories. We have recently attempted to develop tests of this aspect of memory, and we describe these below.

A further source of variability that we consider is age. Whereas a simple model might suggest that individual differences for children at a particular age are paralleled by differences across age, we conclude that these issues may be dissociated. Explaining age differences on the one hand, and individual differences within an age group on the other, may require separate theoretical accounts. However, we also acknowledge that age as a variable is at best a proxy measure for some underlying change, psychological or biological, which takes place.

We discuss recent research that has examined individual differences of response-timing processes. Different phases of the recall process are sensitive to the configuration of working memory tests, and they relate to overall memory scores and external ability measures. Response timing offers clues to some of the variation that exists in working memory tests.

It is apparent, therefore, that we believe it is necessary to think about multiple sources of variability in working memory.

GOING BEYOND SPAN SCORES PER SE IN UNDERSTANDING WORKING MEMORY

Recently, together with Nelson Cowan and other colleagues, we have considered children's working memory span from an alternative and potentially complementary perspective, that of the chronometry of recall responses (Cowan et al., 2003; see also Towse & Cowan, 2005). As well as assessing the quality of memory recall responses, we also considered the timing of the successful response sequences. Over repeated trials (being a span procedure, this varied across participants), we partitioned every correctly recalled response sequence into separate segments. Past research has established distinct components in a recall string in immediate-memory tasks (e.g., Cowan et al., 1998). These include the preparatory interval (the initial delay between the recall cue and the onset of the participants' recall), word durations (the time taken to articulate each recalled item), and the inter-word intervals (the pauses between each response). On the basis of this previous research we measured the durations of the corresponding segments in recall in various working memory span tasks.

Cowan et al. (2003) considered response timing in both children and adults on different measures of memory. In two separate studies, participants were assessed on reading span, counting span, and listening span (participants listened to a sentence, decided whether it was true or not, and remembered the last word in the sentence). A digit span test was incorporated within one experiment also, providing a contrast between short-term memory and the various working memory measures. Various cognitive measures were also collected. These included reading- and numerical-skills attainment and high-school grade percentiles (for counting span and listening span).

One of the most striking aspects of the results was that response timing did not clearly differentiate digit span from counting span, although it did differentiate listening span and reading span from counting span. The principal differences were in the inter-word pauses, which were almost an order of magnitude slower in the two working memory span tasks that involved

language comprehension. Thus, children were doing something very different in listening span and reading span compared with counting span. One suggestion is that children were using a strategy of recalling information about the sentences and using this to identify their final words. No equivalent of this strategy would be possible in the case of counting span insofar as the processing, array counting, is not distinctive. Moreover, the different working memory spans also produced different patterns of correlations with scholastic measures, providing further evidence that they are not strictly equivalent. This view indicates that working memory span is dependent on the content of processing and, to a different degree across different span tasks, raises further challenges for the theory that the resource cost of processing is critical to performance.

A second major finding was that response time measures could account for additional variance in scholastic measures over and above variance associated with working memory spans. Thus, for reading span, response time measures correlated with standardized tests of reading and number skills and this was separable from their relationship with memory performance per se. These observations offer further confirmation that response time measures afford a different and distinctive insight into memory processes.

In summary, Cowan et al. (2003) provide further evidence for the complexity of working memory span, by pointing to some of the additional variables that contribute to performance. The timing of recall is a valuable source of information, capable not only of revealing substantial differences in the way various span tasks are performed but also unique variation in scholastic attainment. These observations move us further away from the idea of working memory span as a simple, domain-free measure.

Additional Measures of Working Memory

As we have just argued, the analysis of response timing can help to build a theoretical picture of working memory, revealing certain commonalities with short-term memory (in the general pattern of specific phases of recall), some striking differences from short-term memory, and indeed differences among working memory tasks themselves (in the duration of the recall phase). The approach is also relevant to individual-difference issues, especially since some but not other phases of recall are associated with working memory span scores. Response-timing analysis serves another useful purpose, however, in demonstrating the value of taking measures other than just the number of recallable items as a way of informing us about working memory.

This is particularly relevant in the context of the task-switching account of children's working memory and its development. We have been arguing that forgetting results from the requirement to hold recent information while completing processing activities. Processing operations that take a long time can be detrimental for working memory performance because memories can degrade. Moreover, there may be individual differences in the performance of processing operations and, separately, there may also be individual differences in the resilience of memory representations. That is, even assuming that a memory is initially formed at the same strength in two individuals, the course of forgetting may be more rapid for one of them. Even if these ideas are only partly accurate, it follows that there is more to working memory than just the number of independent items that can be remembered.

There are several different ways of exploring whether there are individual differences in the durability of representations in working memory. We have recently attempted to operationalize this issue by examining whether the endurance of memories can be measured in a meaningful way for children (Towse, Hitch, Hamilton, Peacock, & Hutton, 2005). We devised a task in which children completed a fixed number of problems that involved "processing + memory," as in complex span. However, instead of increasing the number of problems over successive sets of trials to determine span, we increased the time required to complete the processing operations for the given number of problems. We then derived a measure called *working memory period*, which represented the furthest point in the test at which items could be successfully remembered. In particular, we studied a reading-period task, in which children completed three sentences and then remembered the words that they generated, and operation period task, in which children calculated the answer to four arithmetic problems and then remembered these solutions. As should be apparent from the description, the objective was to attempt to assess the functional duration of working memory for a fixed number of items, rather than the limit on the number of items that can be recalled.

The results indicated that the period score had reasonable test-retest stability, in that it was at least comparable with span (and in one analysis, exceeded the reliability of span). Moreover, the period score had predictive power: operation period correlated with children's reading and number skills. Reading period likewise correlated with these cognitive skills, but particularly with reading. Towse et al. (2005) argued that working memory period was a potentially useful experimental device; the use of fixed length lists makes it amenable to addressing specific theoretical questions. That in itself makes it an interesting approach. However, in the context of a chapter on individual differences, it is the overlap in variance between the working memory period score and cognitive ability that is of particular relevance. Thus the length of the interval over which children could maintain a small number of items was significantly related to the ability to identify words or complete mathematical operations. We believe that this speaks to the value of asking questions about the limits of working memory that go beyond the almost ubiquitous, "How many?"

It should also be noted that we do not assume that the passage of time *causes* forgetting in working memory. Such an interpretation would be consistent with the data: as sentence length increases, there is more forgetting caused by temporal decay. However, it could equally be the case that longer processing events (such as sentences) put additional strain on the ability to inhibit non-target information and increase the likelihood of inhibitory failure (see Chapter 9). It might also be the case that more protracted sentences generate greater representational overlap with the target memory items, and that representational distinctiveness is an important component of memory (Saito & Miyake, 2004). Since we are not in a position to discriminate between these and other possibilities, our proposals are more modest: the endurance of representations is a relevant attribute for working memory, and the endurance can be tested by varying the exact processing events that accompany or produce the memory stimuli.

LIMITS OF THE TASK-SWITCHING ACCOUNT

We have described a series of experiments that provide a variety of evidence for the view that children's working memory performance is affected by the retention duration of the memory stimuli. The idea that memories are perishable, and that delaying the point of recall can impair the quality of recall, seems to us to have much merit, and forms the basis of the task-switching model we advocate here. It is consistent with a very large research literature on immediate memory (i.e., short-term memory) and makes intuitive sense. It is also consistent with data from the experiments designed to test whether it is credible. It helps to explain experimental phenomena and to account for individual differences. And it can be complemented by other findings—for example, with respect to the contribution of recall processes, and situations where processing and memories are mutually supportive, since even where processing scaffolds later recall, one can anticipate that that forgetting takes place during the execution of processing activity. Thus, the task-switching model avoids the need to draw a sharp distinction between processing (for example, that which occurs when a sentence is read for comprehension) and memory (that which enables certain items to be retained for subsequent recall). Such distinctions are inherent in the notion of a trade-off between processing and memory.

At the same time, the task-switching model does not offer a full or comprehensive account of working memory span. We have repeatedly sought to note this. Towse and Hitch (1995) considered conceptual limits. Making the processing task shorter might improve span scores, but of course eliminating a concurrent processing task, akin to a short-term memory task, does not eliminate capacity constraints. Clearly, therefore, there must be other factors to consider. Furthermore, Hitch et al. (2001) noted that controlling for processing speed did not eliminate age differences in working memory, which implies that additional factors influence developmental change. Towse et al. (2000) found that adults' working memory was not related to their processing speed (see also Engle, Cantor, & Carullo, 1992) and thus, while processing delays did affect performance, working memory variation was primarily influenced by some other variable. Towse, Hitch, and Hutton (2002), using an interpolated-task paradigm, argued that the task-switching model did not easily account for age differences in memory performance, nor did it offer a clear explanation for, in one experiment, memory performance being equivalent when the retention intervals were (unexpectedly) different. Response timing analyses from Cowan et al. (2003) also suggest that working memory performance is shaped at recall, and not only during "retention" (see also Haarmann, Davelaar, & Usher, 2003).

Thus, it is important to distinguish our position that retention delay is important for working memory performance (perhaps especially among children) from any straw man that suggests working memory is purely determined by task-processing time. Moreover, we regard both the inadequacy of task switching as a complete account and the proposal that working memory is multifaceted and multidetermined to be both realistic and exciting. The conclusion is realistic because working memory span is a complex task that may well resist being satisfactorily captured by a single mechanism. The conclusion is exciting because it provides a challenge in determining how the account can best be augmented, and also because the account need not be exclusive; other hypotheses may comfortably coexist alongside the ideas we have proposed.

Some recent work, published as this chapter was first drafted, has called into question the task-switching account of working memory. Barrouillet, Barnadin, and Camos (2004) devised span tasks in which the processing operations were discrete and externally paced. By altering the speed of pacing they were able to separate out effects of the total duration of processing from the number of processing operations performed. Among their findings was the observation that, for a given number of processing operations, spans were higher when the duration of processing was longer. Barrouillet et al. (2004) point out that this observation goes against a simple task-switching account in which "there is no active maintenance of stored totals that competes with the execution of counting operations" (Hitch et al., 2001, p. 185). As we have seen, this latter account predicts that span should decline as the total duration of processing increases. Barrouillet et al. argue for a more sophisticated form of task switching in which participants switch attention between processing and maintenance *during* intervening activity. Thus, when the external pacing of such switching is high, this reduces the time available for active maintenance in the gaps between processing operations, resulting in lower spans. Barrouillet and colleagues also show that spans are lower in their paradigm when the difficulty of the processing operations is increased (e.g., retrieving a digit from long-term memory as in "$4 + 1 = ?$" as opposed to simply reading the digit as in "$4 + 1 = 5$"). This leads them to suggest that the attention-switching process is resource limited. To account for these findings they propose a hybrid "time-based resource-sharing model" as an alternative to simple task switching.

We have a number of comments to make about this interesting and ingenious work. The first is that we of course agree on the need to elaborate on the simple task-switching model; we have been arguing here that it is not enough. Towse et al. (2005) have noted the importance of considering the retention function of each memorandum, rather than just the entire memory set, while Cowan et al. (2003) have pointed

to processes during recall that affect working memory performance. Towse et al. (2002) also recognize the possibility that memory "consolidation" might occur with interpolated tasks, that is, rehearsal between presentation and recall of memory stimuli. In short, we have moved beyond the simple task-switching account that Barrouillet et al. argue against.

Second, we have concerns about the generality of their results. Thus, if one paces a processing task slowly enough it is entirely unsurprising that participants will use any unfilled gaps to maintain the memory items (leading to issues grappled with by Jarrold & Bayliss in Chapter 6). We suggest that participants are less likely to switch to memory maintenance when processing involves a continuous chain of interdependent operations (e.g., as in reading a sentence) than when operations are discrete and sequentially independent. Third, we note that Barrouillet et al. studied adults. It is not clear that their results and interpretation would necessarily apply to children (nor that their emphasis on the resource demand of recall activity fits entirely comfortably with the focus on controlled attention in retention [Chapter 2], or representational overlap at recall, see Saito & Miyake, 2004 in adults). Children may show the same effects, yet we caution against any presumption that children and adults must be alike.

Thus, in summary, Barrouillet and colleagues show that simple task switching cannot explain adult performance in particular versions of the working memory span task where processing is discrete and externally paced. We have no problem accepting this. However, we do question the degree to which one would want to generalize from such tasks to other working memory span tasks, to situations where processing and storage may be integrated rather than in competition, and to children. Moreover, we think it is important to recognize the degree of alignment in the different views, and not just focus on differences. There is agreement in suggesting some role for task switching, that is, alternation between processing and memory activities; similarly, there is agreement too that memories may not be continuously maintained throughout an experimental trial, but subject to loss and reactivation. Moreover, we agree that participants may be tempted to insert episodes of rehearsal, as and when they can into an experimental trial (Towse et al., 2002). This could produce task switching at two different grain sizes of analysis; at a micro level within a processing episode and a macro level between separate episodes.

QUESTION 3: CONSIDERATION OF OTHER SOURCES OF VARIATION IN WORKING MEMORY

Do you find other sources of working memory variability proposed in this volume to be applicable to your target population of study? Are these sources of working memory variation compatible or incompatible with your view of your target population?   Our contention is that working memory in general, and working memory span in particular, is affected by several factors. A corollary of this position is that we anticipate that several additional sources of working memory variation will be identified, and their relationship to known factors will need to be clarified and specified. We make no claim about the sufficiency of our theoretical account as a description of working memory. Indeed, we provide evidence in this chapter that there are aspects of developmental change in particular that are not explained by processes that we know about, and we describe other gaps in our account of what determines working memory span. Consequently, we expect that a more complete account of children's working memory will draw upon a range of sources of variation in working memory.

One of our proposals, set out in this chapter, is that the temporal dynamics of working memory span are critical for explaining children's performance. We have chosen to frame this within a "task-switching" account. We find that this is a helpful way of trying to understand the circumstances under which working memory span tasks can be difficult for children. Essentially, the argument is that children's ability to complete successfully a working memory span trial is sensitive to the time spent on the processing phase, since this affects the amount of

forgetting that accrues. The attempt to go beyond a general notion of resource sharing, according to which a central workspace is entirely flexible in the allocation of resources to cognitive tasks, is a thread shared with Caplan, Waters, and DeDe (Chapter 11), who point to language-specific processes in comprehension that are separable from working memory constraints.

More generally, we have viewed resource sharing as a rather crude theoretical entry point, often used evasively and in the abstract. In this context, while we are somewhat skeptical of some attempts to revive resource-sharing ideas (e.g., Barrouillet et al., 2004) and wonder about their capacity to explain relevant developmental phenomena, we greatly welcome the much greater theoretical specificity and precision that these ideas bring, which makes theory comparison more feasible.

With respect to different accounts of working memory variation, it should be noted that we recognize that time itself (i.e., temporal decay of memory traces) may not be the material cause of forgetting. For example, the processing phase of the task may lead to forgetting because of the increase in interference among memory items, and/or because inhibition of irrelevant material cannot be sustained effectively. Thus, to focus on the impact of processing time as we do, is not inherently incompatible with proposals that, for example, inhibition failures produce recall errors—especially since it might make sense to argue that interference or inhibition failures are more likely to occur when there is a longer retention duration, because there is more opportunity for "confusions" to arise.

Accordingly, we are sympathetic to the notion that inhibitory control plays a significant role in working memory performance (Chapter 9). The attempt to tease apart the processing and retention constraints in a task with a fixed-duration processing window is an important enterprise (Chapter 6), and we view the conclusion that retention ability contributes to complex span independently of processing as both plausible and consistent with the ideas expressed here (thus, our focus on the impact of processing activities for working memory span should not be taken to mean that memory has no independent role; rather our view is that at some of the properties of working memory tasks can be attributed to processing differences instead of just memory; see Hutton & Towse, 2001). Furthermore, we agree with Hale and colleagues (Chapter 7) that processing speed is important for working memory, and we share with them as well as with Jarrold and Bayliss the view that working memory comprises both domain-general and domain- or task-specific components. Our inventory of functions that fall under these two headings differs somewhat from that of these authors, but this reflects as much the choice of issues to focus on as it does an allegiance to a limited set of variables.

Another of our proposals is that response time processes (that is, examining the chronometry of recall) can be informative not only for how children carry out working memory tasks, but also for revealing some of the strategies and skills that differentiate those children who show particular strengths at the task. We view response-timing variables partly as markers for other cognitive processes, and we discuss what these processes might represent.

We argue that not all working memory span tasks are the same. Although we agree that most span tasks show impressive and sometimes similar correlational profiles, and we recognize that they may share some core cognitive properties, we review several pieces of evidence that indicate nontrivial differences between working memory span tasks. We interpret these differences as evidence that working memory span reflects a combination of domain-specific and domain-general factors. We discuss how these differences might have an impact on variation in working memory, in particular considering age-related changes in span.

We also believe that accounts of long-term working memory are potentially relevant to understanding working memory and developmental change (see, e.g., Ericsson & Delaney, 1999). The notion that networks of long-term knowledge representations can facilitate the efficient structuring and integration of target memories is a view that appears consistent with the ideas we analyze in this chapter. For example, it provides one way of conceptualizing

the domain specificity of different working memory span tasks.

An important question that we feel requires investigation (i.e., remains unresolved) is the overlap between working memory as measured by span tests, and working memory as understood within concepts of mental control (an issue developed by Reuter-Lorenz and Jonides in Chapter 10). We regard this question as relevant within a developmental context because notions of executive control extend to issues such as theory of mind and conflict resolution (Towse & Cowan, 2005).

WHAT DOES A WORKING MEMORY SPAN TASK MEASURE?

In this chapter, we have drawn evidence from a number of sources, principally our own, to illustrate some of the cognitive processes measured by working memory span tests. What have we learned? In working memory span tasks, it is self-evident that the participant cannot completely and continuously focus effort on the retention of information because there are processing requirements, such as the need to comprehend a sentence. This processing task is influential in a number of ways. It increases the likelihood that information will be forgotten since memory representations may not be actively maintained (Towse & Hitch, 1995; Towse et al., 1998). The processing task itself may require information to be remembered, adding further stress of the system's ability to retain the experimentally identified memory items (Towse et al., 2002). In the case of reading span, the processing task provides a temporal and semantic context for the memory items, such that recall may involve consideration of the entire processing episode (Copeland & Radvansky, 2001; Cowan et al., 2003; Osaka, Nishizaki, Komori, & Osaka, 2002). Of course, the contribution from processing may vary substantially with the type of working memory test—outside of language-based spans, processing events may offer primarily a temporal context for discriminating memory items.

We believe these recent perspectives increase the attractiveness of the principle of an episodic-buffer component of working memory (Baddeley, 2000), insofar as it establishes a venue for bringing together different types of representation (including semantic, in the sense of thematic, information). It also dissociates executive control from memory functions as part of the central executive, and is thereby highly compatible the task-switching account, as well as a perspective that incorporates domain-specific views of memory. An episodic buffer offers a structural alternative to the long-term working memory framework (e.g., Ericsson & Delaney, 1999).

A dominant assumption driving theoretical research into working memory and variation in working memory is that it is legitimate to ask the simple question of how people carry out working memory tasks. At issue, then, is *which* theoretical account is the most satisfactory. Towse and Cowan (2005) have recently suggested that a more pluralist approach might be appropriate. That is, given the complexity of working memory, and the richness of the data from working memory studies, individuals may differ not only in information-processing capacities but also in the type of strategy that they call upon. That is, perhaps there are several qualitatively different ways in which a task can be completed, just as there are different theories of working memory represented in this volume. There are several sources of evidence for this position. For example, recent analysis has examined recall timing in reading span as a function of task experience. Towse, Cowan, Horton & Whytock (2006) compared how children recalled correct sequences on two separate occasions and compared recall when the trial format was either unfamiliar, or followed exposure to similar trials. Of relevance to the present argument, it was found that the timing of recall changed even in circumstances where overall span levels were equivalent. Furthermore, there were changes in the patterns of correlations between memory and ability as children wcrc exposed to reading span trials. Thus, rather than performance just improving, it seems as though experience at the reading span task led to changes in performance strategy. The results underline the possibility that there is more flexibility in the way that the task

is accomplished than many theoretical positions would concede.

Furthermore, as we noted earlier, Cowan et al. (2003) report important differences among working memory tasks. Preparatory intervals and inter-word pauses are longer for reading span and listening span than for counting span. One explanation for this is that the sentence frames in the reading and listening span tasks provide much more in the way of a distinct representation than for counting span (where the counting process for different arrays is really pretty much alike), and these sentence representations are accessed during recall. Therefore, some working memory span tests may involve integration between processing and memory instead of simply competition. If one accepts this perspective, it seems a small step to the argument that *some* individuals might approach span tasks by attempting to integrate the different requirements, while others choose not to do so.

Finally, we have noted that both children and adults are affected by the retention duration of memory stimuli. However, individual differences in adults' working memory span are not correlated with on-line processing speed, although the correlation is reliable among primary-school children. Thus, there is a qualitative difference. This conclusion could be rephrased as adults' strategies on the working memory span tasks can be differentiated from those of children, despite some underlying continuities. Since adults and children differ in this way, it would not be surprising to discover that some adults have a performance profile that is indistinguishable from that of children, and some children have a profile that is indistinguishable from that of adults. In other words, there are qualitative differences in the way that individuals approach the task.

QUESTION 4: CONTRIBUTIONS TO GENERAL WORKING MEMORY THEORY

What does the variability within your target population of study tell us about the structure, function, and/or organization of working memory in general? Variability is of course inherent to a developmental perspective on working memory. The challenge is to understand and explain developmental change, and assess the correspondence between variation in working memory both within and across age groups. Task performance shows clear changes with age, accompanied by profound changes in the skills and experience that older children and adults can bring to bear on cognitive tasks. Our research identifies both qualitative and quantitative changes in working memory span performance across age, and we attempt to integrate these into a model of the task in which multiple processes are seen to be relevant

Although research is still very much building up a picture of the nature and mechanisms underlying differences between children and adults, it is already apparent that what is true for adult working memory is not necessarily true in every case for children's working memory, though it may be in some. Certainly, one needs to be cautious in assuming that conclusions from children will apply to adults, or vice versa, and we attempt to provide illustrations of such developmental differences. We note that some of the contemporary challenges to the arguments we put forward come from research with adults (Barrouillet et al., 2004; Saito & Miyake, 2004). That is not cause to dismiss these critical findings, of course, but it does mean that they need to be evaluated in their context.

One of the aspects of many, though not all, complex working memory tasks is that the completion of processing is under the control of the participant. Therefore, as children vary in their ability to carry out relevant processing operations (within and between ages), their ability to interleave these activities with memory requirements is affected.

With respect to the value of individual difference, we argue that experimental and correlational approaches are best seen as having an interactive and iterative relationship in the specification of theory about working memory. They are often suited to investigating different types of issues, though they work best when they provide convergent evidence for a particular conclusion.

We use our research into working memory span to exemplify the gains from both research methodologies. Our initial collaborative work on counting span adopted an experimental approach to assess the veracity of the dominant theory of working memory mechanisms. Subsequent work (see also Barrouillet & Camos, 2001; Barrouillet et al., 2004; Saito & Miyake, 2004) has pursued an experimental approach in an attempt to understand the cognitive building blocks of the working memory span paradigm. At the same time, the implications of our early findings feed into issues such as domain specificity of processes, the impact of processing speed on the determination of working memory ability, and the relationship between working memory and high-level cognitive abilities. Individual-difference analyses offer a highly suitable vehicle for addressing these questions. In turn, these approaches have led to further predictions for experimental work, and indeed have encouraged the development of alternative and potentially complimentary measures of working memory (Towse et al., 2005).

TOWARD A CONCLUSION

Our studies of working memory span in children point to a number of general observations that seem to apply across different working memory span tasks. One set of these observations relates principally to what we have called the *temporal dynamics* of working memory. Thus, the time durations for which temporary information must be held are important, such that the longer the interval the lower the working memory span. This is evident both in experimental manipulations (where the sequence of processing operations is varied so that different patterns of durations are experienced) and in the finding that children who process information faster tend to have higher spans. The speed–span relationship is found both across age groups and across individuals when effects of age are partialed out (Hitch et al., 2001; Towse et al. 1998), but it is not found in adults (Towse et al., 2000). The importance of time intervals is consistent with task switching, according to which one factor limiting working memory span is the rapid forgetting of temporary information while performing a sequence of operations. In contrast, we found only very modest experimental support for the common explanation of span as reflecting a limit on the capacity for resource sharing. Thus, children's spans were unaffected by a substantial difference in the difficulty of processing operations (Towse & Hitch, 1995), and there was only limited support for the prediction that fewer resources remain available to sustain processing operations as memory load increases. Nevertheless, there was some evidence for an interaction between memory load and processing efficiency, underlining our view that task switching does not give complete account of the limit on working memory span.

At the same time as finding commonalities across various working memory span tasks, significant and substantial differences were revealed in some analyses of individual differences. Thus, while different span tasks did tend to correlate with one another, they also showed different patterns of correlation with children's performance on tests of reading and arithmetic and with their scores on tests of processing speed. As we have noted, these observations point to a role for domain-specific processes in any particular test of working memory span. To develop a fuller theoretical account of the complexities of span, we take the view that it is necessary to tease apart the domain-specific component of any particular working memory span task from the domain-free component common to all such tasks. We suggest that task switching is an important factor in the domain-free component of working memory span. From our evidence it seems more important and pervasive than resource sharing, but we cannot rule out resource sharing or indeed other factors as components of the domain-free component of working memory span.

As regards the domain-specific component of working memory span, we note that this has two orthogonal dimensions, corresponding to modality of information and information content, as in Fodor's (1983) horizontal vs. vertical classification scheme. In the present context, *modality* refers chiefly to whether information is verbal or visuospatial, whereas *content* refers to the knowledge domain to which the information relates, such as reading or arithmetic.

The span tasks we have studied in detail all involve a substantial verbal component. As a consequence, we interpret our empirical evidence for domain specificity in terms of differences between the knowledge domains tapped by each span task. One way of thinking about this type of specificity is in terms of the concept of long-term working memory (Ericsson & Delaney, 1999), whereby the organization of knowledge structures within a domain influences the operation of working memory. We note, however, that other investigators have found evidence for domain specificity in span tasks that seems more appropriately interpreted in terms of modality. For example, in the study of Bayliss et al. (2003), evidence for domain specificity came from working memory span tasks that involved different combinations of visuospatial and verbal processing and storage. Modality specificity of this type fits more neatly with the multicomponent model of working memory (Baddeley, 1986; Baddeley & Hitch, 1974; see also Hale, Bronik, & Fry, 1997). The notion of an episodic buffer provides an additional domain-specific constraint that can help account for differences between tasks, particularly complex memory tasks likely to involve integrated or multiple representations incorporating thematic information from processing. In turn, this suggests that working memory span or period tasks are not just dual-task paradigms. Moreover, the four-component working memory model may allow for an explanation of both vertical and horizontal domain specificity.

We find complementary evidence from experimental and individual-differences approaches to determining mechanisms of working memory span in children. The two approaches converge on our main conclusion, namely that working memory is constrained by a temporal dynamic. A second conclusion stems mostly from studies of individual differences, that working memory span is multifaceted and involves domain-free and domain-specific sources of variation. A more specific example of this conclusion is the argument we pursue that working memory can require the integration of task requirements, and not just resolution of the competition between them. We attribute the sensitivity of working memory to temporal factors to the domain-free component of span, given that we find consistent effects over a variety of span tasks. We speculate that the domain-specific component of span has two orthogonal dimensions, one of which reflects the modality of information storage, as in Baddeley's (1986) account of the structure of working memory, the other of which is knowledge based, as in Ericsson & Kintsch's (1995) view of long-term working memory.

Our central goal is to develop a more satisfactory and complete account of working memory and its development. In this regard, we value the methodological control that is available from experimental research, and which provides a foundation from which an understanding of cognitive systems can be understood through classical hypothesis testing. Insofar as working memory span tasks correlate well with complex cognitive skills, there are reasons to believe that our interest in working memory has applications. Yet, appreciating the forces that drive this and other individual differences relationships is for us a means toward our central goal, and not an end in itself. Individual differences provide a complementary perspective on working memory and provide another way of testing theoretical accounts, sometimes with greater purchase than is possible experimentally. Likewise, mapping out the differences in the way that younger children and older children carry out working memory tasks is a staging post on the road toward appreciating why the mature system takes the form it does, and how developmental change takes place.

BOX 5.1. SUMMARY ANSWERS TO BOOK QUESTIONS

1. THE OVERARCHING THEORY OF WORKING MEMORY

Working memory is a limited-capacity system that maintains and operates on fragile representations in complex thought. We regard working memory as a multicomponent system that comprises a central executive, a phonological loop, a visuospatial sketchpad, and possibly an episodic buffer. We view working memory span as a truly complex measure, yet our data lead us to believe that the interaction between processing and memory is an important ingredient that distinguishes it from many other tasks. This interaction occurs in different and subtle ways, with elements of both competition and cooperation.

2. CRITICAL SOURCES OF WORKING MEMORY VARIATION

We argue that variation in working memory in normally developing children arises from several factors. These include differences in the rate at which information can be processed, the ability to sustain information in accessible form while engaged in a separate processing task, response-timing processes, and the parameters of specific subsystems. A further source of variability is age. However, we suggest that separate theoretical accounts may be required to explain age differences on the one hand, and individual differences within an age group on the other. We acknowledge that age is at best a proxy measure for some underlying psychological or biological change.

3. OTHER SOURCES OF WORKING MEMORY VARIATION

We anticipate that several additional sources of working memory variation will be identified besides those we have identified in our own research. We recognize that processing time itself may not be the material cause of forgetting in working memory tasks and that differences in susceptibility to interference or the ability to inhibit irrelevant material may also contribute. We share with others the view that working memory comprises both domain-general and domain-specific components. We suggest that far from memory activities occurring in isolation, the processing context and long-term knowledge contribute to working memory performance.

4. CONTRIBUTIONS TO GENERAL WORKING MEMORY THEORY

Our data lead us to suggest that information processing and storage interact in working memory through task switching. This account identifies the fragility of representations as a limiting factor in working memory, and is a counterweight to the usual assumption of a limit on resource sharing. We propose that task switching is a general feature of working memory but that the balance between task switching and other limiting factors varies across individuals and during development. Other data suggest that working memory has the same multicomponent structure in children as in adults. Overall, working memory appears to serve a similar function in adults and children, given that variation in working memory in children is related to cognitive skills and their acquisition.

Note

1. Close examination of this study reveals an ambiguity. The plotted figure in Case et al.'s (1982) article suggests that adults were counting objects at a rate of 450 ms per item, yet the Results section records a rate of 490 ms. The value used here is taken from the text, although this may be a typographical error, since it makes the adult data appear more discrepant from the children's speed–span function than one might expect from other aspects of the study.

References

Alloway, T. P., Gathercole, S. E., Willis, C., & Adams, A. (2004). A structural analysis of working memory and related cognitive skills in young children. *Journal of Experimental Child Psychology*, 87(2), 85–106.

Baddeley, A. D. (1986). *Working memory*. Oxford: Clarendon Press.

Baddeley, A. D. (2000). The episodic buffer: a new component of working memory. *Trends in Cognitive Sciences*, 4, 417–423.

Baddeley, A. D. (1994). Working memory: The interface between memory and cognition. In D. L. Schacter & E. Tulving (Eds.), *Memory systems 1994* (pp. 351–367). Cambridge, MA: MIT Press.

Baddeley, A. D., & Hitch, G. J. (1974). Working memory. In G. H. Bower (Ed.), *The psychology of learning and motivation: Advances in research and theory* (Vol. 8, pp. 47–89). New York: Academic Press.

Baddeley, A. D., & Lieberman, K. (1980). Spatial working memory. In R. Nickerson (Ed.), *Attention and performance* (pp. 521–539). Hillsdale, NJ: Lawrence Erlbaum Associates.

Baddeley, A. D., Lewis, V. J., & Vallar, G. (1984). Exploring the articulatory loop. *Quarterly Journal of Experimental Psychology*, 36, 233–252.

Barrouillet, P., Bernadin, S., & Camos, V. (2004). Time constraints and resource sharing in adults' working memory span. *Journal of Experimental Psychology: General*, 133, 83–100.

Baddeley, A. D., Thomson, N., & Buchanan, M. (1975). Word length and the structure of short-term memory. *Journal of Verbal Learning and Verbal Behavior*, 9, 176–189.

Barrouillet, P., & Camos, V. (2001). Developmental increase in working memory span: Resource sharing or temporal decay? *Journal of Memory and Language*, 45, 1–20.

Bayliss, D. M., Jarrold, C., Baddeley, A. D., Gunn, D. M., & Leigh, E. (2005). Mapping the developmental constraints on working memory span performance. *Developmental Psychology*, 41(4), 579–597.

Bayliss, D. M., Jarrold, C., Gunn, D. M., & Baddeley, A. D. (2003). The complexities of complex span: Explaining individual differences in working memory in children and adults. *Journal of Experimental Psychology: General*, 131, 71–92.

Case, R. (1985). *Intellectual development: Birth to adulthood*. New York: Academic Press.

Case, R., Kurland, M., & Goldberg, J. (1982). Operational efficiency and the growth of short-term memory span. *Journal of Experimental Child Psychology*, 33, 386–404.

Copeland, D. E., & Radvansky, G. A. (2001). Phonological similarity in working memory. *Memory & Cognition*, 29, 774–776.

Cowan, N., Towse, J. N., Hamilton, Z., Saults, J. S., Elliott, E. M., Lacey, J. F., Moreno, M. V., & Hitch, G. J. (2003). Children's working memory processes: A response-timing analysis. *Journal of Experimental Psychology: General*, 132, 113–132.

Cowan, N., Wood, N. L., Wood, P. K., Keller, T. A., Nugent, L. D., & Keller, C. V. (1998). Two separate verbal processing rates contributing to short-term memory span. *Journal of Experimental Psychology: General*, 127, 141–160.

Daneman, M., & Blennerhassett, A. (1984). How to assess the listening comprehension skills of prereaders. *Journal of Educational Psychology*, 76, 1372–1381.

Daneman, M., & Carpenter, P. A. (1980). Individual differences in working memory and reading. *Journal of Verbal Learning and Verbal Behavior*, 19, 450–466.

Ekstrom, R. B., French, J. W., Harman, H. H., & Dermen, D. (1976). *Manual for kit of factor-referenced cognitive tests*. Princeton, NJ: Educational Testing Service.

Emerson, M. J., Miyake, A., & Rettinger, D. A. (1999). Individual differences in integrating and coordinating multiple sources of information. *Journal of Experimental Psychology: Learning, Memory, and Cognition*, 25, 1300–1321.

Engle, R. W., Cantor, J., & Carullo, J. J. (1992). Individual differences in working memory and comprehension: A test of four hypotheses. *Journal of Experimental Psychology: Learning, Memory and Cognition*, 18, 972–992.

Ericsson, K. A., & Delaney, P. F. (1999). Long-term working memory as an alternative to capacity models of working memory in everyday skilled performance. In A. Miyake & P. Shah (Eds.), *Models of working memory* (pp. 257–297). New York: Cambridge University Press.

Ericsson, K. A., & Kintsch, W. (1995). Long-term working memory. *Psychological Review*, 102, 211–245.

Fodor, J. A. (1983). *The modularity of mind*. Cambridge, MA: MIT Press.

Hale, S., Bronik, M. D., & Fry, A. F. (1997). Verbal and spatial working memory in school-age chil-dren: Developmental differences in susceptibility to interference. *Developmental Psychology*, 33, 364–371.

Haarmann, H. J., Davelaar, E. J., & Usher, M. (2003). Individual differences in semantic short-term memory capacity and reading comprehension. *Journal of Memory and Language*, 48, 320–345.

Halliday, M. S., & Hitch, G. J. (1988). Developmental applications of working memory. In G. Claxton (Ed.), *New directions in cognition* (pp. 193–222). London: Routledge and Keegan Paul.

Hitch, G. J. (1978). The role of short-term working memory in mental arithmetic. *Cognitive Psychology*, 10, 302–323.

Hitch, G. J., & Halliday, M. S. (1983). Working memory in children. *Philosophical Transactions of the Royal Society of London (B) 302*, 325–340.

Hitch, G. J., Halliday, M. S., & Littler, J. E. (1989). Item identification time and rehearsal rate as predictors of memory span in children. *Quarterly Journal of Experimental Psychology*, 41A, 321–337.

Hitch, G. J., & McAuley, E. (1991). Working memory in children with specific arithmetical learning difficulties. *British Journal of Psychology*, 82, 375–386.

Hitch, G. J., Towse, J. N., & Hutton, U. M. Z. (2001). What limits working memory span? Theoretical accounts and applications for scholastic development. *Journal of Experimental Psychology: General*, 130, 184–198.

Hitch, G. J., Woodin, M. E., & Baker, S. (1989). Visual and phonological components of working memory in children. *Memory & Cognition*, 17, 175–185.

Hulme, C., Thomson, N., Muir, C., & Lawrence, A. (1984). Speech rate and the development of short-term memory span. *Journal of Experimental Child Psychology*, 38, 241–253.

Hutton, U. M. Z., & Towse, J. N. (2001). Short-term memory and working memory as indices of children's cognitive skills. *Memory*, 9, 383–394.

Klatzky, R. L. (1980). *Human memory: Structures and processes* (2nd ed.). San Francisco: Freeman.

Leather, C. V., & Henry, L. A. (1994). Working memory span and phonological awareness tasks as predictors of early reading ability. *Journal of Experimental Child Psychology, 58,* 88–111.

Osaka, M., Nishizaki, Y., Komori, M., & Osaka, N. (2002). Effect of focus on verbal working memory: Critical role of the focus word in reading. *Memory and Cognition, 30,* 562–571.

Quinn, J. G., & McConnell, J. (1996). Irrelevant pictures in visual working memory. *Quarterly Journal of Experimental Psychology, 49A,* 200–215.

Ransdell, S., & Hecht, S. A. (2003). Time and resource limits on working memory: Cross age consistency in counting span performance. *Journal of Experimental Child Psychology, 86,* 303–313.

Saito, S., & Miyake, A. (2004). On the nature of forgetting and the processing-storage relationship in reading span performance. *Journal of Memory and Language, 50,* 425–443.

Siegel, L. S., & Ryan, E. B. (1989). The development of working memory in normally achieving and subtypes of learning disabled children. *Child Development, 60,* 973–980.

Towse, J. N., & Cowan, N. (2005). Working memory and its relevance for cognitive development. In W. Schneider, R. Schumann-Hengsteler & B. Sodian (Eds.), *Young children's cognitive development: Interrelationships among executive functioning, working memory, verbal ability, and theory of mind* (pp. 9–37). Mahwah, NJ: Lawrence Erlbaum Associates.

Towse, J. N., Cowan, N., Horton, N., & Whytock, S. (2006). Task experience and children's working memory performance: A perspective from recall timing. Manuscript submitted for publication.

Towse, J. N., & Hitch, G. J. (1995). Is there a relationship between task demand and storage space in tests of working memory capacity? *Quarterly Journal of Experimental Psychology, 48A,* 108–124.

Towse, J. N., Hitch, G. J., Hamilton, Z., Peacock, K., & Hutton, U. M. Z. (2005). Working memory period: The endurance of mental representations. *Quarterly Journal of Experimental Psychology, 58A,* 547–571.

Towse, J. N., Hitch, G. J., & Hutton, U. M. Z. (1998). A reevaluation of working memory capacity in children. *Journal of Memory and Language, 39,* 195–217.

Towse, J. N., Hitch, G. J., & Hutton, U. M. Z. (2000). On the interpretation of working memory span in adults. *Memory & Cognition, 28,* 341–348.

Towse, J. N., Hitch, G. J., & Hutton, U. M. Z. (2002). On the nature of the relationship between processing activity and item retention in children. *Journal of Experimental Child Psychology, 82,* 156–184.

Towse, J. N., & Houston-Price, C. M. T. (2001). Combining representations in working memory: A brief report. *British Journal of Developmental Psychology, 19,* 319–324.

Walker, P., Hitch, G. J., Dewhurst, S. A., Whiteley, H. E., & Brandimonte, M. A. (1997). The representation of nonstructural information in visual memory: Evidence from image combination. *Memory & Cognition, 25,* 484–491.

Yee, P. L., Hunt, E., & Pellegrino, J. W. (1991). Coordinating cognitive information: Task effects and individual differences in integrating information from several sources. *Cognitive Psychology, 23,* 615–680.

6

Variation in Working Memory Due to Typical and Atypical Development

CHRISTOPHER JARROLD and DONNA M. BAYLISS

Studies of working memory performance in adults have shown that the ability to hold information in mind while manipulating or processing other material is a reliable predictor of a range of other skills. For example, in a seminal study, Daneman and Carpenter (1980) presented adult undergraduate participants with a reading span task in which they were required to read a series of sentences and remember the final words from each of these sentences for subsequent serial recall. The maximum number, or span, of final words that individuals could successfully hold in mind was found to be related to verbal comprehension skills and to individuals' verbal Scholastic Aptitude Test (SAT) scores. Subsequent research has confirmed that performance on this kind of working memory measure, namely a task that combines the need to process information with the apparently simultaneous requirement to store the product of that processing for subsequent recall, can predict adult participants' verbal abilities (see Daneman & Merikle, 1996) as well as their spatial skills (Shah & Miyake, 1996), mathematics competence (Daneman & Tardif, 1987), reasoning abilities (Kyllonen & Christal, 1990), and general fluid intelligence (Conway, Cowan, Bunting, Therriault, & Minkoff, 2002; Engle, Tuholski, Laughlin, & Conway, 1999).

Given these findings, a better grasp of the causes of variation in working memory performance would clearly have important implications, both in terms of the theoretical understanding of the processes involved in higher-order cognitive abilities such as reading and mathematics, and in terms of potential educational benefits. It is possible, of course, that certain sources of variance in working memory task performance are irrelevant to the prediction of other abilities (see Maybery & Do, 2003). However, the factors that mediate the link between working memory measures and other cognitive skills must be a subset of those factors that constrain performance on working memory tasks. Consequently, one can ask two specific research questions about variance in working memory that are linked to the general theoretical questions addressed in each chapter of this volume. The first is: what are the critical sources of variation in working memory task performance? The second, which has clear implications for theoretical accounts of general working memory theory, is: what aspect of this variance mediates the relationship between task performance and abilities such as reading and math?

The aim of our research is to address these two research questions by exploring the working memory abilities of typically and atypically developing individuals. Both of these populations have the potential to provide informative answers to these questions for two main reasons. First, these samples are associated with relatively greater variation in ability and performance than undergraduate participants, who are necessarily drawn from a much narrower intellectual range. This larger range increases the power of an individual-differences approach to highlight the different constraints on task performance and the patterns of association between constructs. Of course, a representative sample of typically developing children will, by definition, vary in IQ to the same extent as a similarly representative sample of adult participants from the general rather than student population. This is not the case, however, for individuals undergoing atypical development. A greater degree of variation in intelligence is possible among individuals with generalized learning difficulties, although in such a sample the degree of covariation among different aspects of intellectual functioning (for example, verbal and nonverbal ability) is likely to be no greater than that seen in the typical population. Work with individuals experiencing specific learning difficulties provides the potential for teasing apart domains of functioning. For example, verbal and nonverbal abilities might appear to play a similar role in determining performance on a range of working memory tests in the typical population, but this might simply reflect the degree of correlation between these abilities. Assessing individuals with specific verbal or nonverbal learning difficulties might indicate that verbal and nonverbal skills are in fact potentially independent constraints on performance on certain tasks.

It could be argued that this kind of issue could be addressed equally easily among a typical adult sample by impairing a domain of functioning through the use of selective dual-task interference (cf., Baddeley, 1993; although see Hegarty, Shah, & Miyake, 2000). The second advantage of employing developmental groups is that one can explore causal relationships, in terms of either constraints on working memory task performance or associations between working memory measures and academic achievement, in a way that adult experimental methods do not allow, simply because children's abilities change so rapidly over time. Such developmental studies do not necessarily require the use of longitudinal designs, although these are particularly informative (Bishop, 1997); rather, differences in age or ability *between* individuals can be used to explore the causal links between domains of ability and working memory performance (e.g., Case, Kurland, & Goldberg, 1982; Fry & Hale, 1996). One can then determine the factors that lead to age-related change in working memory, which need not necessarily be the same as those factors that underpin individual differences within an age group (Conway et al., 2002; Jenkins, Myerson, Hale, & Fry, 1999; Towse, Hitch, & Hutton, 1998), as well as the consequences of working memory development. Once again, work with individuals experiencing atypical development can provide a strong test of the causal relationships between domains of cognitive functioning, thus enabling the separation of factors that are collinear in the typical case. For example, in a recent study, Jarrold, Baddeley, Hewes, Leeke, and Phillips (2004) examined verbal short-term memory performance among children with learning difficulties who had an equivalent level of vocabulary knowledge but differed in rate of vocabulary attainment, to determine the likely causal relation between these measures. More generally, determination of whether working memory problems are a cause or a consequence of an individual's learning difficulties is central to a proper understanding of the broader educational implications of such difficulties.

CRITICAL SOURCES OF VARIATION IN WORKING MEMORY

In working with these populations, our approach starts from a principled analysis of the construct of working memory and the type of measures used to index this construct. If *working memory* is defined as the storage of to-be-remembered information during the simultaneous processing or manipulation of other, perhaps related, information, then broadly speaking there are two obvious sources of potential variation in working memory ability. Individuals may vary in terms of their ability to hold information in mind (storage), and/or in their ability to simultaneously manipulate information (processing). In other words, individuals' performance on the type of complex span task used by Daneman and Carpenter (1980) might be expected to depend on their ability to remember the list of to-be-recalled target words, and to read the sentences that provide these words to be remembered.

In fact, a focus on this type of measure shows how likely it is that storage constraints operate to limit working memory performance. Because the dependent variable in a complex-span procedure is typically the number of items successfully recalled, it is almost a truism to suggest that performance will depend on storage capacity. Indeed, the evidence of word length and phonological similarity effects in complex span tasks (La Pointe & Engle, 1990; Tehan, Hendry, & Kocinski, 2001) indicates that short-term storage factors are operating in these working memory tests (cf., Baddeley, Thomson, & Buchanan, 1975; Conrad, 1964). At the same time, working memory measures are seen by most investigators to capture something more than short-term memory tasks. Clearly, the difference between complex span measures and simple span tests such as digit span and word span is that the former involve a degree of active manipulation or processing of information not present in the latter; this, we would argue, is what distinguishes working from short-term memory. The fact that complex span tasks tend to be stronger predictors of other skills than corresponding simple span tasks (e.g., Conway et al., 2002; Daneman & Carpenter, 1980; Engle, Tuholski, et al., 1999; Kail & Hall, 2001; Oberauer, Schulze, Wilhelm, & Süß, 2005) suggests that the processing requirements of the task do affect working memory performance in a meaningful way.

The storage and processing requirements of the complex span task are therefore two plausible sources of variation in working memory performance and, in turn, potential mediators of the link with higher-level cognitive abilities. However, a third possible source of variance could arise from the need to combine, coordinate, or integrate these two component aspects of the task. Duff and Logie (2001) compared the effect of combining the processing and storage operations of a complex span task, relative to performance on these components considered in isolation. They showed a small but reliable cost on span performance when these two components were combined, which they attributed to the demands of coordinating these operations. As noted above, this result in itself does not imply that the link between complex span performance and higher-level abilities is mediated to any meaningful extent by individual differences in coordination ability, whatever that entails. However, Towse and Houston-Price (2001) showed that the ability to coordinate two sets of representations in a short-term memory paradigm was related to educational ability, even when performance on the two separate aspects of the combined task was accounted for.

In short, therefore, working memory span tasks involve both storage of to-be-remembered information and the processing of other information, and possibly also the coordination or combination of the two. Consequently, there are at least three potential sources of variation in working memory performance that we aim to consider in our work.

OVERARCHING THEORY

These three sources of variation in working memory can be integrated within a theoretical framework, namely Baddeley's (1986) working memory model. This model distinguishes between the short-term storage of information and the executive control of those systems involved in this storage (see also Baddeley & Hitch, 1974). As a result, it is consistent with the notion that storage demands can operate as a potentially independent constraint on working memory performance. In addition, the model posits functionally independent storage systems, the phonological loop and the visuospatial sketchpad, dedicated to the short-term mainte-nance of verbal and visuospatial information respectively. The capacity of these subsystems is thought to be tapped by simple span tasks that require the relatively passive maintenance of information without its transformation, such as digit span and Corsi span tasks (Corsi, cited in Milner, 1971).

Evidence for the potential distinctiveness of these two systems comes from a number of sources. Verbal and visuospatial dual tasks have been shown to have selective interference ef-fects on the short-term maintenance of ver-bal and visuospatial information (Hale, Bronik, & Fry, 1997; Hale, Myerson, Rhee, Weiss, & Abrams, 1996; Logie, Zucco, & Baddeley, 1990; see Chapter 7, this volume), and functional imaging studies have implicated different neu-roanatomical substrates for these systems (e.g., Smith, Jonides, & Koeppe, 1996; see Chapter 10, this volume). Consistent with these findings, selective deficits of verbal and visuospatial short-term memory have been observed in neuro-psychological patients (see Vallar & Papagno, 1995) and among individuals with specific learning difficulties and/or developmental dis-orders. For example, verbal short-term memory deficits have been documented among in-dividuals with specific language impairment (see Montgomery, 2003) and Down syndrome (see Jarrold, Baddeley, & Phillips, 1999), while specific impairments of visuospatial short-term memory have been reported among indi-viduals with nonverbal learning disabilities (Cornoldi, Della Vecchia, & Tressoldi, 1995) and Williams syndrome (Vicari, Carlesimo, Brizzolara, & Pezzini, 1996). Indeed, it has been suggested that the contrast in short-term memory skills of individuals with the genetic conditions of Down syndrome and Williams syndrome represents a double dissociation in short-term memory impairments (Wang & Bellugi, 1994; see also Jarrold, Baddeley, & Hewes, 1999).

From our standpoint, these data do not necessarily indicate that verbal and visuospatial short-term memory are subserved by entirely distinct and encapsulated systems, as Badde-ley's working memory model would suggest. There are likely to be a number of processes that are common to both verbal and visuospa-tial short-term memory tasks (Chuah & May-bery, 1999; Jones, Farrand, Stuart, & Morris, 1995; Pickering, Gathercole, & Peaker, 1998; Smyth & Scholey, 1996a, 1996b). However, it is also the case that these tasks differ in ways that allow them to be dissociated in certain circumstances. One possible source of this difference is in terms of the representations held in short-term memory; Baddeley's distinction between the phonological loop and visuospa-tial sketchpad may reduce to a fundamental difference in the nature of verbal and visuo-spatial information and the ways in which these different representations can be encoded, maintained, and retrieved (see Chapter 10). If so, then evidence of short-term memory deficits in developmental disorders may, in some cases at least, reflect a more fundamental difficulty in dealing with verbal or visuospatial repre-sentations in general (see Hulme & Roodenrys, 1995; Jarrold, 2001). Nevertheless, regardless of the source of these impairments, it does appear that the nature of to-be-remembered informa-tion, or the *content* of working memory, will be a potentially important constraint on complex span performance (cf., Oberauer, Süß, Schulze, Wilhelm, & Wittmann, 2000).

What is less clear is how one would map the notion of processing demands as a constraint on complex span performance onto the work-ing memory model. In the early instantiation of this model, Baddeley and Hitch (1974) refer to a "central processor . . . [that] forms the core of working memory" (p. 81), which might suggest that the "central executive" of the current work-ing model is responsible for what we have termed the *processing* portion of a complex span task. Indeed, Engle and colleagues (e.g., Engle, Tuholski, et al., 1999) have suggested that what differentiates complex and simple span tasks, and hence working memory from short-term mem-ory, is central-executive functioning. However, even in the original Baddeley and Hitch model, and more clearly in the more recent versions of this account (Baddeley, 1986, 2000), the cen-tral executive's role is really one of "control processing" of the kind required in monitoring and coordination of memory activities (e.g., Baddeley, 1996). There is no obvious sense in which the processing component of a complex task—that is, the task that is interleaved between storage episodes—involves control of this form, and consequently we would argue that the processing aspect of a complex span task need not be executive in nature.

Evidence to support this view comes from a study by Russell, Jarrold, and Henry (1996), who examined the working memory abilities of individuals with autism. Autism is thought to be associated with executive difficulties (Pennington & Ozonoff, 1996; Russell, 1997), and consequently one might expect impaired working memory in this condition (see also Bennetto, Pennington, & Rogers, 1996). As a test of this account, Russell et al. employed three complex span tasks, each of which contained two conditions that varied the level of complexity of the processing involved, the prediction being that individuals with autism would be particularly impaired when complex span tasks involved more complex processing (cf., Braver et al., 1997). However, on one task, individuals with autism showed a significantly *smaller* complexity effect than controls. In this counting span task (cf., Case et al., 1982) participants were required to count the number of dots on a series of screens and then recall the series of totals. "Easy" processing involved counting dots arranged in a canonical pattern, as seen on dice, while "difficult" processing involved counting distributed patterns of dots that also contained distractor items to prevent subitizing.

Analysis of the time taken to complete the counting component of these tasks showed that individuals with autism, unlike controls, were not aided by the canonical representation of dots (Jarrold & Russell, 1997). Indeed, rather than simply reading off the total from this canonical representation, individuals with autism tended to count the dots one by one. This relative difficulty in carrying out the processing component of this condition of the counting span task led to impaired working memory performance. However, Jarrold and Russell (1997) argued that this failure to perceive the global

form reflected a low-level bias toward local processing of visual stimuli known to be associated with autism (see Frith & Happé, 1994), rather than any form of higher-level executive problem.

These data, along with similar evidence from studies employing complex span tasks with other individuals with learning difficulties (e.g., Hitch & McAuley, 1991; Siegel & Ryan, 1989), show, unsurprisingly, that an individual's ability to perform the processing component of a complex span task will affect their overall performance. However, to the extent that that component itself is non-executive in nature, processing constraints on performance need not be executive. Similarly, there is no reason to suspect that such constraints on performance need necessarily be domain general in nature. The processing components of different tasks may share common aspects—they may, for example, be limited by general speed of processing (Fry & Hale, 1996; Salthouse, 1996; Salthouse & Babcock, 1991)—but an individual might still struggle on one kind of processing task while finding another relatively easier, as the Russell et al. (1996) data indicate.

This is not to say that Engle is incorrect to suggest that there are executive aspects to complex span tasks that are not present in simple span tests. The working memory model would suggest that working memory differs from short-term memory in terms of the added need for executive control. However, by definition this control must reflect the higher-level combination of the processing and storage components of the task, rather than the ability to perform these components in isolation. As Kyllonen and Christal (1990) argue, the executive aspect of working memory reflects "concurrent processing and storage efficiency, independent of both the concurrent operations and the efficiency of nonconcurrent storage" (p. 425). Consequently, if Baddeley's (1986) central executive is involved in mediating complex span performance, it must be through some executive requirement associated with combining or coordinating the processing and storage aspects of the task. Furthermore, for the executive to be a meaningful system it must be domain general in its operation; it makes little sense to have a central control system that can only coordinate a limited set of tasks. Of course, it may be possible that certain combinations of storage and processing overlap or interact in different ways (cf., Shah & Miyake, 1996), but if Baddeley's model of the central executive is correct, then one would expect the executive coordination of processing and storage to be common to all complex span tasks (cf., Emerson, Miyake, & Rettinger, 1999).

In sum, the theoretical structure provided by Baddeley's (1986) working memory model is broadly consistent with the three potential sources of variation in working memory ability outline above. Performance on a complex span task may depend on an individual's ability to store the memory *content* of the task, to carry out the *process* interleaved between storage episodes, and to *control* the simultaneous operation of these two aspects of the test. In addition, we would argue that constraints of content and of process are potentially domain specific, although there may be common aspects to each of these constraints across tasks. In contrast, control constraints must be domain general if they are to be interpreted as evidence of any higher-level executive activity (Engle, Tuholski, et al., 1999).

CONSIDERATION OF OTHER ACCOUNTS

These points are not particularly contentious; most theorists would accept that complex span tasks differ from short-term memory tests by the addition of a processing component that involves manipulation of material, while at the same time sharing the need to store to-be-remembered target information (Dixon, Le-Fevre, & Twilley, 1988; Engle, Kane, & Tuholski, 1999; Waters & Caplan, 1996). Where accounts differ is over the question of which of these potential constraints mediates the link between complex span performance and other abilities, and of how these various constraints interrelate. Clearly the processing component of the complex span task plays a role in determining its predictive power, because this is what differentiates working memory from

short-term memory measures, but it is not obvious why the addition of processing has this effect.

Traditional resource-sharing accounts (Case et al., 1982; Daneman & Carpenter, 1980) argue that processing and storage demands draw on a common, limited-capacity pool of working memory resources (cf., Baddeley & Hitch, 1974). Given this trade-off between storage and processing requirements, relatively efficient processing frees up relatively greater resources for storage; indeed, individual differences in storage capacity and processing efficiency are collinear in this account. According to this view, "processing efficiency not storage is the real locus of individual differences in working memory capacity" (Daneman & Carpenter, 1987, p. 494). Similarly, the development of complex span performance need not reflect a change in overall working memory capacity, but rather a change in the efficiency with which one can carry out the processing requirements of the task (Case et al., 1982).

Alternative, resource switching accounts (e.g., Hitch & Towse, 1995; Chapter 5, this volume) accept that processing plays a role in constraining complex span performance, but argue that this role is less direct and is mediated instead by the influence that processing time has on the storage demands of a task. Towse and colleagues emphasize the commonalities between short-term and working memory measures and note that the storage requirements of any immediate recall paradigm will vary with the total duration of that test. In the context of complex span measures, where the onset of successive processing intervals is typically self-paced, relatively less efficient processing will lead to the task taking relatively longer overall, with consequently greater likelihood of forgetting to-be-remembered information. The key difference between this account and resource-sharing theories is that although it accepts that processing time does affect storage demands, there is no inevitable relationship (or sharing of resources) between processing and storage constraints. Instead, the suggestion that the participant switches between these phases of the task means that they are potentially independent. Indeed, in a situation where processing time is held constant, processing difficulty should have no effect on task performance (Towse, Hitch, & Hutton, 2002). This account accepts that developmental improvements in complex span performance follow from changes in processing efficiency, and individual differences in processing efficiency play a role in mediating the link between complex span performance and other abilities (Hitch, Towse, & Hutton, 2001). Remaining questions in this account are whether changes in storage capacity moderate age-related change in complex span performance, and whether variance in storage capacity is seen as a further, independent factor underlying the relationship between complex span performance and higher-level abilities (see Chapter 5).

This relationship may, of course, by driven by variation in the ability to combine the storage and processing phases of a complex span task. Engle and colleagues argue that complex span tasks tap executive "controlled attention," and one reason for this may be that they require participants to coordinate their component operations. In line with this suggestion, when Engle, Tuholski, et al. (1999) partialed out short-term memory ability from an estimate of individuals' working memory ability as measured by complex span tasks, they found that the residual variance correlated with an index of general fluid intelligence. As noted, this approach does not conclusively demonstrate that this residual variance represents the executive ability to coordinate storage and processing, because it fails to control for basic variance in processing efficiency. However, Conway et al. (2002) showed that residual variance in working memory performance, having accounted for short-term memory ability, was not related to an index of general speed of processing. This is consistent with the view that this residual variance captures more than the ability to carry out the processing aspects of complex span tasks. Indeed, Kyllonen and Christal (1990) found that an estimate of working memory ability that controlled for the ability to carry out both the processing and storage aspects of the component working memory tasks (Experiment 1, model 1x) was closely related to an index of individuals' reasoning ability.

Our analysis of the possible constraints on complex span performance shares features with all three of the accounts outlined above, and therefore differs to some extent from each of them. We concur with the resource-switching account's emphasis on the storage constraints on complex span performance and would argue, contrary to resource-sharing views, that these are potentially independent of the effects of processing efficiency. Indeed, although complex span tasks tend to be stronger predictors of higher-level abilities than simple span measures, there are occasions when simple storage measures are equally strong and reliable predictors of these other skills (Bayliss, Jarrold, Baddeley, & Gunn, 2005; Cowan et al., 2003; Hutton & Towse, 2001; Oakhill & Kyle, 2000; Shah & Miyake, 1996; see also Maybery & Do, 2003). In some cases this might reflect the fact that the processing requirements of the complex span task are not sufficiently demanding to reliably reduce span levels relative to simple span (Myerson, Jenkins, Hale, & Sliwinski, 2000; although see Shah & Miyake, 1996). Nevertheless, because simple span measures do predict these other abilities in these instances, storage constraints may play some role in mediating the relationship between complex span performance and higher-level abilities (see also Cantor, Engle, & Hamilton, 1991; Engle, Tuholski, et al., 1999). In addition, studies in which the domain of the content of simple and complex span tasks has been manipulated have often shown higher correlations between pairs of short-term and working memory tasks that share content than those observed between pairs of working memory tasks that do not share content (Kane, Hambrick, Tuholski, Wilhelm, Payne, & Engle, 2004; Maybery & Do, 2003; Oberauer & Süß, 2000; Shah & Miyake, 1996; although see Oberauer, Süß, Wilhelm, & Wittman, 2003). In other words, tasks that share storage constraints but differ in processing requirements tend to have more in common than tasks that differ in storage constraints yet share processing requirements.

Like the resource-sharing account but somewhat at odds with the resource-switching and controlled-attention views, we accept that the ability to carry out the particular processing component of any complex span task may influence performance. Part of this ability may reflect the effect of variation in processing time on overall storage demands, as Towse and colleagues suggest, but we are open to the possibility that processing constraints affect performance even under fixed time conditions. Finally, we predict a potentially executive aspect to complex span tasks that arises from the need to combine storage and processing operations and, in line with Kyllonen and Christal (1990), would argue that one should assess this by partialing out uncontaminated estimates of *both* storage and processing abilities from complex span performance.

OUR METHODOLOGICAL APPROACH

Our approach to identifying the constraints on working memory has been to examine the extent to which variation in complex span performance can be attributed to individual differences in the ability to perform the processing and storage requirements of the complex span task in isolation. This involves partitioning the variance in complex span performance into the unique and shared contributions associated with each component of working memory. Although this technique for examining individual differences in working memory abilities is not uncommon (Kane et al., 2004; Salthouse & Babcock, 1991; Shah & Miyake, 1996), the novelty of our approach is in the design of our complex span tasks. Across a series of studies we have used a common methodology in which we systematically vary the domain of processing and storage involved in each task. To do this, we first developed two processing tasks that share the same basic characteristics but differ in the content of the information to be manipulated (verbal and visuospatial). We then integrated these tasks with two types of storage (verbal and visuospatial) to create four complex span tasks in which the processing and storage components are factorially combined across the verbal and visuospatial domains. Another important aspect of our design is careful control of the timing of processing and storage episodes so that

the duration of the trials within each task is always the same.

The strength of this design is that it allows us to directly compare performance across the processing and storage domains of complex span tasks. It also allows us to examine whether the constraints on complex span performance are largely domain general in nature and show a consistent pattern of results across all complex span tasks, or are domain specific and therefore dependent on the particular combination of processing and storage involved. Perhaps the most important aspect of this design, however, is that it allows us to take *independent* measures of the processing and storage involved in each complex span task and account for the variance in performance that is associated with these. Theoretically, this leaves us with a relatively pure estimate of any potentially executive contribution to complex span performance that follows from combining the processing and storage components of the task. As a result, this approach has allowed us to address the two questions central to our work: what are the various constraints on complex span performance, and how do these constraints mediate the link between complex span performance and higher-level cognition?

WHAT ARE THE CONSTRAINTS ON COMPLEX SPAN PERFORMANCE?

Two Initial Studies

We first explored this question in two studies that examined the nature of constraints underlying complex span performance in both children and adults (Bayliss, Jarrold, Gunn, & Baddeley, 2003). In the first study, 75 children aged 8 and 9 years completed a battery of four complex span tasks—two independent measures of processing efficiency and two independent measures of storage capacity. Consistent display characteristics were used across all four complex span tasks: nine different-colored circles were presented in a random arrangement on the screen, with one of the digits 1 to 9 shown in the center of each circle. In addition, one of the circles was presented with a beveled edge, the location of which varied on successive trials. In the tasks involving verbal processing, the children were presented with a verbal object name (i.e., "milk") and were asked to find the circle that corresponded to the color of the object as quickly as possible. This was thought to involve verbal processing in that the child was required to first associate the object name with the object and then retrieve the color most often identified with that object. Clearly efficiency of target detection could depend on a number of factors such as lexical semantic knowledge and visual imagery, a point we return to below. In the tasks involving visuospatial processing, the children were asked to find the circle with a beveled edge as quickly as possible. Both processing tasks led the children to an appropriate target circle, at which point they were asked to remember either the number in the center of the target circle (verbal storage) or the location of the target circle (visuospatial storage) for later recall. The timing of each processing and storage interval was fixed so that if a child found the target circle relatively quickly they did not move on to the next processing episode of the trial until this set interval had elapsed. In contrast, if a child failed to find the appropriate target within the available time, the correct storage item was shown to them before the presentation of the next processing episode. The number of processing and storage episodes in each list increased in a span procedure until the child could no longer recall the storage items in correct serial order.

In addition to the four complex span tasks described above, we also took independent measures of the processing and storage requirements of each task. The processing tasks corresponded to the processing involved in the complex span tasks but were presented without any associated storage requirements. They were designed as search tasks, and required the participant to either decide what color a verbally presented object was and touch the appropriately colored circle as quickly as possible (verbal), or scan the array of circles for the circle with the beveled edge (visuospatial). By varying the number of distractor items present in these search displays, we were able to confirm that target detection in our visuospatial processing task depended on the number of distractors present, a finding that suggests that participants were actively scanning the visual display. In contrast, in the verbal processing task, performance was not affected by number of distractors. This finding suggests that regardless of the precise processes involved in determining the typical color of a named object, these do not lead to visuospatial searching of the display. Similarly, our independent measures of individuals' storage capacity were taken by replicating the storage demands of the complex span tasks but without any concurrent processing requirements. Consequently, these corresponded to a digit span (verbal storage) and a Corsi span (visuospatial storage) task. Analysis of the relationship among these independent measures of processing and storage ability showed that the verbal and visuospatial processing measures were highly correlated ($r = .75$), suggesting that there may be a common factor driving performance on these measures. In contrast, the correlation between the verbal and visuospatial storage measures was not as strong ($r = .32$), and was in fact comparable to the correlations between storage and processing measures.

These suggestions were borne out by an exploratory factor analysis on the data from our four complex span tasks, our two processing tasks and our two storage tasks, which produced three factors that together accounted for 72% of the total variance. The first factor corresponded to a general processing factor with strong loadings from both measures of processing efficiency. The second factor showed loadings from digit span and the two complex span tasks involving verbal storage, results suggesting that it corresponded to a verbal storage factor. In contrast, the third factor showed loadings from the two complex span tasks involving visuospatial storage and Corsi span, which suggests that this factor was best interpreted as a visuospatial storage factor. Consistent with the Baddeley (1986) model, these results provide further support for separation of the systems responsible for the storage of verbal and visuospatial information. However, they also suggest the involvement of a domain-general processing component, which is largely driven by both measures of processing efficiency. Given the simplicity of these processing tasks, we would argue that this general processing factor is non-executive in nature, and instead reflects the constraints imposed by individual differences in the ability to perform the processing component of the complex span task.

To explore the relative importance of each of these constraints, we examined the extent to which individual variation in both processing efficiency and storage capacity determined performance on each complex span task. To do this, we used a variance partitioning procedure to identify the unique and shared variance attributable to the processing and storage components (cf., Salthouse & Babcock, 1991). A series of hierarchical multiple-regression analyses showed that the domain-appropriate measures of storage capacity contributed unique variance to performance on each complex span task (between 8.5% and 18.9% of the total variation). The independent measures of processing efficiency also accounted for significant unique variance in the two complex span tasks incorporating verbal processing (14.6% and 19.3% when entered together) but not in the two tasks involving visuospatial processing. We argue that this result may be due to the visuospatial processing task not being demanding enough to influence performance on the complex span tasks incorporating this type of processing. Indeed, the two complex span tasks involving verbal processing showed a greater drop in performance relative to simple span performance than the two complex span tasks involving visuospatial processing (cf., Oberauer & Süß, 2000). In addition, there was very little shared variance between the processing and storage measures, indicating that most of the variation in span performance was accounted for by unique contributions. These results suggest that, in children, complex span performance is constrained by variation in both processing efficiency and storage capacity, and furthermore, that these contributions are largely independent of one another.

In our second study, we were interested to see if this pattern would replicate in an adult sample. The tasks from our first experiment were modified to make them more appropriate for adult participants; however, the basic characteristics of each task remained the same. The one significant change that we did make was to convert the simple visuospatial search task from the initial study into a conjunctive search task. This involved changing the display screen to an array of big and small squares, half of which were presented with a beveled edge and half of which were not. The visuospatial processing task involved searching the array to locate the big square with a beveled edge as quickly as possible. Only one of these squares was presented in each display, thus making the search task more difficult, as the target could not be distinguished from the distractors by the presence or absence of a single feature. A sample of 48 adults completed the four complex span tasks, the two independent measures of processing and the two independent measures of storage. An exploratory factor analysis performed on the data from the complex span tasks and the independent measures of storage and processing revealed a three-factor structure similar to that found with the initial sample of children. The first factor corresponded to a visuospatial storage factor with strong loadings from Corsi span and the two complex span tasks incorporating visuospatial storage. The second factor showed loadings from the two measures of processing efficiency, suggesting that this was a general processing factor. The third factor showed high loadings of the two complex span tasks involving verbal storage and the digit span task, results suggesting that this factor corresponded to a verbal storage factor. These results closely replicated the pattern found previously with children and provided further support for the existence of distinct verbal and visuospatial storage systems and a domain-general processing component.

Also consistent with our initial results was the finding that the independent measures of verbal and visuospatial storage capacity each contributed significant unique variance to the corresponding complex span tasks (between 12% and 41%). The independent measures of processing efficiency uniquely accounted for 12% of the variance in the complex span task combining verbal processing with verbal storage; however, this was the only significant contribution of processing efficiency to complex span performance in the adult sample. Nonetheless, the finding that processing efficiency was a significant predictor of performance in one of the tasks indicates that an individual's processing ability can be, but is not necessarily, a constraint on complex span performance even under conditions where the duration of each trial is held constant. On the basis of these findings, we argue that individuals could potentially vary in terms of both their ability to perform the processing activity of the complex span task and their ability to maintain the storage items in mind. Furthermore, we argue that it is the balance of these constraints within an individual that will determine their complex span performance (cf., Hitch et al., 2001).

A third source of potential variation that we were interested in exploring was whether the coordination of the processing and storage episodes of the complex span task required an additional executive ability, independent of the processing and storage abilities themselves. Borrowing from the approach of Kyllonen and Christal (1990; see also Engle, Tuholski, et al., 1999), we examined the residual variance in complex span performance once variance associated with the independent measures of processing efficiency and storage capacity was removed. In line with the arguments advanced above, we maintain that if there is an executive ability involved in complex span performance that is reflected in the residual variance, then this should be domain general and should be observed on all tasks that involve the combination of storage and processing requirements. In other words, residual variance should correlate across our different complex span tasks. The correlations between the residuals derived from our first two studies are shown in

Table 6.1. Although only two of these correlations were significant in the children's data, all but one of the residuals were significantly correlated in the adult data. This finding is important because it indicates that these residuals do not simply reflect measurement error but instead index an additional ability that contributes consistent variance to complex span performance (cf., Emerson et al., 1999). Moreover, the fact that the residuals from all four complex span tasks were correlated to a certain degree in the adult sample suggests that this ability is domain general (cf., Oberauer et al., 2003), as one would expect if it is executive in nature. Indeed, in the adult sample, the residuals from the two same-domain complex span tasks (verbal–verbal and visuospatial–visuospatial) shared 13% variance and the two cross-domain tasks (verbal–visuospatial and visuospatial–verbal) shared 11% variance, despite the fact that these pairs of tasks share none of their processing or storage elements.

A DEVELOPMENTAL STUDY

Consistent with our original hypotheses, the results of these first two experiments provide evidence for three independent sources of working memory variation: storage capacity (whether it is verbal or visuospatial), processing efficiency, and executive ability. More recently, we have turned our attention to exploring the factors that drive age-related increases in working memory performance. The results from the two experiments reported by Bayliss et al. (2003) highlight some important similarities between children and adults, but also some important differences

TABLE 6.1. Correlational Analysis of Complex Span Residuals from Samples of Children (to the Bottom Left of the Leading Diagonal) and Adults (to the Top Right of the Leading Diagonal).

Residuals	1.	2.	3.	4.
1. Verbal verbal	—	.296*	.399**	.364*
2. Verbal visuospatial	.126	—	.329*	.399**
3. Visuospatial verbal	.124	.233*	—	.239
4. Visuospatial visuospatial	.174	.293*	.033	—

**$p < .01$; *$p < .05$. These data were not previously reported in Bayliss et al. (2003).

(i.e., processing efficiency seems to be a more important predictor of complex span performance in children than in adults). It is possible that the constraints imposed on complex span performance may follow different developmental trajectories and, consequently, the relative importance of these constraints may change across different stages of development (cf., Conway et al., 2002; Cowan et al., 2005). The capacity of working memory has been shown to increase with development (Case et al., 1982; Hale et al., 1997; Towse et al., 1998) and decline during older adulthood (Salthouse & Babcock, 1991). A number of researchers have argued that this age-related change in working memory capacity is directly related to changes in processing speed. For example, Fry and Hale (1996) found that developmental increases in processing speed accounted for most of the age-related increases in working memory capacity (cf., Salthouse & Babcock, 1991). However, the findings from our previous work suggest that developmental increases in the capacity for short-term storage may also be important in driving age-related improvements in complex span performance.

We addressed these issues in a developmental study (Bayliss, Jarrold, Baddeley, Gunn, & Leigh, 2005) examining the complex span performance of 120 typically developing children aged 6, 8, and 10 years. To assess the claims of Fry and Hale (1996) and of Salthouse and colleagues (Salthouse, 1994, 1996; Salthouse & Babcock, 1991), that speed of processing mediates most of the age-related change in working memory performance, we included a number of verbal and visuospatial speed tasks designed to measure various levels of speeded performance. The most basic measures were designed as forced-choice reaction-time tasks that were broadly linked to the verbal and visuospatial domains. In both tasks, a fixation cross was displayed in the center of the screen, with a picture of a bird on one side and a frog on the other. In the auditory speed task, the children were presented with either a short, high-pitch tone, which they were told corresponded to the bird, or a short, low-pitch tone, which corresponded to the frog. They were told that they had to listen to the tones and touch

the corresponding picture on the screen as quickly as they could without making mistakes. In the visual speed task, the participants were presented with a picture of either the bird or the frog in the center of the screen and were told to touch the correct picture on the screen as quickly as possible. Reaction times for correct touch-responses were taken as a measure of basic auditory and visual speed.

In addition, we also included tasks designed to measure verbal and visuospatial maintenance rate, which we thought might underlie some of the age-related variation in storage capacity. In the verbal domain, it is commonly assumed that storage items are maintained in the phonological loop by means of a subvocal rehearsal process and that the rate at which one can articulate a list of items provides a good approximation of the rate of covert rehearsal (Baddeley, Lewis, & Vallar, 1984; Baddeley et al., 1975). In line with this research, we took a measure of each child's articulation rate as a surrogate for the rate at which they were able to maintain the verbal storage items. In the visuospatial domain, Logie (1995) has suggested that the maintenance of spatial patterns may be supported by a spatially based system termed the "inner scribe." The most common method of disrupting the spatial storage system in a dual-task paradigm is spatial tapping (Logie, 1995). Performance on this task is not generally taken as an index of the ability to maintain visuospatial material in short-term memory, however. So in contrast, we designed a mental rotation task as our measure of visuospatial maintenance rate. Various mental rotation tasks have been used as a measure of the speed with which a target figure can be spatially manipulated (Hegarty et al., 2000; Miyake, Friedman, Rettinger, Shah, & Hegarty, 2001). We argued that a mental rotation task would provide a suitable visuospatial analogue of articulation rate. In line with our previous work, we also took independent measures of the verbal and visuospatial processing involved in the complex span tasks, as well as independent measures of each child's verbal and visuospatial storage capacity by means of a digit span and a Corsi span task, respectively. For practical reasons, we chose to include only two of the complex span tasks described above—the task combining verbal processing with verbal storage and the task combining visuospatial processing with visuospatial storage. As expected, clear age trends were evident in each of the measured variables.

One of our interests was to evaluate whether there was a common speed factor underlying performance on all of the processing and storage variables, or whether there were a number of factors corresponding to the different types of speeded tasks. To explore this issue, we performed an exploratory factor analysis on the data from the six processing speed tasks and the two measures of storage capacity. Analysis of the results suggested a two-factor solution, which accounted for 70% of the total variance. The first factor showed strong loadings of the two basic speed measures, and moderate to strong loadings of the two measures of processing efficiency and the two measures of maintenance rate, results suggesting a link to a general processing speed factor. The second factor can best be described as a storage factor with high loadings of the two storage tasks and a moderate loading of articulation rate. This finding suggests the presence of a general factor related to processing speed as well as a separate storage-related factor. In contrast to our previous findings, there was no evidence of domain-specific storage, as both the verbal and visuospatial storage measures loaded on the same factor. We argue that this may reflect the independence of developmental and individual differences in working memory capacity. To a large extent, verbal and visuospatial storage abilities develop in parallel (Chuah & Maybery, 1999; Gathercole, 1999) and so are both closely associated with age. Thus, across a large developmental sample, dissociations between the two storage systems are likely to be swamped by strong correlations between the two factors driven by age-related improvements in both. However, within a specific age group, when age does not have such an overriding influence, it is possible to isolate the specific constraints that each imposes on complex span performance.

To assess the adequacy of the two-factor model, we performed a confirmatory factor analysis. Digit span, Corsi span, and articulation rate were linked to one latent *storage* variable, while the verbal and visuospatial processing measures, the auditory and visual speed variables, rotation rate, and articulation rate were all linked to a second latent variable named *speed*. Initially, this model did not provide a good fit to the data. However, modification indices suggested that the errors from the two processing tasks and the two basic speed tasks should be linked, reflecting the fact that there was some task-specific variance associated with these measures. With this adjustment, the two-factor model provided an excellent fit to the data, as indicated by all the measures of fit considered. Parameter estimates for the final model are presented in Figure 6.1. The two factors were correlated, as indicated by the double-headed arrow connecting the two latent variables. However, a subsequent analysis of a one-factor model, which is equivalent to assuming a perfect correlation between the two factors, did not provide a satisfactory fit to the data. This discrepancy provided further support that two factors were needed to describe the data. To explore the relationship between each of these latent variables and age-related variance in complex span performance, we constructed a structural-equation model linking each of the latent variables to a third latent variable drawn from the two complex span variables. On the basis of increasingly popular hypothesis that speed of processing mediates most of the age-related change in working memory performance, we specified direct paths from the speed variable to the storage variable and the complex span variable. We also specified a direct path from the storage variable to the complex span variable and direct paths from age to each latent variable. This initial model provided a good fit to the data; however, a number of the paths were nonsignificant. These paths were deleted and the model was reanalyzed. On the basis of the fit statistics, the revised model also provided a good fit to the data. This final structural equation model is presented in Figure 6.2. For clarity, the observed variables contributing to the speed and storage latent variables have been omitted from the diagram.

As expected, the speed and storage variables both have direct effects on complex span performance, and age has direct effects on the

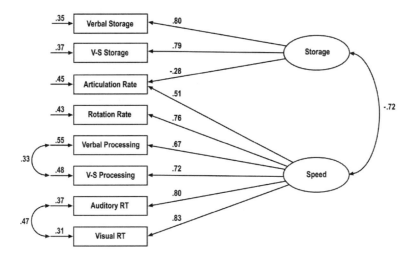

Figure 6.1. Parameter estimates for the final two-factor model following confirmatory factor analysis. RT = reaction time; V-S = visuospatial. (Adapted with permission from Bayliss, D. M., Jarrold, C., Baddeley, A. D., Gunn, D. M., & Leigh, E., Mapping the developmental constraints on working memory span performance, *Developmental Psychology*, 41, p. 588, 2005, American Psychological Association.)

speed and storage variables. Thus age-related changes in both speed of processing and storage capacity may contribute to age-related improvements in complex span performance. Indeed, the absence of a direct link between age and complex span indicates that these two effects account for most age-related variance in working memory performance. The key finding, however, is that there was no link between the speed and storage variables. That is, the age-related effect of storage capacity on complex span performance was not entirely mediated by age-related changes in speed of processing. This finding is in contrast with the developmental cascade hypothesis of Fry and Hale (1996) and suggests that processing speed and storage-related factors provide separable constraints on age-related changes in complex span performance. The model presented in Figure 6.2, however, does appear to be consistent with our

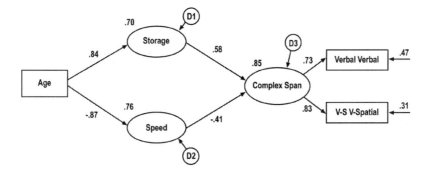

Figure 6.2. Structural-equation model of relations among age and components of complex span performance. V-S = visuospatial. (Adapted with permission from Bayliss, D. M., Jarrold, C., Baddeley, A. D., Gunn, D. M., & Leigh, E., Mapping the developmental constraints on working memory span performance, *Developmental Psychology*, 41, p. 590, 2005, American Psychological Association.)

own finding that processing efficiency and storage capacity impose independent constraints on complex span performance.

Taken together, the evidence from the studies reported here suggests that there are at least three sources of variation in working memory performance. We have clearly shown the importance of individual differences in domain-specific storage and domain-general processing to complex span performance in children and adults. Furthermore, there is evidence of a third source of potentially executive variation. Examination of the factors driving age-related changes in complex span performance also revealed two sources of independent variation, processing speed and storage capacity. The implication of these findings is that complex span performance is multidetermined; one or all of these independent sources of variation may be important in mediating the relation between complex span performance and cognitive skills such as reading and mathematics.

WHAT MEDIATES THE LINK BETWEEN COMPLEX SPAN PERFORMANCE AND HIGHER-LEVEL COGNITION?

Predictors of Higher-Level Cognition in Typically Developing Individuals

Having identified at least three independent sources of variation in complex span performance, we were interested in exploring the relationship between these factors and level of educational attainment. A subsequent analysis of the data from our initial work (Bayliss et al., 2003) showed that the scores from the general processing factor accounted for unique variance in children's reading and mathematics performance (7% and 6%, respectively). In addition, scores from the visuospatial storage factor uniquely accounted for an additional 13% of the variation in children's mathematics performance. In the adult sample, scores from the verbal storage factor uniquely accounted for over 25% of the variance in reading performance. These findings suggest that variation in children's general processing efficiency may be

an important mediator of the relationship between their complex span performance and reading and mathematics ability. Moreover, it seems that variance related to visuospatial storage abilities is particularly important for mathematics performance in children (cf., McLean & Hitch, 1999; although see Bull, Johnston, & Roy, 1999), whereas in adults, verbal storage ability may be an important mediator of reading performance. Converging evidence for the importance of storage abilities to academic attainment comes from our developmental study in which scores from the storage factor contributed unique variance to reading and mathematics performance across development (10% and 11%, respectively). Developmental differences in general speed of processing also contributed significant unique variance to reading and math performance in this study (5% in both cases).

Residual variation independent of individuals' ability to carry out the processing and storage components of complex span tasks was also found to be an important predictor of reading and math skills in both children and adults in our initial studies (Bayliss et al., 2003). In our first study, the residuals from the two complex span tasks involving verbal storage were significantly correlated with children's reading and mathematics performance. Furthermore, in the adult sample assessed in our second study, most of the correlations between the residuals from the complex span tasks and the measures of reading, mathematics, and performance on the Raven's Standard Progressive Matrices were either significant or approaching significance. These findings provide further evidence that there is a third, potentially executive, source of variation in complex span performance. If these residuals do reflect variation in some executive ability, then the fact that this variation is an important predictor of academic abilities is consistent with the findings of Engle, Tuholski, et al. (1999) and Conway et al. (2002), who argued that controlled attention was the component of working memory responsible for the predictive power of the complex span task. However, what our results suggest is that individual differences in general processing speed and storage ability may also mediate the relationship between complex span performance and reading and mathematics ability. To address this issue further, we have begun to examine how different sources of working memory variation map onto task variance in reading.

Predictors of Higher-Level Cognition in Atypically Developing Individuals

To gain a greater understanding of the relationship between the various components of working memory and reading skills, we assessed reading ability on three different levels: the ability to recognize written letters, the ability to decode and recognize written words, and the ability to make sense of sentences (cf., Baddeley, Gathercole, & Spooner, 2003). To maximize the variation in reading abilities assessed by these tests, we examined the performance of 80 children with moderate learning difficulties. By examining the working memory abilities of these children, we expected to gain a clearer picture of how the various components of working memory influence different aspects of reading skill. Each child completed a battery of our working memory tasks: two complex span tasks combining verbal processing with verbal storage in one case and visuospatial storage in the other, two independent measures of storage (digit span and Corsi span), and an independent measure of verbal processing efficiency. In addition, we also included two measures of phonological awareness (rhyme detection and initial phoneme deletion) taken from the Phonological Abilities Test (Muter, Hulme, & Snowling, 1997) (see Bayliss, Jarrold, Baddeley, & Leigh, 2005, for full details).

A series of hierarchical regression analyses were performed on each reading test to examine the unique contribution of these various measures to the prediction of different aspects of reading ability. The storage measures were the only variables to contribute significant unique variance to the letter decision task, explaining just over 10% of the total variance when entered together. In contrast, in the word decision task, the two storage measures failed to independently account for any significant unique variance in performance, whereas the

two measures of phonological awareness together accounted for approximately 10% of the variance uniquely and the two complex span measures uniquely accounted for approximately 7% of variance when entered together. The measures of phonological awareness also accounted for a significant amount of variance in performance on the sentence decision task (12%) independently of the other variables. The storage measures again accounted for very little variance when entered after the other variables, whereas the complex span measures uniquely explained 5% of the variance in performance on the sentence decision task.

Consequently, across these three levels of reading, the relative importance of each aspect of working memory performance varied (cf., Swanson & Berninger, 1995, 1996). Examination of the differential contribution of variables from the more basic letter recognition skills through to the more comprehensive level of reading skill required in the word and sentence decision tasks revealed a decrease in the contribution of basic storage ability and an increase in the contribution of complex span performance. These findings suggest that complex span performance is more than just the sum of its parts. The complex span measures contributed variance to the word and sentence decision tasks over and above that accounted for by measures of storage ability, processing efficiency, and phonological skills. Thus, complex span performance may tap an additional working memory ability, possibly a controlled attention or executive component, an ability involved in key aspects of reading skill. This idea is consistent with numerous studies from the Engle lab, which have emphasized the controlled-attention component as the driving force behind the predictive power of the complex span task. However, the finding that other components of working memory are important at more basic levels of reading ability suggests that if one of these components of working memory fails to develop normally, these early stages of learning to read may not be navigated successfully. A deficit of this form could have repercussions not only for later stages of reading but also numerous other areas of a child's development that are either directly dependent on or in some way linked to reading ability (cf., Bishop, 1997). Thus, each source of working memory variation may have its own role to play at different stages of development. An understanding of how these various sources interact to constrain performance is crucial to understanding the link between working memory and cognition.

SUMMARY OF AND IMPLICATIONS FOR GENERAL WORKING MEMORY THEORY

Summary

The aim of the program of research described above was to answer two questions concerning variation in working memory: that of the sources of variance in complex span performance, and determining which of these sources of variance mediate the link between task performance and other measures of higher-level cognition such as reading and mathematics ability. Our starting point for the first of these questions was a logical task analysis suggesting that storage, processing, and some potentially executive factor associated with combining these two might all constrain complex span performance.

In addition, we couched these constraints within the framework provided by Baddeley's (1986) model of working memory. This model is consistent with the notion that storage demands might be independent of other influences on performance, and implies that these demands will be domain specific. In other words, the content of the to-be-remembered information in a complex span task will play a role in determining performance; variation in the ability to store verbal material may be unrelated to variance in the ability to maintain visuospatial information. This model also argues explicitly for an executive-control aspect to working memory tasks, such as the complex span procedure, which differentiates these tasks from short-term memory measures such as simple span. However, we have argued that the processing component of a complex span task—the operations that are interleaved between storage episodes—need not be executive in nature. Rather, we

suggest that one would need to add the notion of processing to the working memory model to properly explain complex span performance. From our standpoint, we would expect processing constraints to be relatively task specific, as one operation may be harder than another for any given individual, although processing efficiency may also be constrained by general factors such as processing speed. In contrast, any executive aspect to complex span performance should, almost by definition, operate as a domain-general constraint on performance on all tasks.

The empirical results of our research tend to support this theoretical analysis. The two initial studies that we conducted with groups of a limited age or ability range showed that individual differences in storage ability relate to complex span performance. In itself this is not a particularly surprising finding, given that complex span tasks require serial recall of to-be-remembered information in the same way as simple span tasks (cf., La Pointe & Engle, 1990; Tehan et al., 2001). Indeed, the design of our tasks is such that the storage requirements of these complex span tests are deliberately matched to those of the corresponding simple span task. However, two other aspects of our findings on storage constraints are of crucial importance. The first is that these are domain specific, as we would predict; the factor analysis of our data from these two studies confirms that storage constraints are best conceived of as separate verbal and visuospatial factors rather than as a single, domain-general factor. This is not to say that the mechanisms or systems underpinning verbal and visuospatial storage in short-term or working memory paradigms are entirely independent; indeed they may share a number of common features (see Chuah & Maybery, 1999; Jones et al., 1995; and see below). Nevertheless, individual differences in ability to maintain verbal and visuospatial content are clearly not collinear, and can be differentiated in both children and adults.

Second, and perhaps even more crucially, our work shows that these storage constraints can operate independently of processing effects. In general in our tasks, the influence of processing demands on performance is not substantial. This may reflect the fact that our measures are designed primarily for use with children, and in some cases have been used with children as young as 6 years. Children of this age tend to have digit spans of between four and five items (Dempster, 1981); consequently, one is limited in the degree of difficulty of processing one can impose in a complex span task without producing floor performance. Nevertheless, in both of our initial studies a processing factor emerged from exploratory factor analysis which received reasonable loadings from some complex span tasks, notably those involving verbal as opposed to visuospatial processing. Furthermore, explicit analysis of the shared and unique contributions to variance in complex span performance showed that, for these complex span tasks, there was a reliable and independent contribution of processing efficiency to performance over and beyond that accounted for by variation in storage ability. Somewhat contrary to our predictions, this influence of processing demand appeared domain general in these data. Both measures of processing efficiency (assessed independently of the need for storage) shared substantial variance and loaded on the same factor in the data structure. Consequently, although the verbal and visuospatial processing manipulations employed in our tasks do differ in certain respects (see Bayliss et al., 2003), they appear to share variance which itself is related to complex span performance. One possibility, alluded to above, is that both tasks involve a degree of visual processing, because to complete our verbal processing task one might need to create a visual image of the object to determine its typical color. However, even if this is the case, one might argue that this visual processing is somewhat different from the more *visuospatial* processes required to detect a target in a display (cf., Logie & Marchetti, 1981). Whatever the case, clearly a range of other processing tasks needs to be employed before one can conclude that processing constraints on complex span performance are necessarily domain general.

A final source of individual differences in working memory that emerged from these initial studies and which is again consistent with our theoretical analysis is related to whatever is involved in combining processing and storage operations in a complex span task. By partialing out from overall task performance estimates of the variance attributable to both storage and processing constraints, using independent measures that are directly matched to the storage and processing components of the task, any remaining residual variance should be a relatively pure index of individual differences in this ability. The fact that this residual variance correlates reliably across tasks, particularly among adult participants, shows that it represents more than measurement error, and suggests that there may be a domain-general constraint on complex span performance associated with the combination of storage and processing demands.

The question that then arises is, which, or which combination, of these sources of variation in complex span performance accounts for the power of the measure to predict other abilities? Here, again, our findings are consistent with existing work suggesting that each of the influences of content, process, and control may play a role in mediating these relationships. In our first study the composite scores from processing and visuospatial storage factors accounted for unique variance in children's mathematics performance, while in our second, adult, study, a composite verbal storage factor accounted for unique variance in reading ability. The fact that the residual variance that remains, having accounted for estimates of processing efficiency and storage capacity, which by definition is itself unrelated to both of these measures, predicted reading and mathematics performance shows that this third, combinatorial constraint can also play an independent role in driving these associations.

These conclusions are strengthened and extended by the data that come from our study of typical development and our assessment of reading abilities in individuals with moderate learning difficulties. As noted at the outset of this chapter, developmental populations provide a means of testing the causal priority of associations and of the possible consequences of problems in particular areas. Our study of reading abilities among individuals with learning difficulties provides further evidence that different sources of variance in complex span performance play a role in the association between working memory ability and other skills, and provides some indication of what these roles might be. Among these individuals, an index of short-term memory capacity was a stronger predictor of reading at the letter level than was complex span performance. In contrast, word and sentence comprehension were more closely related to complex span performance than to storage capacity or processing efficiency. These findings support the suggestion that making sense of text involves higher-order and potentially executive processes associated with the combination of the storage and processing requirements of reading (Turner & Engle, 1989). These findings also indicate, however, that lower-order factors may constrain other, more basic aspects of reading (Swanson & Berninger, 1995, 1996). In turn, as individuals develop, the relationships between different aspects of working memory on the one hand and of skills such as reading and mathematics on the other may change. As noted above, this may not be a simple progression with different associations developing in parallel, rather, the interaction between working memory and reading at one level may constrain the development of associations at another. For example, one would clearly need to have developed beyond the stage of single-word reading to be in a position to integrate meaning across words in a sentence.

This potential interdependency of stages of learning highlights the need to look at the *developmental* progression of working memory and investigate the predictors, and predictive power, of age- (or ability-) related variance. This was the aim of our third study, which assessed complex span performance in individuals from a relatively large age range. A key finding from this study was the confirmation that storage and processing constraints on complex span performance are separable at the level of developmental differences. Figure 6.2 shows that the age-related change in complex span performance was mediated by two separate pathways. One of these was driven by variance in a storage-latent variable, while the other rested on developmental change in a speed construct, which was closely linked to all measures of processing speed. This model seems to suggest that a more general index of the speed with which children can perform processing operations is what constrains performance on these tasks. Consequently, these data suggest that as children develop, two age-related but potentially dissociable improvements in performing the component aspects of the task lead to increases in complex span.

Implications

The finding that processing and storage constraints are, to some extent, independent of one another at both the level of individual and developmental differences has clear implications for existing theoretical accounts of complex span performance. As noted above, general resource-sharing theories would argue that variance in storage and processing should be collinear; as more efficient processing leads directly to increased storage capacity. A basic reading of the resource-switching account, by contrast, would seem to predict that effects of processing be eliminated in tasks such as ours, that keep total time duration constant. In all of our complex span tests, individuals who take relatively longer to complete the processing operations of the task do not have to store information for relatively longer overall. Consequently, from our observations on complex span performance, the effects of processing on individuals' ability to remember information cannot reflect differences in the overall retention time of to-be-remembered information.

Having said this, processing time clearly does vary in an important sense at a more microlevel of our tasks. An advantage of our design is that by fixing the pace with which successive processing and storage episodes are presented, we remove the inevitable association between processing and storage demands that Towse and colleagues have highlighted in traditional, self-paced tasks. However, the use of a fixed time window for processing in our procedures does not mean that individuals are engaged in processing during this entire time period. Indeed, the duration of processing within this window can, and does, vary across individuals. There are two possible consequences of variation at this microlevel that mirror the resource-sharing and resource-switching accounts of complex span at the task level. On the one hand, engagement in processing may affect the ease with which individuals can simultaneously engage in other activities such as maintenance operations. Alternatively, processing may prevent individuals from carrying out any other activity at all.

Our data do not rule out the possibility that processing disrupts one's ability to share resources for the reactivation or rehearsal of to-be-remembered material. However, other findings indicate that an explanation of the processing effect in terms of its blocking of maintenance activities may be preferable. The crucial support for this form of account comes from studies that have attempted to separate duration and difficulty of processing by asking individuals to continuously perform processing tasks for a fixed interval. For example, Halford, Maybery, O'Hare, and Grant (1994, Experiment 4) compared the effects of a fixed duration of either forward or backward counting on the recall of a digit list, and found that while both processing tasks reduced recall relative to a baseline condition, the size of this effect was comparable in each case. Similar results have been reported by Towse et al. (2002). These findings are clearly inconsistent with the notion that individuals are sharing resources during processing phases, and instead suggest that any form of processing will block maintenance regardless of its cognitive demand. If one extrapolates these findings to our complex-span situation, then one would predict that individual differences in processing efficiency would not relate to performance if individuals used up all of the available time for processing. If so, then any effect of processing that we do see in our tasks would be due to the duration of the processing within this fixed time window, rather than its difficulty (cf., Conway & Engle, 1996).

Other studies have provided somewhat different results from those of Halford et al. (1994) and Towse et al. (2002), and have suggested that processing difficulty can have an effect on item retention, independent of duration effects (e.g., Barrouillet, Bernardin, & Ca-

mos, 2004; Barrouillet & Camos, 2001; Posner & Rossman, 1965). It seems possible, however, that in these cases where apparent processing difficulty effects are observed the tasks involved allowed space for individuals to carry out other activities while completing processing. In other words, a form of micro–resource switching might occur during these processing tasks (Barrouillet & Camos, 2001; Barrouillet et al., 2004; Gavens & Barrouillet, 2004). In fact, if this suggestion is correct, then it might not be so much the demand of a processing task that determines whether switching to retention-based activities can be carried out alongside processing, but rather the rate at which that task is presented (Barrouillet & Bernardin, 2002). Barrouillet and Bernardin (2002) reported data showing that relatively undemanding processing tasks can have a severe impact on complex span performance if presented at a rapid pace (see also Barrouillet et al., 2004). If this is the case, then provided that a processing task is rapid enough to keep participants busy it will prevent switching to retention-based activities, and the duration but not the difficulty of that processing will be what determines degree of forgetting. In contrast, if the task allows participants to slow the rate at which they perform processing to the point at which it can be temporarily interrupted, then a reduced effect of processing difficulty may appear to occur, even though it may more accurately reflect an increase in the time spent switching away from processing to maintenance activity. Towse et al.'s (2002) manipulation may have been successful in preventing this form of switching because of the way in which processing operations were continuously repeated (although see Halford et al., 1994, Experiment 1, for contradictory results).

A MODEL

These points lead us to propose a novel account of complex span performance that is consistent with Baddeley's working memory model and Towse and colleagues' resource-switching hypothesis. It also extends these approaches by considering the potentially independent effects of storage and processing constraints, as well as the possibly executive requirements of combining these operations. One of our main claims is that variation in the rate at which individuals can complete the processing operations of our tasks leads to variation in the extent of forgetting to-be-remembered information, as maintenance operations are prevented for the duration of processing. However, a key difference between our complex span procedure and the design employed by Towse et al. (2002) is that our fixed-time window procedure leads not only to periods when maintenance is prevented but also to those when reactivation of the to-be-remembered information can occur (cf., Cowan, 1992; Cowan et al., 1998), presumably by some form of rehearsal. This potential for reactivation, we would argue, is what accounts for the importance of storage constraints in our procedures. Of course, our design is such that variation in time available for reactivation is collinear with variation in processing duration. As a result, one might expect that processing and storage influences could not be separated in the way that we have demonstrated in our studies. However, while the extent of information loss from immediate memory in the absence of maintenance operations depends on time elapsed, the success of these maintenance operations depends on the rate at which individuals can reactivate to-be-remembered information. Consequently, provided this rate of reactivation is not determined by the same factors that limit speed of completion of processing operations, these effects can be independent in our design. That is, although individuals who process quickly will have more time available for maintenance activities, the extent to which they benefit from this time will also be determined by the rate at which they can reactivate the to-be-remembered information in that period (cf., Oberauer & Kliegl, 2001).

This explanation is strongly supported by the results of our developmental study, which provide evidence that rate of reactivation of stored information can be dissociated from an individual's general speed of processing (see also Cowan, 1999; Cowan et al., 1998; Jarrold, Hewes, & Baddeley, 2000). In modeling these data it was shown that although articulation rate was associated with a general index of processing speed, it shared additional variance with measures of storage. This finding suggests that the storage construct that emerges in this model captures variance in rate of reactivation of to-be-remembered information. One possibility is that this variance represents speed of subvocal rehearsal. A central tenet of Baddeley's (1986) model is that immediate serial recall of verbal information is determined by the rate at which individuals can articulate and thereby rehearse this material (e.g., Baddeley et al., 1975). However, the storage construct shown in Figure 6.1 is drawn from tasks that involve either verbal or visuospatial storage. Consequently, it seems unlikely that this indexes verbal subvocal rehearsal rate specifically. Instead, it may reflect a common reactivation mechanism that operates on different domains of content in verbal and visuospatial immediate-recall tasks (cf., Jones et al., 1995). Indeed, other studies have shown that articulation rate is an equally strong predictor of visuospatial and verbal short-term memory performance (Chuah & Maybery, 1999; Smyth & Scholey, 1992, 1996a). This is not to say that all variance in storage ability is domain general in nature; as noted above, our other studies show that the content of to-be-remembered information is an important source of variability in some instances. Taken together, therefore, our data indicate that verbal and visuospatial storage abilities can dissociate and give rise to separable variance at the level of individual differences (see also Jarrold, Baddeley, & Hewes, 1999; Smith et al., 1996), but that the factor driving development in verbal and visuospatial storage is common to both domains (Chuah & Maybery, 1999).

The one source of variability left unexplained by the above analysis is the residual variance in complex span performance that we observe when we partial out independent estimates of individuals' storage and processing abilities. This factor may reflect the executive cost of coordinating these aspects of the task, which in our terms would correspond to the switch between phases of processing, during which maintenance is blocked, and periods of reactivation. One way of testing this proposal would be to examine the residuals that arise

BOX 6.1. SUMMARY ANSWERS TO BOOK QUESTIONS

1. THE OVERARCHING THEORY OF WORKING MEMORY

We are guided by Baddeley's (1986) model of working memory that distinguishes between domain-specific short-term storage of verbal and visuospatial information and domain-general executive-control processes. We argue, however, that the distinction between short-term storage systems may reflect a distinction in content rather than process, and that age-related change in verbal and visuospatial storage may be mediated by a common mechanism. We also suggest that the processing operations involved in traditional working memory tasks are typically not in and of themselves executive in nature. Rather, we argue, in line with Engle and colleagues (e.g., Engle, 2002), that executive control may well be required in complex span tasks as a result of the *combination* of storage and processing demands.

2. CRITICAL SOURCES OF WORKING MEMORY VARIATION

Our principled analysis of the demands of complex span tasks suggests that variation in working memory performance might arise for three main reasons. First, individuals might differ in their storage capacity, whether in the verbal or visuospatial domain. Second, variation might arise due to differences in the efficiency with which individuals carry out the processing operations of the task. Finally, the requirement to combine storage and processing operations gives rise to a third potential source of variance in performance. Our data support this analysis by providing evidence that all three of these factors operate to constrain working memory performance and can play a role in mediating the relationship between working memory and other higher-level abilities.

3. OTHER SOURCES OF WORKING MEMORY VARIATION

Our approach is at odds with resource-sharing accounts of working memory variation, in that we emphasize and find support for separable influences of processing efficiency and storage capacity on complex span performance. This finding might also appear problematic for a basic resource-switching hypothesis, as variation in processing efficiency affects performance without affecting the time-dependent storage demands of our tasks. Our model of complex span performance is in fact consistent with a resource-switching account if one accepts that reactivation of memory items occurs in pauses between processing. In addition, we suggest that individuals may vary in the rate at which they forget information during processing activities. This may well reflect variation in individuals' ability to resist interference, as argued by a number of authors in this volume.

4. CONTRIBUTIONS TO GENERAL WORKING MEMORY THEORY

There are three main implications of our research that follow, at least in part, from our use of typically and atypically developing populations. First, our data support a model that sits somewhere between previous accounts that have emphasized either the processing or storage aspects of complex span. Our data also confirm that complex span performance is more than the sum of its parts, and suggest ways of testing what is involved in combining storage and processing operations. Second, they show that the factors leading to differences across individuals of different ages need not be the same as those that cause variation among individuals of the same age. Finally, in addition to confirming that complex span is multiply determined, our findings show that the constraints on working memory performance and the ways in which these mediate the relationship with other higher-level abilities can vary among individuals of different ages and levels of ability.

from complex span–type tasks in which the ordering of processing and storage episodes was varied to manipulate the number of switches between these phases of the task.

An alternative and intriguing suggestion is that this residual variance reflects differences in the rate at which individuals forget information while engaged in processing (Barrouillet et al., 2004; Hitch et al., 2001; Lépine, Barrouillet, & Camos, 2005). In our analysis the effect of processing reflects the time during which re-activation is prevented. However, it is possible that individuals vary in the rate at which information is lost during that period. Crucially, this variation will only be observed when storage is combined with a processing requirement, and so would represent an emergent property of the complex span design. Indeed, variation in rate of forgetting during processing might arise as a result of executive factors that determine individuals' resistance to interference (see Chapters 2 and 9). Alternatively, individual differences in forgetting-rates might simply reflect variation in a relatively low-level decay parameter (Oberauer & Kliegl, 2001), which would remove the need to view this emergent constraint in executive terms. Future research could separate these possibilities by comparing the residuals, once processing efficiency and storage capacity are accounted for, from complex span tasks that vary in the extent to which they give rise to distracting interference (cf., Lustig, May, & Hasher, 2001). Our work builds on previous research using complex span tasks (e.g., Engle, Tuholski et al., 1999; Kyllonen & Christal, 1990) to show that one can derive meaningful and predictive residuals that capture more than the ability to complete the component aspects of the task alone. Having demonstrated this, the challenge for our future research is to properly specify exactly what this residual variance really represents.

Acknowledgments

The research described in this chapter was supported by a cooperative group component grant from the United Kingdom Medical Research Council to Christopher Jarrold and Alan D. Baddeley (Grant G0000258, within Cooperative Group Grant G9901359). Deborah Riby (ne Gunn) and Eleanor Leigh also contributed considerably to this work.

References

Baddeley, A. (1986). *Working memory*. New York: Oxford University Press.

Baddeley, A. (1993). Working memory or working attention. In A. Baddeley & L. Weiskrantz (Eds.), *Attention: selection, awareness, and control. A tribute to Donald Broadbent* (pp. 152–170). Oxford: Clarendon Press.

Baddeley, A. (1996). Exploring the central executive. *Quarterly Journal of Experimental Psychology, 49A*, 5–28.

Baddeley, A. D., Gathercole, S. E., & Spooner, A. (2003). *The reading decision test*. Hove, UK: Psychology Press.

Baddeley, A. D., & Hitch, G. J. (1974). Working memory. In G. H. Bower (Ed.), *The psychology of learning and motivation: Advances in research and theory* (Vol. 8, pp. 47–89). New York: Academic Press.

Baddeley, A. D., Lewis, V., & Vallar, G. (1984). Exploring the articulatory loop. *Quarterly Journal of Experimental Psychology, 36A*, 233–252.

Baddeley, A. D., Thomson, N., & Buchanan, M. (1975). Word length and the structure of short-term memory. *Journal of Verbal Learning and Verbal Behavior, 14*, 575–589.

Barrouillet, P., & Bernardin, S. (2002). *Working memory spans in adults depend on the pace of the secondary task*. Presented at the First European Working Memory Symposium, Ghent, September.

Barrouillet, P., Bernardin, S., & Camos, V. (2004). Time constraints and resource sharing in adults' working memory spans. *Journal of Experimental Psychology: General, 133*, 83–100.

Barrouillet, P., & Camos, V. (2001). Developmental increase in working memory span: Resource sharing or temporal decay? *Journal of Memory and Language, 45*, 1–20.

Bayliss, D. M., Jarrold, C., Baddeley, A., & Gunn, D. (2005). The relationship between short-term memory and working memory: Complex span made simple? *Memory, 13*, 414–421.

Bayliss D. M., Jarrold, C., Baddeley, A. D., Gunn, D. M., & Leigh, E. (2005). Mapping the developmental constraints on working memory span performance. *Developmental Psychology*, *41*, 579–597.

Bayliss, D. M., Jarrold, C., Baddeley, A. D., & Leigh, E. (2005). Differential constraints on the working memory and reading abilities of individuals with learning difficulties and typically developing children. *Journal of Experimental Child Psychology*, *92*, 76–99.

Bayliss, D. M., Jarrold, C., Gunn, D. M., & Baddeley, A. D. (2003). The complexities of complex span: Explaining individual differences in working memory in children and adults. *Journal of Experimental Psychology: General*, *132*, 71–92.

Bennetto, L., Pennington, B. F., & Rogers, S. J. (1996). Intact and impaired memory functions in autism. *Child Development*, *67*, 1816–1835.

Bishop, D. V. M. (1997). Cognitive neuropsychology and developmental disorders: Uncomfortable bedfellows. *Quarterly Journal of Experimental Psychology*, *50A*, 899–923.

Braver, T. S., Cohen, J. D., Nystrom, L. E., Jonides, J., Smith, E. E., & Noll, D. C. (1997). A parametric study of prefrontal cortex involvement in human working memory. *Neuroimage*, *5*, 49–62.

Bull, R., Johnston, R. S., & Roy, J. A. (1999). Exploring the roles of the visual-spatial sketch pad and central executive in children's arithmetical skills: Views from cognition and developmental neuropsychology. *Developmental Neuropsychology*, *15*, 421–442.

Cantor, J., Engle, R. W., & Hamilton, G. (1991). Short-term memory, working memory, and verbal abilities: How do they relate? *Intelligence*, *15*, 229–246.

Case, R., Kurland, D. M., & Goldberg, J. (1982). Operational efficiency and the growth of short-term memory span. *Journal of Experimental Child Psychology*, *33*, 386–404.

Chuah, Y. M. L., & Maybery, M. T. (1999). Verbal and spatial short-term memory: common sources of developmental change? *Journal of Experimental Child Psychology*, *73*, 7–44.

Conrad, R. (1964). Acoustic confusions in immediate memory. *British Journal of Psychology*, *55*, 75–84.

Conway, A. R. A., Cowan, N., Bunting, M. F., Therriault, D. J., & Minkoff, S. R. B. (2002). A latent variable analysis of working memory capacity, short-term memory capacity, processing speed, and general fluid intelligence. *Intelligence*, *30*, 163–183.

Conway, A. R. A., & Engle, R. W. (1996). Individual differences in working memory capacity: More evidence for a general capacity theory. *Memory*, *4*, 577–590.

Cornoldi, C., Dalla Vecchia, R., & Tressoldi, P. E. (1995). Visuo-spatial working memory limitations in low visuo-spatial high verbal intelligence children. *Journal of Child Psychology and Psychiatry*, *36*, 1053–1064.

Cowan, N. (1992). Verbal memory span and the timing of spoken recall. *Journal of Memory and Language*, *31*, 668–684.

Cowan, N. (1999). The differential maturation of two processing rates related to digit span. *Journal of Experimental Child Psychology*, *72*, 193–209.

Cowan, N., Elliot, E. M., Saults, J. S., Morey, C., Mattox, S., Hismjatullina, A., et al. (2005). On the capacity of attention: Its estimation and its role in working memory and cognitive abilities. *Cognitive Psychology*, *51*, 42–100.

Cowan, N., Towse, J. N., Hamilton, Z., Saults, J. S., Elliott, E. M., Lacey, J. F., et al. (2003). Children's working-memory processes: A response-timing analysis. *Journal of Experimental Psychology: General*, *132*, 113–132.

Cowan, N., Wood, N. L., Wood, P. K., Keller, T. A., Nugent, L. D., & Keller, C. V. (1998). Two separate verbal processing rates contributing to short-term memory span. *Journal of Experimental Psychology: General*, *127*, 141–160.

Daneman, M., & Carpenter, P. A. (1980). Individual differences in working memory and reading. *Journal of Verbal Learning and Verbal Behavior*, *19*, 450–466.

Daneman, M., & Merikle, P. M. (1996). Working memory and language comprehension: A meta-analysis. *Psychonomic Bulletin & Review*, *3*, 422–433.

Daneman, M., & Tardif, T. (1987). Working memory and reading re-examined. In M. Coltheart (Ed.), *Attention and performance XII* (pp. 491–508). Hillsdale, NJ: Lawrence Erlbaum Associates.

Dempster, F. N. (1981). Memory span: Sources of individual and developmental differences. *Psychological Bulletin*, *89*, 63–100.

Dixon, P., LeFevre, J.-A., & Twilley, L. C. (1988). Word knowledge and working memory as predictors of reading skill. *Journal of Educational Psychology, 80*, 465–472.

Duff, S. C., & Logie, R. H. (2001). Processing and storage in working memory span. *Quarterly Journal of Experimental Psychology, 54A*, 31–48.

Emerson, M. J., Miyake, A., & Rettinger, D. A. (1999). Individual differences in integrating and coordinating multiple sources of information. *Journal of Experimental Psychology: Learning, Memory, and Cognition, 25*, 1300–1321.

Engle, R. W. (2002). Working memory capacity as executive attention. *Current Directions in Psychological Science, 11*, 19–23.

Engle, R. W., Kane, M. J., & Tuholski, S. W. (1999). Individual differences in working memory capacity and what they tell us about controlled attention, general fluid intelligence, and functions of the prefrontal cortex. In A. Miyake & P. Shah (Eds.), *Models of working memory: Mechanisms of active maintenance and executive control* (pp. 102–134). Cambridge, UK: Cambridge University Press.

Engle, R. W., Tuholski, S. W., Laughlin, J. E., & Conway, A. R. A. (1999). Working memory, short-term memory, and general fluid intelligence: A latent-variable approach. *Journal of Experimental Psychology: General, 128*, 309–311.

Frith, U., & Happé, F. (1994). Autism: Beyond "theory of mind." *Cognition, 50*, 115–132.

Fry, A. F., & Hale, S. (1996). Processing speed, working memory, and fluid intelligence: Evidence for a developmental cascade. *Psychological Science, 7*, 237–241.

Gathercole, S. E. (1999). Cognitive approaches to the development of short-term memory. *Trends in Cognitive Sciences, 3*, 410–419.

Gavens, N., & Barrouillet, P. (2004). Delays of retention, processing efficiency, and attentional resources in working memory span development. *Journal of Memory and Language, 51*, 644–657.

Hale, S., Bronik, M. D., & Fry, A. F. (1997). Verbal and spatial working memory in school-aged children: Developmental differences in susceptibility to interference. *Developmental Psychology, 33*, 364–371.

Hale, S., Myerson, J., Rhee, S. H., Weiss, C. S., & Abrams, R. A. (1996). Selective interference with the maintenance of location information in working memory. *Neuropsychology, 10*, 225–240.

Halford, G. S., Maybery, M. T., O'Hare, A. W., & Grant, P. (1994). The development of memory and processing capacity. *Child Development, 65*, 1338–1356.

Hegarty, M., Shah, P., & Miyake, A. (2000). Constraints on using the dual task methodology to specify the degree of central executive involvement in cognitive tasks. *Memory & Cognition, 28*, 376–385.

Hitch, G. J., & McAuley, E. (1991). Working memory in children with specific arithmetical learning difficulties. *British Journal of Psychology, 82*, 375–386.

Hitch, G. J., & Towse, J. (1995). Working memory: What develops? In F. Weinert & W. Schneider (Eds.), *Memory performance and competencies: Issues in growth and development* (pp. 3–21). Mahwah, NJ: Lawrence Erlbaum Associates.

Hitch, G. J., Towse, J. N., & Hutton, U. M. Z. (2001). What limits children's working memory span? Theoretical accounts and applications for scholastic development. *Journal of Experimental Psychology: General, 130*, 184–198.

Hulme, C., & Roodenrys, S. (1995). Practitioner review: verbal working memory development and its disorders. *Journal of Child Psychology and Psychiatry, 36*, 373–398.

Hutton, U. M. Z., & Towse, J. N. (2001). Short-term memory and working memory as indices of children's cognitive skills. *Memory, 9*, 333–348.

Jarrold, C. (2001). Applying the working memory model to the study of atypical development. In J. Andrade (Ed.), *Working memory in perspective* (pp. 126–150). Hove, UK: Psychology Press.

Jarrold, C., Baddeley, A. D., & Hewes, A. K. (1999). Genetically dissociated components of working memory: Evidence from Down's and Williams syndrome. *Neuropsychologia, 37*, 637–651.

Jarrold, C., Baddeley, A. D., Hewes, A. K., Leeke, T., & Phillips, C. (2004). What links verbal short-term memory performance and vocabulary level? Evidence of changing relationships among individuals with learning disability. *Journal of Memory and Language, 50*, 134–148.

Jarrold, C., Baddeley, A. D., & Phillips, C. (1999). Down syndrome and the phonological loop: The evidence for, and importance of, a specific verbal short-term memory deficit. *Down Syndrome Research and Practice, 6,* 61–75.

Jarrold, C., Hewes, A. K., & Baddeley, A. D. (2000). Two separate speech measures constrain verbal short-term memory in children. *Journal of Experimental Psychology: Learning, Memory, and Cognition, 26,* 1626–1637.

Jarrold, C., & Russell, J. (1997). Counting abilities in autism: Possible implications for central coherence theory. *Journal of Autism and Developmental Disorders, 27,* 25–37.

Jenkins, L., Myerson, J., Hale, S., & Fry, A. F. (1999). Individual and developmental differences in working memory span across the life span. *Psychonomic Bulletin & Review, 6,* 28–40.

Jones, D., Farrand, P., Stuart, G., & Morris, N. (1995). Functional equivalence of verbal and spatial information in serial short-term memory. *Journal of Experimental Psychology: Learning, Memory, and Cognition, 21,* 1008–1018.

Kail, R., & Hall, L. K. (2001). Distinguishing short-term memory from working memory. *Memory & Cognition, 29,* 1–9.

Kane, M. J., Hambrick, D. Z., Tuholski, S. W., Wilhelm, O., Payne, T. W., & Engle, R. W. (2004). The generality of working memory capacity: A latent-variable approach to verbal and visuospatial memory span and reasoning. *Journal of Experimental Psychology: General, 133,* 189–217.

Kyllonen, P. C., & Christal, R. E. (1990). Reasoning ability is (little more than) working memory capacity?! *Intelligence, 14,* 389–433.

La Pointe, L. B., & Engle, R. W. (1990). Simple and complex memory spans as measures of working memory capacity. *Journal of Experimental Psychology: Learning, Memory and Cognition, 16,* 1118–1133.

Lépine, R., Barrouillet, P., & Camos, V. (2005). What makes working memory spans so predictive of high level cognition? *Psychonomic Bulletin & Review, 12,* 165–170.

Logie, R. H. (1995). *Visuo-spatial working memory.* Hillsdale, NJ: Lawrence Erlbaum Associates.

Logie, R. H., & Marchetti, C. (1991). Visuo-spatial working memory: Visual, spatial or central executive? In R. H. Logie & M. Denis (Eds.), *Mental images in human cognition* (pp. 105–115). Amsterdam: Elsevier.

Logie, R. H., Zucco, G. M., & Baddeley, A. D. (1990). Interference with visual short-term memory. *Acta Psychologia, 75,* 55–74.

Lustig, C., May, C. P., & Hasher, L. (2001). Working memory span and the role of proactive interference. *Journal of Experimental Psychology: General, 130,* 199–207.

Maybery, M. T., & Do, N. (2003). Relationships between facets of working memory and performance on a curriculum-based mathematics test in children. *Educational and Child Psychology, 20,* 77–92.

McLean, J. F., & Hitch, G. J. (1999). Working memory impairments in children with specific arithmetic learning difficulties. *Journal of Experimental Child Psychology, 74,* 240–260.

Milner, B. (1971). Interhemispheric differences in the localisation of psychological processes in man. *British Medical Bulletin, 27,* 272–277.

Miyake, A., Friedman, N. P., Rettinger, D. A., Shah, P., & Hegarty, M. (2001). How are visuospatial working memory, executive functioning, and spatial abilities related? A latent-variable analysis. *Journal of Experimental Psychology: General, 130,* 621–640.

Montgomery, J. W. (2003). Working memory and sentence comprehension in children with specific language impairment: What we know so far. *Journal of Communication Disorders, 36,* 221–231.

Muter, V., Hulme, C., & Snowling, M. (1997). *The Phonological Abilities Test.* San Antonio, TX: The Psychological Corporation.

Myerson, J., Jenkins, L., Hale, S., & Sliwinski, M. (2000). Stocks and losses, items and interference: A reply to Oberauer and Süß (2000). *Psychonomic Bulletin & Review, 7,* 734–740.

Oakhill, J., & Kyle, F. (2000). The relation between phonological awareness and working memory. *Journal of Experimental Child Psychology, 75,* 152–164.

Oberauer, K., & Kliegl, R. (2001). Beyond resources: Formal models of complexity effects and age differences in working memory. *European Journal of Cognitive Psychology, 13,* 187–215.

Oberauer, K., Schulze, R., Wilhelm, O., & Süß, H.-M. (2005). Working memory and intelligence—their correlation and their relation: Comment on Ackerman, Beier, and Boyle (2005). *Psychological Bulletin, 131*, 61–65.

Oberauer, K., & Süß, H.-M. (2000). Working memory and interference: A comment on Jenkins, Myerson, Hale, and Fry (1999). *Psychonomic Bulletin & Review, 7*, 727–733.

Oberauer, K., Süß, H.-M., Schulze, R., Wilhelm, O., & Wittmann, W. W. (2000). Working memory capacity—facets of a cognitive ability construct. *Personality and Individual Differences, 29*, 1017–1045.

Oberauer, K., Süß, H.-M., Wilhelm, O., & Wittmann, W. W. (2003). The multiple faces of working memory: Storage, processing, supervision and coordination. *Intelligence, 31*, 167–193.

Pennington, B. F., & Ozonoff, S. (1996). Executive functions and developmental psychopathology. *Journal of Child Psychology and Psychiatry, 37*, 51–87.

Pickering, S. J., Gathercole, S. E., & Peaker, S. M. (1998). Verbal and visuo-spatial short-term memory in children: Evidence for common and distinct mechanisms. *Memory & Cognition, 26*, 1117–1130.

Posner, M. I., & Rossman, E. (1965). Effect of size and location of informational transforms upon short-term retention. *Journal of Experimental Psychology, 70*, 496–505.

Russell, J. (1997). *Autism as an executive disorder.* Oxford, UK: Oxford University Press.

Russell, J., Jarrold, C., & Henry, L. (1996). Working memory in children with autism and with moderate learning difficulties. *Journal of Child Psychology and Psychiatry, 37*, 673–686.

Salthouse, T. A. (1994). How many causes are there of aging-related decrements in cognitive functioning? *Developmental Review, 14*, 413–437.

Salthouse, T. A. (1996). The processing-speed theory of adult age differences in cognition. *Psychological Review, 103*, 403–428.

Salthouse, T. A., & Babcock, R. L. (1991). Decomposing adult age differences in working memory. *Developmental Psychology, 27*, 763–776.

Shah, P., & Miyake, A. (1996). The separability of working memory resources for spatial thinking and language processing: An individual differences approach. *Journal of Experimental Psychology, 125*, 4–27.

Siegel, L. S., & Ryan, E. B. (1989). The development of working memory in normally achieving and subtypes of learning disabled children. *Child Development, 60*, 973–980.

Smith, E. E., Jonides, J., & Koeppe, R. A. (1996). Dissociating verbal and spatial working memory using PET. *Cerebral Cortex, 6*, 11–20.

Smyth, M. M., & Scholey, K. A. (1992). Determining spatial span: The role of movement time and articulation rate. *Quarterly Journal of Experimental Psychology, 45A*, 479–501.

Smyth, M. M., & Scholey, K. A. (1996a). The relationship between articulation time and memory performance in verbal and visuospatial tasks. *British Journal of Psychology, 87*, 179–191.

Smyth, M. M., & Scholey, K. A. (1996b). Serial order in spatial immediate memory. *Quarterly Journal of Experimental Psychology, 49A*, 159–177.

Swanson, H. L., & Berninger, V. (1995). The role of working memory in skilled and less skilled reader's comprehension. *Intelligence, 21*, 83–108.

Swanson, H. L., & Berninger, V. W. (1996). Individual differences in children's working memory and writing skill. *Journal of Experimental Child Psychology, 63*, 358–385.

Tehan, G., Hendry, L., & Kocinski, D. (2001). Word length and phonological similarity effects in simple, complex and delayed serial recall tasks: Implications for working memory. *Memory, 9*, 333–348.

Towse, J. N., Hitch, G. J., & Hutton, U. M. Z. (1998). A reevaluation of working memory capacity in children. *Journal of Memory and Language, 39*, 195–217.

Towse, J. N., Hitch, G. J., & Hutton, U. M. Z. (2002). On the nature of the relationship between processing activity and item retention in children. *Journal of Experimental Child Psychology, 82*, 156–184.

Towse, J. N., & Houston-Price, C. M. T. (2001). Combining representations in working memory: A brief report. *British Journal of Developmental Psychology, 19*, 319–324.

Turner, M. L., & Engle, R. W. (1989). Is working memory capacity task dependent? *Journal of Memory and Language, 28*, 127–154.

Vallar, G., & Papagno, C. (1995). Neuropsychological impairments of short-term memory. In A. D. Baddeley, B. A. Wilson, & F. Watts (Eds.), *Handbook of memory disorders* (pp. 135–165). Chichester: John Wiley & Sons.

Vicari, S., Carlesimo, G. A., Brizzolara, D., & Pezzini, G. (1996). Short-term memory in children with Williams syndrome: A reduced contribution of lexical-semantic knowledge to word span. *Neuropsychologia, 34,* 919–925.

Wang, P. P., & Bellugi, U. (1994). Evidence from two genetic syndromes for a dissociation between verbal and visual-spatial short-term memory. *Journal of Clinical and Experimental Neuropsychology, 16,* 317–322.

Waters, G. S., & Caplan, D. (1996). The measurement of verbal working memory capacity and its relation to reading comprehension. *Quarterly Journal of Experimental Psychology, 49A,* 51–79.

7

Developmental and Computational Approaches to Variation in Working Memory

YUKO MUNAKATA, J. BRUCE MORTON,
and RANDALL C. O'REILLY

You've lost your keys and are searching around the house for them. To find them, you must keep in mind the goal of searching for the keys as you wander from room to room, searching pockets, hooks, and containers. And you want to keep track of where you have already searched and where you have yet to search. Although we are not perfect at these skills, we are reasonably good at them (as evidenced by the fact that typically keys are ultimately found!).

In this chapter, we consider the working memory processes that contribute to our abilities to handle these kinds of tasks, and differences that lead to variations in these working memory processes. We focus on two processes, active maintenance and information updating, that are central to working memory abilities. We do not mean to claim that these are the *only* processes involved in working memory, but they are important processes that other working memory processes likely tap or build on. We describe computational models and behavioral studies designed to test the mechanisms subserving active maintenance and infor-

mation updating. We discuss how variations in these processes may contribute to variations in working memory observed across development, across diseases and disorders, and across typical adults. Understanding such variation may help us to understand working memory in general. We close with a discussion of the relation between our approach to working memory and others' in this volume (see Box 7.1 for summary).

Before turning to these substantive issues, we provide a brief overview of the particular computational approach that we take. Our modeling work fits within the growing field of *computational cognitive neuroscience* (O'Reilly & Munakata, 2000), which focuses on the use of computational models to help understand the relation between the brain and behavior. We use artificial neural network models that mathematically simulate biological neurons. These networks can be manipulated and tested in very specific and precise ways, to assess theories of how biological neural networks function to produce our thoughts and behaviors.

Such models can be crucial for helping us to understand complex, nonlinear interactions of the sort that characterize brain–behavior relations. Moreover, such models assist in theory comparison and evaluation by requiring theories to be specific and plausible enough that they can lead to working models, and by generating testable predictions. For these reasons and others, many researchers argue that such modeling work is essential for advancing theorizing about cognitive functioning (e.g., Elman et al., 1996; O'Reilly & Munakata, 2000; Rumelhart & McClelland, 1986; Seidenberg, 1993).

In the domain of working memory, computational models can help us to understand the specializations required for the functions of activation maintenance and information updating. This kind of approach can inform an understanding of how and why different neural regions subserve different functions. For example, converging evidence from a number of methods indicates that the prefrontal cortex and basal ganglia play an important role in working memory (e.g., Bell & Fox, 1992; Braver et al., 1997; Brown & Marsden, 1990; Goldman & Rosvold, 1972; Miller, Erickson, & Desimone, 1996; Petrides, 1994; Smith & Jonides, 1998; Stuss & Benson, 1984). What is it about these brain regions that supports these specializations? Why, for example, doesn't parietal cortex play more of a role than prefrontal cortex? Why doesn't all of the neocortex contribute equally to working memory? A computational approach can help answer these kinds of questions, as described in the next section.

OVERARCHING THEORY OF WORKING MEMORY

Our overarching theory of working memory focuses on the computational mechanisms underlying the active maintenance and updating of information. *Active maintenance* refers to holding information "in mind" in a robust form, for example, when it is no longer present in the environment, across delays, and in the face of distraction caused by ongoing processing. For example, to find your keys, you must actively keep this goal in mind throughout the search, rather than being distracted by what you come across in the environment (e.g., a stack of bills that need to be paid!). Active maintenance can be subserved by the sustained firing of neurons, as observed in prefrontal cortex during working memory tasks (e.g., Fuster, 1989; Miller et al., 1996).

Updating of information in working memory refers to the process of interrupting the active maintenance of current information, so that new information can be represented in working memory. This updating process is critical for flexible behavior. For example, in searching for your keys, if you are actively maintaining the goal of searching yesterday's pants pockets but the keys are not there, you want to interrupt the maintenance of that location and move on to other possibilities. Updating may be guided by specialized systems that signal whether information should be maintained or interrupted (knowing "when to hold 'em and when to fold 'em"). Such signals might be mediated by signals from the basal ganglia to the prefrontal cortex (e.g., Frank, Loughry, & O'Reilly, 2001; O'Reilly & Frank, 2006).

We focus on these complementary processes of maintenance and updating in our investigations of working memory for two related reasons. First, active maintenance and updating may be relatively amenable to computational investigation, because they can be defined, implemented, and manipulated in computational models in relatively straightforward ways. Other aspects of working memory, such as the manipulation of information (e.g., when mentally computing 42×17), are more complicated and may be more difficult to link directly to underlying neural mechanisms initially. Second, we believe that active maintenance and updating of information may form the bases for other processes related to working memory. In some cases (e.g., mental multiplication), additional mechanisms may be required, building on maintenance and updating. In other cases, a process that may appear distinct from maintenance and updating (e.g., inhibition) may actually emerge from these basic processes without requiring additional mechanisms. In either case, maintenance and updating are likely to play an important role (e.g., Miyake & Shah, 1999), so we focus our current efforts on these processes.

We are particularly interested in the kinds of representations and learning that allow systems to specialize in active maintenance and information updating. We use neural network models to investigate the relation between relevant brain areas (specifically prefrontal cortex and basal ganglia) and working memory processes. Much of this work is guided by a consideration of *computational trade-offs* in different memory demands, as described next.

Computational Trade-offs in Active Maintenance

A computational perspective can provide insight into how and why neural regions are specialized for different functions (reviewed in O'Reilly & Munakata, 2000). Such specializations can be understood in terms of computational trade-offs, whereby two objectives cannot be achieved simultaneously. That is, as a system specializes on its ability to achieve one objective, it must relinquish its ability to achieve another objective. For example, there is a computational trade-off between fast learning and slow learning; a system that specializes in learning rapidly is not well suited to learning gradually and vice versa. Thus, if there are demands on a system for both fast and slow learning, these functions are likely to depend on distinct neural regions with unique specializations. Similarly, there is a computational trade-off between representations that are highly overlapping and representations with little overlap, so that if both are desired, they too are likely to rely on specialized neural systems.

These kinds of computational trade-offs, between distinct types of learning and representations, can provide insight into the specializations of neural systems subserving working memory functions. We first explore such trade-offs in very simple models, to see how specializations are required to maintain information in an active form across time and to update information (O'Reilly, Mozer, Munakata, & Miyake, 1999; O'Reilly & Munakata, 2000). We later consider the elaboration of such models to simulate performance on specific tasks and explore sources of working memory variability.

Consider the simple network in Figure 7.1 (O'Reilly & Munakata, 2000). This network contains input and hidden units that represent a monitor, speakers, and keyboard. Weights connect hidden units that represent semantically related information; in this case, each hidden unit is connected to the other two. Such interactive representations confer semantic benefits, such as allowing a system to go from incomplete information to activate related information. This kind of connectivity could subserve semantic networks of the sort observed in posterior cortical regions (e.g., McClelland & Rogers, 2003; Lambon-Ralph, Patterson, Garrard, & Hodges, 2003).

However, such interactive representations also come with a price: loss of information when it is supposed to be maintained across delays. When this network is presented with a monitor and speakers, the network correctly activates the

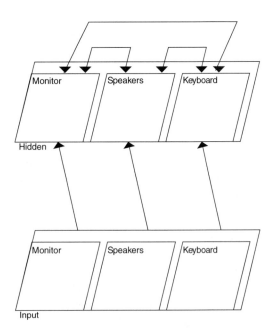

Figure 7.1. Interconnected network. Weights connect hidden units that represent semantically related information. Such connectivity could subserve semantic networks of posterior cortical areas. (Adapted from O'Reilly & Munakata [2000], Figure 9.18, p. 301. Copyright 2000 MIT Press.)

corresponding hidden units (top half of Fig. 7.2). However, when the input is removed, the activation spreads across the hidden units via the weights connecting all of the units (bottom half of Fig. 7.2). As a result, during the maintenance period, it is no longer clear what the network was initially presented with; the network has failed to cleanly maintain this information. Such failures to reliably maintain activation are observed in posterior cortical areas (e.g., Miller & Desimone, 1994; Steinmetz, Connor,

Constantinidis, & McLaughlin, 1994). Transient maintenance may be observed in these areas, but it is much less robust than that in prefrontal cortex, for example, failing to sustain activity in the face of interfering stimuli.

The simple network in Figure 7.1 can be elaborated to improve its active maintenance abilities. For example, higher-order representations can be added, which connect with lower-level features that go together (Fig. 7.3). This improves the network's ability to maintain information after it is removed. Instead of the activation simply spreading from Monitor and

cycle	trial	Event	Input	Hidden
9	0	Input		
19	0	Input		
29	0	Input		
39	0	Input		
49	0	Input		
59	0	Input		
69	0	Input		
79	0	Input		
89	0	Input		
99	0	Input		
9	1	Maintain		
19	1	Maintain		
29	1	Maintain		
39	1	Maintain		
49	1	Maintain		
59	1	Maintain		
69	1	Maintain		
79	1	Maintain		
89	1	Maintain		
99	1	Maintain		

Figure 7.2. Input and hidden-unit activity as the interconnected network in Figure 7.1 is presented with two inputs (top half of figure), and then those inputs are removed (bottom half of figure). Each row corresponds to one time-step of processing. Each unit's activity level is represented by the size of the corresponding black square. The network correctly activates the corresponding hidden units when the inputs are present, but fails to maintain this information alone when the input is removed, because of interactive representations. (Adapted from O'Reilly & Munakata [2000], Figure 9.19, p. 301. Copyright 2000 MIT Press.)

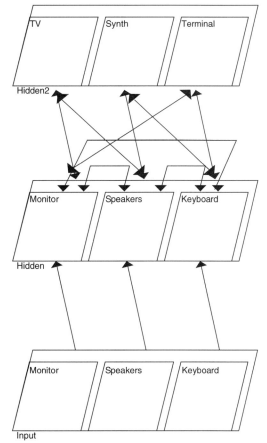

Figure 7.3. Semantic network with higher-order representations. Weights connect hidden units that represent semantically related information, with a layer of higher-order representations that connect with lower-level features. (Adapted from O'Reilly & Munakata [2000], Figure 9.20, p. 302. Copyright 2000 MIT Press, used with permission.)

Speakers to Keyboard, for example, the higher-order representation of TV is preferentially activated in the second hidden layer, and this preferentially activates Monitor and Speakers. However, because the system is still relatively interconnected (e.g., Monitor also connects to Terminal and Speakers also connects to Synth), this solution is not particularly robust. When a small amount of noise is introduced into the network processing (of the sort that our brains likely contend with on a regular basis), activation again spreads beyond the initial input, because of the connections with other units.

More isolated representations may be required for systems to maintain representations over delays, in the absence of input, and in the face of noise (e.g., for working memory). An extreme form of such isolated representations is shown in Figure 7.4. In this network, each input unit is connected to its corresponding hidden unit, and each hidden unit is connected only to itself, rather than to the other semantically related hidden units. When this network is presented with a monitor and speakers, the network correctly activates the corresponding hidden units (top half of Fig. 7.5). When the input is removed, the activation is maintained in these units (bottom half of Fig. 7.5), because there is no way for the activation to spread from these units to any other units. As a result, this network successfully maintains the previously presented information during the maintenance period. This solution is robust to noise in the network processing. This kind of isolated connectivity could subserve active maintenance abilities of prefrontal cortical regions.

Dynamic Gating and Information Updating in the Basal Ganglia

What about the process of updating information in working memory? We can again explore this

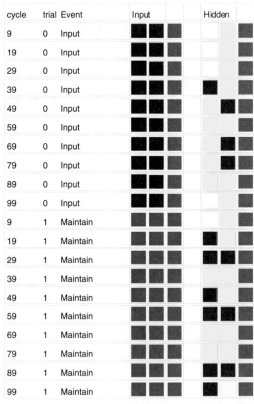

Figure 7.5. Input and hidden-unit activity as the network in Figure 7.4 is presented with two inputs (top half of figure), and then those inputs are removed (bottom half of figure). The network activates the corresponding hidden units when the inputs are present, and maintains this information when the input is removed, because of isolated representations.

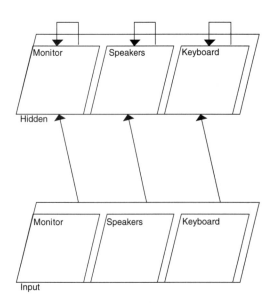

Figure 7.4. Network with isolated representations. Each hidden unit connects to only itself, rather than to other semantically related units. Such connectivity could subserve active maintenance abilities of prefrontal cortical areas.

issue first through simple simulations. Consider a revised set of inputs presented to the network in Figure 7.4. As in Figure 7.5, these inputs start with a stimulus that is presented and then removed, but then a new input pattern is presented and then removed. In some cases, the goal might be to ignore the second stimulus and maintain the first stimulus throughout the delay and the second input (e.g., when the first stimulus represents a location to search for keys and the second stimulus represents a stack of bills to be paid). In other cases, the goal might be to update with the second stimulus (e.g., when the first stimulus represents a location to search for keys that turns out to be empty, and the second stimulus represents a new location to search).

One parameter that affects whether the network maintains or updates is the strength of its recurrent connections. When these are relatively weak, the network updates instead of maintaining. When these are relatively strong, the network maintains instead of updating. However, such static systems, set either to consistently maintain or to consistently update information, would not be particularly useful for working memory. For example, a system that always maintained information would fail to ever move beyond whatever it represented first (e.g., to search in pants pockets). On the flip side, a system that always updated information would fail to withstand interference from distractors (e.g., the stack of bills to be paid). Thus, to be useful, the working memory system instead needs to be dynamic, maintaining and updating information as required across different situations and with different inputs.

This dynamic switching between maintaining and updating can be achieved via a *gating* mechanism (Fig. 7.6A) (e.g., Cohen, Braver, & O'Reilly, 1996; Hochreiter & Schmidhuber, 1997; O'Reilly, Braver, & Cohen, 1999). When the gate is open, working memory representations can be updated (e.g., from incoming sensory inputs), and when it is closed, working memory representations are protected from interference from such inputs, leading to robust maintenance. The basal ganglia have a number of neural specializations that appear ideally suited to serve as a gating mechanism to the prefrontal cortex (PFC) working memory sys-

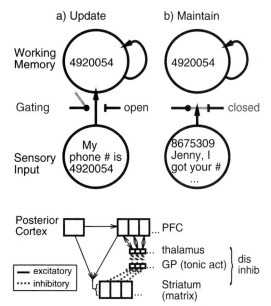

Figure 7.6. A: Illustration of dynamic gating. When the gate is open, sensory input can rapidly update working memory, but when it is closed, it cannot, thereby preventing other distracting information from interfering with the maintenance of previously stored information. B: The basal ganglia (striatum, globus pallidus [GP], and thalamus) are interconnected with frontal cortex through a series of parallel loops. Direct-pathway striatal neurons disinhibit prefrontal cortex (PFC) by inhibiting tonically active GP internal–segment (and substantia nigra pars reticulata, not shown) neurons, releasing thalamic neurons from inhibition. This disinhibition provides a modulatory or gating-like function (Go signal). There are also indirect-pathway neurons (not shown) that provide a counteracting inhibitory (NoGo) signal.

tem; we have captured these mechanisms in an integrated prefrontal–basal ganglia working memory (PBWM) model (Frank et al., 2001; O'Reilly & Frank, 2006). First, the basal ganglia are strongly interconnected with the PFC. Second, the output of the basal ganglia is *modulatory* on PFC, in that it disinhibits prefrontal neurons, instead of directly exciting them. This disinhibition interaction is one way that neural systems can achieve gating, which is a fundamentally modulatory interaction. Third, there are a number of parallel loops interconnecting PFC and the basal ganglia (Alexander,

DeLong, & Strick, 1986), so that the basal ganglia can provide multiple independent gating signals (i.e., *selective* gating), so that some areas of PFC can be maintaining while others are updating.

Figure 7.6B provides a more detailed (but still simplified; see Frank et al., 2001; O'Reilly & Frank, 2006, for fuller details), anatomical picture of the PFC–basal ganglia system, showing the *direct pathway* through the dorsal striatum, globus pallidus (GP), thalamus, and back to PFC. This pathway produces disinhibitory modulation of PFC. The GP neurons are tonically active and thus tonically inhibit the thalamus. When a striatal neuron fires (they are usually inactive), it inhibits the GP neurons to which it projects, thus disinhibiting the thalamus, which is reciprocally interconnected with the frontal cortex via excitatory connections. This thalamic disinhibition thus enables, but does not directly cause (i.e., gates), a loop of excitation into the frontal cortex. The effect of this excitation in the PBWM model is to toggle the state of bistable currents in the prefrontal neurons. Thus, when prefrontal neurons are in the *up* state, they have a persistent excitatory current that helps them remain active over time, while other neurons in the *down* state lack this extra excitation (Durstewitz, Kelc, & Gunturkun, 1999; Durstewitz, Seamans, & Sejnowski, 2000; Fellous, Wang, & Lisman, 1998; Wang, 1999). This bistable maintenance is further supported by recurrent excitatory connections among other such prefrontal neurons, and the combination provides important computational advantages (Frank et al., 2001; O'Reilly & Frank, 2006).

In short, the firing of a direct-pathway neuron, which we refer to as a Go signal, toggles the maintenance of information in PFC in the PBWM model. These Go neurons are activated directly by stimulus inputs contextualized by descending PFC projections, via learned weights. If a PFC neuron is not maintaining information, and a Go signal is received, it will start maintaining its current representation. If it is already maintaining something, then the Go signal will turn off this maintenance, allowing it to start maintaining something else. To clear an existing representation and store a different one (i.e., an update), two Go signals are required. This toggling pattern of behavior has been observed in prefrontal neurons in vitro (J. Seamans, personal communication, January 2002). There are also striatal neurons that project via an *indirect* pathway, with the effect of increasing the level of inhibition on the thalamic pathway. We refer to these as the *NoGo* neurons in the PBWM model—they compete with the Go neurons and enable the PFC to continue to maintain currently stored information. Interestingly, these NoGo neurons only have their effect by preventing (out-competing) Go neuron firing; they do not result in any kind of direct effect on the PFC.

In other work, we have shown that the appropriate patterns of Go and NoGo firing in the basal ganglia gating system can be *learned* via powerful reinforcement-learning mechanisms that are widely thought to be supported by other aspects of the basal ganglia system (Contreras-Vidal & Schultz, 1999; Houk, Adams, & Barto, 1995; Joel, Niv, & Ruppin, 2002; O'Reilly & Frank, 2006; Schultz, Dayan, & Montague, 1997; Suri & Schultz, 2001). We will describe these learning mechanisms in greater detail later. The resulting model was able to learn complex working memory tasks, including those requiring multiple levels of maintenance and updating of working memory operating in parallel, and thus serves as an initial platform for developing biologically based cognitive models of working memory function. Work is currently under way in applying this model to a wide range of working memory tasks that have previously been modeled with a variety of other existing working memory models (e.g., AX-CPT, Stroop, Wisconsin Card Sorting task, Erikson Flanker task), with the goal of developing a "unified model" of working memory function.

Summary

These simulations demonstrate computational trade-offs in active maintenance, which provide a strong computational foundation for our overall theory of working memory function. Interactive representations can support semantic knowledge and isolated representations can subserve active maintenance of information across delays, of the sort required for working memory. Both types of representations are useful, but there is a computational trade-off between them; a single system cannot simultaneously specialize in interconnected and isolated representations. As a result, one neural system (posterior cortex) may specialize in interconnected representations, while another system (prefrontal cortex) may specialized in isolated representations. This computational approach is consistent with (and may help to make sense of) findings from neuroscience on the anatomy (Levitt, Lewis, Yoshioka, & Lund, 1993) and physiology (Rao, Williams, & Goldman-Rakic, 1999) of PFC, which may suggest more isolated representations in this region.

Further, the system that specializes in active maintenance must also be able to dynamically switch between robust maintenance and rapid updating with new information. This switching requires a dynamic gating mechanism, and the basal ganglia have appropriate specialized neural mechanisms to achieve this dynamic gating function through extensive disinhibitory connections with the PFC. Furthermore, the basal ganglia also contain learning mechanisms capable of training the dynamic gating mechanisms in task-relevant ways. Thus, we think our integrated PBWM model has the elements in place for a fully self-contained theory of both maintenance and control of working memory, without relying on unexplained "homunculi" such as a central executive.

We have investigated to varying degrees these components of our overarching theory—isolated representations for active maintenance, and a gating system for information updating—and their relevance to variation in working memory. In what follows, we describe findings from this research, and we consider avenues for further exploration within this framework.

CRITICAL SOURCES OF WORKING MEMORY VARIATION

There are many potential sources of working memory variation within our framework, which we have investigated to varying degrees. For example, people could differ in the degree of isolation and strength of working memory representations, the learning of working memory representations, and the efficiency of gating processes. After briefly presenting some of these possibilities, we will focus our discussion on contributions from variations in the strength of working memory representations, the main source of variation we have explored to date.

Gating and Learning of Representations

We expect that our models will provide a rich source of predictions regarding the specific contributions of the basal ganglia dynamic gating system to individual variability. Differences in gating abilities should be important both in the "mature" trained form of the networks and over the developmental time course of learning tasks. By virtue of having numerous anatomically specified mechanisms, our full PBWM model has the potential for exploring a wide range of sources of individual variability in working memory function, which could in principle be independently assessed through various neuroscience measurement techniques. This potential has yet to be realized, however, as we are just at the initial stages of exploring these models. Nevertheless, we can provide some examples of what these differences might look like.

Diseases of the basal ganglia provide one extreme source of variability. For example, Parkinson patients can exhibit working memory difficulties similar to those of frontal patients (e.g., Brown & Marsden, 1990). However, our model would predict that a more careful analysis would reveal some differences. Specifically, we would expect that Parkinson patients should not be impaired on raw maintenance of working memory information per se, but rather they should be impaired on updating working memory. This can be manifest in cases where one needs to change (e.g., reverse) prior patterns of responding. Consistent with this prediction, evidence in both humans and animals suggests that basal ganglia damage produces selective deficits in reversal learning (e.g., Brown & Marsden, 1990; Ragozzino, Ragozzino, Mizumori, & Kesner, 2002). Another example of the potential spectrum of phenomena that could be addressed with our model comes from the detailed analysis of a set of cognitive control tasks in populations with schizophrenia, Sydenham chorea, Tourette syndrome, and attention-deficit hyperactivity disorder (ADHD) (Casey, Durston, & Fossella, 2001). Casey et al.'s (2001) framework for understanding the PFC and basal ganglia system has much in common with our PBWM model; they were able to interpret behavioral patterns across tasks and populations in terms of deficits in Go–NoGo dynamics contributed by the basal ganglia. Our PBWM model may provide increasingly detailed and mechanistically explicit explanations and predictions of this sort.

Another source of variability that arises in our computational models is variability in the kinds of representations that develop over learning. Even with fixed learning mechanisms and parameters, the complex interactions between these mechanisms, random initial weights, and simulated environmental experiences can produce different representations after learning. These differences in representations, particularly in the PFC and basal ganglia systems, could then substantially affect a whole range of working memory–related behaviors. We have recently explored one aspect of representational development in a PFC model, looking at how the PFC component of the network was able to develop more discrete, abstract, rule-like representations of stimulus dimensions than the posterior-cortex component. These more abstract representations then greatly facilitated cross-task generalization, where experience with items in one task context generalized to other related task contexts (Rougier, Noelle, Braver, Cohen, & O'Reilly, 2005). The development of these representations interacted critically with three factors: (1) the presence of neural specializations associated with both the PFC and basal ganglia; (2) the need to maintain stimulus dimensions over contiguous trials; and (3) the breadth of experience across multiple different task contexts. Thus, individual variability in any of these factors could lead to important differences in the kinds of representations that develop, and consequently in the ability to perform more abstract forms of generalization or transfer. Having explicit computational models enables us to explore complex interactions such as these, which might be too difficult to manage in purely verbal terms.

Variations in Strength of Working Memory Representations

The main source of variation we have explored to date is the strength of actively maintained representations. These explorations are based on the idea that representations are graded in nature rather than being all-or-nothing, present or absent (reviewed in Munakata, 2001). That is, instead of simply remembering or knowing something or not knowing it, we remember and know things to differing degrees. In the case of working memory representations, this gradedness might be instantiated in terms of the number of neurons contributing and the firing rates of those neurons. This graded-representations approach has been applied to understanding variation with development and following brain damage (e.g., Farah, Monheit, & Wallace, 1991; Farah, O'Reilly, & Vecera, 1993; Joanisse & Seidenberg, 2003; Munakata, McClelland, Johnson, & Siegler, 1997; Plaut & Booth, 2000). The developmental work has demonstrated how the strengthening of working memory representations can lead to variations observed across infants and children at different ages. Relatively weak working memory representations might suffice for tasks that children carry out successfully early on, but stronger representations are required for tasks that children master later in development.

We have focused on the strength of working memory representations as a source of variability for two primary reasons. First, this seems to be a highly plausible candidate source of variability, given that representations can vary in strength in numerous ways and result in variability in performance. Second, this framework may provide a parsimonious, unified account of variability. Much of the variability observed across development has been explained in somewhat piecemeal ways. For example, infants succeed on looking measures of memory before reaching measures because of problem-solving deficits specific to reaching tasks. They then succeed on reaching measures with a single-target location before reaching measures with multiple-target locations, because of inhibition deficits specific to multiple-location reaching tasks. And so on. Although the variety of factors posited across such accounts may be relevant to developmental change, there may also be important contributions from single factors (such as the strength of working memory representations) that change gradually with development. In some cases, consideration of these single factors may obviate the need for the variety of factors posited to explain variability. These ideas have been instantiated in neural-network models, and resulting behavioral predictions have been tested and confirmed.

As reviewed below, these models implement the idea that computational trade-offs demand specialized brain regions, and demonstrate how graded changes in active maintenance can simulate variability across development and tasks. Moreover, these models demonstrate how inhibitory control can arise as a functional consequence of active maintenance. The models provide a framework for understanding variation in cognitive control and attention, across ages and tasks. Specifically, they provide insight into why infants and children often repeat old behaviors that are no longer appropriate, despite apparent knowledge of the correct response, and how this changes with development. We focus on three instances of such variation: in card sorting, object search, and tasks with visible solutions.

Card Sorting

As described earlier, in card-sorting tasks (Zelazo, Frye, & Rapus, 1996), children first sort cards one way (e.g., by color) and are then asked to switch to sort the same cards in a different way (e.g., by shape). Although children correctly answer simple questions about the new sorting rule (e.g., "Where do trucks go in the shape game?"), most 3-year-olds perseverate, by inappropriately sorting the cards in the old way. By age 5 years, children perform at ceiling both sorting cards and answering questions. We used neural-network models to explore how variation in active maintenance mechanisms might lead to this sort of age- and task-related variation (Morton & Munakata, 2002a). In the models,

sorting cards one way leads to a bias for particular features. Switching to a new sorting rule creates a conflict between previously and currently relevant features. Strong, active maintenance of the new rule is required for resolving this conflict, whereas weak maintenance suffices for non-conflict tasks such as answering simple questions about the new rule.

The network consisted of three input layers (visual features, rule, and verbal features), two hidden layers (internal representation and PFC), and an output layer (Fig. 7.7; see also Cohen & Servan-Schreiber, 1992). The visual-features layer encoded the shape (truck or flower) and color (red or blue) of the cards, the verbal-features layer encoded verbal statements

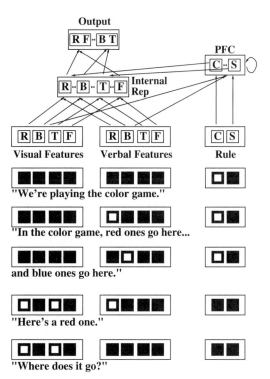

Figure 7.7. Simplified version of the card-sorting network and the elements of a trial. R = red; B = blue; T = truck; F = flower; C − color; S = shape; PFC = prefrontal cortex. In the inputs with "go here," the corresponding output unit was activated for the network to indicate where the card should go. (Adapted from Morton & Munakata [2002], Figure 1, p. 259. Copyright 2002 Wiley Periodicals, Inc., used with permission)

including questions about the current sorting rule (e.g., "Where do trucks go in the shape game?"), and the rule layer encoded the current sorting rule (color or shape). The internal-representation layer summarized available inputs, the PFC layer maintained a representation of the current sorting rule, and the output layer registered the network's response on each trial (toward the tray with the red flower target or the tray with the blue truck target).

Feedforward connections linked relevant units of different layers. For example, the red unit in the visual-features layer was connected to the red unit in the internal-representation layer, which was in turn connected to the red output unit. These connections were excitatory, so that activity in the red input units ultimately led to input to the red output unit. Feedforward connections changed with experience according to a Hebbian learning rule, such that connections between units that showed correlated activity increased in strength. In this way, experience in sorting cards according to a particular feature (e.g., color) led to a bias for that feature. As a result, presenting a red truck (by activating the red and truck units in the visual-features layer) led to greater input to the red unit than to the truck unit of the internal-representations layer. This in turn would bias the network to sort the card as something red rather than as a truck.

Prefrontal cortex units were isolated from one another, with each connecting to itself through excitatory recurrent connections. PFC units could therefore remain active following the removal of external input. This connectivity implemented the notion that different neural regions are specialized to allow incompatible computational demands to be met simultaneously.[1] Top-down connections linked PFC units to the internal-representation units. Specifically, color was connected to blue and red, and shape was connected to truck and flower. These connections were also excitatory, so that activity in a PFC unit led to an increase in the input to its corresponding internal-representation units.

Inhibitory connections were present within PFC, internal representation, and output layers. This connectivity subserved the competi-tion we view as occurring throughout the cortex, via inhibitory interneurons. In this system, inhibition can arise indirectly as a result of active maintenance of certain options leading to the inhibition of other options, rather than through a specific brain area specializing in the inhibition of other areas.

To investigate the effects of graded changes in active maintenance with age, recurrent connections in the PFC were varied continuously in strength. When these connections were weak, PFC units maintained a weak representation of the current sorting rule. As recurrent connections became stronger, PFC units maintained stronger representations of the current sorting rule in the absence of external stimulation.

Networks with weak recurrent connections performed much like 3-year-olds. They correctly answered simple questions about new rules (e.g., "Where do trucks go in the shape game?"), but perseverated on color when required to sort cards by shape. Thus, like 3-year-olds, networks with weak recurrent connections showed apparent discrepancies between knowledge and action. However, the apparent knowledge–action discrepancies were actually based on the amount of conflict that needed to be resolved to succeed. Specifically, the cards to sort contained conflicting information from the previously relevant dimension, tapping the network's bias to respond perseveratively. In contrast, the simple question contained no conflict information from the previously relevant dimension, and so did not tap the network's bias to respond perseveratively. As a result, weak representations of the rule sufficed for the simple questions, but not for sorting cards. Thus, the apparent knowledge–action dissociations disappeared in the network when knowledge and action measures were equated for conflict (e.g., by inserting conflict into the knowledge questions by asking, "Where do red trucks go in the shape game?"). When conflict was equated in this way, similarly strong active maintenance was required for the new rule, so that the network performed similarly on the knowledge and action measures. Consistent with this network prediction, children perform similarly on knowledge and action measures in card sorting when the

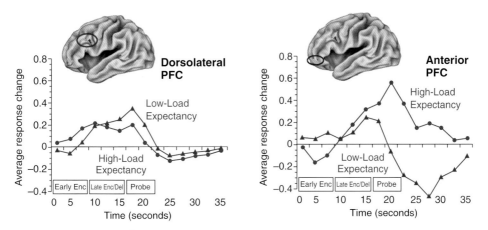

Figure 4.2. Memory strategy effects on prefrontal cortex (PFC) activity (Speer et al., 2003). *Left panel*: Left dorsolateral PFC region showing anticipatory, delay-related activation in low-load expectancy condition. *Right panel*: Left anterior PFC region showing increased probe-related activity in high-load expectancy condition. X-axis refers to the time course of activity. Y-axis refers to average percentage fMRI signal change (from baseline).

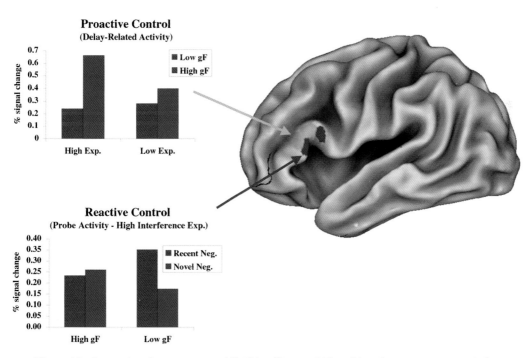

Figure 4.3. Interactions between general fluid intelligence (gF) and interference expectancy in lateral prefrontal cortex (PFC) activity (Burgess & Braver, 2004). *Top panel*: High-gF group shows that high interference expectancy leads to increased delay-related activity in left ventrolateral PFC, whereas the low gF group shows no expectancy effect. *Bottom panel*: In high-expectancy condition, low-gF group shows increased probe-related activity in a nearby left ventrolateral PFC region for recent negatives, but high-gF group does not.

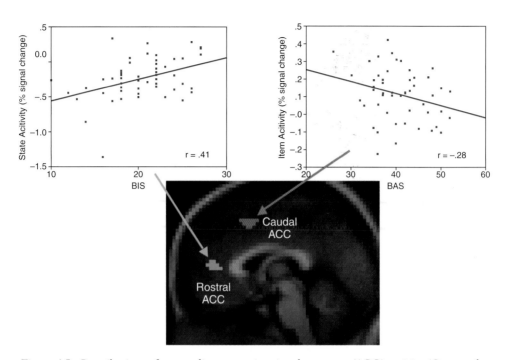

Figure 4.5. Contributions of personality to anterior cingulate cortex (ACC) activity (Gray et al., 2005). *Left panel*: Positive association between behavioral inhibition system (BIS) (punishment-sensitivity) and tonic activity in rostral ACC. *Right panel*: Negative association between behavioral approach system (BAS) (reward-sensitivity) and trial-specific activity in caudal ACC. Y-axis is percentage fMRI signal change (from baseline).

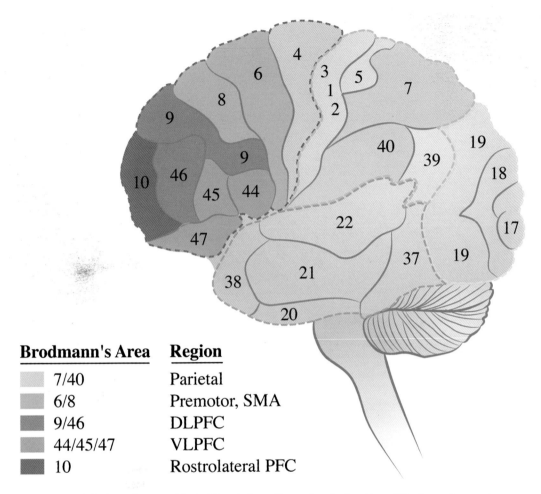

Brodmann's Area	Region
7/40	Parietal
6/8	Premotor, SMA
9/46	DLPFC
44/45/47	VLPFC
10	Rostrolateral PFC

Figure 10.1. Lateral view of the left hemisphere illustrating the location of Brodmann's areas (numerical codes) known to participate in aspects of working memory. Color coding is used to identify the neuroanatomical regions in which these Brodmann's areas are situated. SMA = supplementary motor cortex; PFC = prefrontal cortex; DLPFC = dorsolateral PFC; VLPFC = ventrolateral PFC.

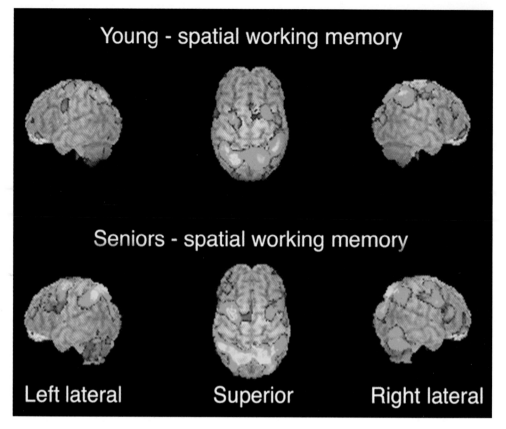

Figure 10.2. Surface-rendered images (left lateral, superior, and right lateral views) of PET activations obtained from younger and older adults performing a verbal working memory task requiring the maintenance only of four letters. The predominance of left-sided activation in the regions of younger adults is evident in contrast to the left- and right-sided activations evident in the older group. For more details see Reuter-Lorenz et al. (2000).

measures are equated for conflict (Munakata & Yerys, 2001).

The network's ability to ultimately overcome bias depended critically on how strongly the PFC units maintained the new rule. When recurrent connections were weak and the shape rule was only weakly maintained, PFC units offered little support to the shape units in the internal-representations layer. Consequently, the color units tended to win the competitive struggle and the network sorted by color. By contrast, when recurrent connections were strong and the shape rule was strongly maintained, PFC units offered considerable support to the shape units in the internal-representation layer. Under these circumstances, the shape units tended to win and the network correctly sorted by shape. These results suggest that the association between age-related advances in cognitive control and development of the frontal lobes may be due to advances in active maintenance mechanisms.

In addition, these results speak to the issue of active maintenance and inhibition discussed earlier. In the model, what might appear to be changes in inhibitory abilities arises as a functional by-product of changes in active maintenance mechanisms. There is no inhibitory system per se in the model, and the model's performance improves without any changes to the inhibitory connections throughout the model.

A-not-B

This framework is general enough to account for age-related changes in cognitive control and attention across various tasks and ages. For example, an earlier version of the model (Munakata, 1998; see also Dehaene & Changeux, 1989) simulated age- and task-related variability in the A-not-B task, in terms of the strength of active maintenance abilities. In this task (Piaget, 1954), infants watch and successfully search for a toy hidden at one location (called the A location) for several trials. The toy is then hidden at an alternate B location. After a brief delay, most infants search perseveratively for the toy at the A location, a phenomenon referred to as the A-not-B error. However, infants show

some sensitivity to the correct location of the toy in their looking behaviors. They occasionally gaze at the correct hiding location while reaching to the previous location (Diamond, 1985; Hofstadter & Reznick, 1996; Piaget, 1954), and they show earlier sensitivity to the correct hiding location in gaze-only versions of the task (Hofstadter & Reznick, 1996) and in violation-of-expectation versions (Ahmed & Ruffman, 1998). In the model of the A-not-B task (Munakata, 1998), weak active maintenance abilities sufficed for success on A trials, because there was no conflict from preceding trials (just as in the first rule trials in the card sorting task). Further, weak active maintenance abilities sufficed for success on gaze and violation-of-expectation versions of the task, but not for the standard reaching task. This looking–reaching dissociation resulted from differences between the two systems in the frequency of updating. The looking system was allowed to update continually throughout the trials (as infants are typically able to do in the A-not-B task), whereas the reaching system was only allowed to update at the end of each trial (as infants are allowed to do when the hiding apparatus is pushed to within their reach). The more frequently updating looking-system was able to make better use of weak representations of the object's hiding location than the less frequently updating reaching system, yielding the same looking–reaching dissociation observed in infants. Ultimately, with stronger active maintenance abilities, the model succeeded on both looking and reaching variants of the A-not-B task. Again, apparent improvements in inhibitory abilities emerged from the development of active maintenance abilities.

Visible Solutions

Some researchers have argued that active maintenance abilities cannot account for problems of control in development, because perseveration occurs even in tasks in which solutions are fully visible. One example is a task in which infants are presented with two towels, one with a distant toy on it and the other with a toy behind it (Aguiar & Baillargeon, 2000). As in the A-not-B task, infants initially pull the correct towel to retrieve the toy (i.e., the one with the toy on it).

Then the towels are switched, for example, so that the towel with the toy on it was on the left and is now on the right. As in A-not-B, infants perseverate, pulling the towel in the old location even though it does not yield the toy. However, unlike A-not-B, the infant can see which towel will yield the toy. How can active maintenance be involved when the solution is fully visible?

To investigate this question, we applied the same neural-network approach used for card sorting and A-not-B to the towel-pulling task (Stedron, Sahni, & Munakata, 2005). Specifically, we investigated the effects of changes in active maintenance when solutions are fully visible. We discovered that the same increases to active maintenance abilities that improved the model's performance on card sorting and the A-not-B task similarly improved performance on the towel-pulling task, by increasing the network's attention to the correct towel.

The network (Fig. 7.8) comprised two input layers encoding the location, identity, and placement of the objects (toy on or attached), internal-representation and PFC layers represented the location of the objects (left or right), and an output layer indicated the network's response. As in the previous models, excitatory connections linked corresponding units, and these connections changed with experience according to a Hebbian learning rule. Inhibitory connections were present within the internal representation, PFC, and output layers. PFC units were linked to themselves through excitatory recurrent connections, allowing them to actively maintain a representation of the current (and visible) location of the towel supporting the toy. Again, these recurrent connections were varied continuously in strength to investigate the effects of graded changes in active maintenance with age.

The simulated task consisted of four A trials in which a toy and a towel were present in both locations (with one toy on its towel and the other toy not on its towel), followed by a B trial in which toy placement was reversed. The network performed well on A trials, which led to a bias for the towel location that supported the toy on A trials. Reversing the toy placement on B trials therefore created a competi-

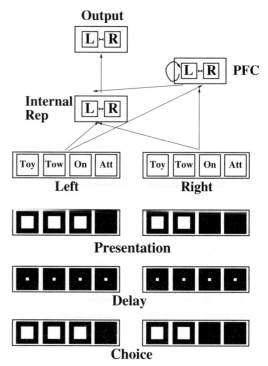

Figure 7.8. Towel-pulling network and the elements of an A trial (Stedron, Sahni, & Munakata, 2005). The input units encode information about the identity of objects (toy and towel) and their placement (on and attached). A toy sitting behind a towel would activate the toy and towel units only (as on the right side of the trial shown). A toy sitting on a towel would activate the toy, towel, and on units (as on the left side of the trial shown). A toy that attached to its supporting towel would activate the toy, towel, on, and attached units; this condition is not be discussed here.

tion between this bias and the current input indicating that the toy was now placed on the opposite towel. Whether the network overcame this bias and responded correctly on B trials therefore depended on input from the PFC and the strength of the recurrent connections. When recurrence was low and PFC only weakly represented information about the new towel supporting the toy, input to the internal-representations layer was weak and the network succumbed to its initial bias. However, when recurrence was high and the PFC formed strong representations, input to the internal-representations layer was comparatively high and the network responded correctly.

Thus, this model demonstrated how a similar mechanism—active maintenance—could subserve performance in both tasks with obvious working memory demands and tasks without such obvious demands. In tasks with fully visible solutions, active maintenance supports attention to relevant information in the environment. This perspective shares much in common with that of Braver, Gray, and Burgess (Chapter 4) and Kane, Conway, Hambrick, and Engle (Chapter 2).

In sum, the card-sorting, A-not-B, and towel-pulling models implement the core assumptions of our working memory theory and explore possible consequences of graded changes in active maintenance abilities. Together, they provide a unified framework for understanding sources of age- and task-related variability in cognitive control.

CONTRIBUTIONS TO GENERAL WORKING MEMORY THEORY

We next address the question of how our approach informs the study of working memory in general, in terms of what we have learned from variation across cognitive development and from the PBWM modeling work outlined above.

We believe that the variability observed across cognitive development is very informative for understanding cognition more generally. First, general cognitive processes likely contribute to the variability observed both across development and in the mature system. Children may simply reveal these processes in more obvious ways (e.g., through their errors), whereas adults show them in more subtle ways (e.g., in their reaction times, and in their errors under demanding conditions). Second, understanding developmental trajectories may be crucial for understanding functioning of the mature system. We elaborate these points and address potential skepticism about the relevance of development.

Finally, the PBWM-modeling work outlined above provides a direct implementation of many aspects of our general working memory theory. We elaborate this model in the final part of this section.

Clearer Windows into Underlying Processes

One example of developmental studies providing a clearer window into underlying processes is in the types of cues children and adults use to reorient themselves after becoming disoriented. Children tend to reorient themselves according to geometric information about the layout of the environment (e.g., that a corner of a room has a long wall to the left of a short wall), while failing to use featural information about the room (e.g., that one wall in the room is blue) (Hermer & Spelke, 1994). Although adults can generally reorient themselves using both geometric and featural information, children's failures to use featural information do not reflect cognitive processing unique to children. Adults show similar patterns of behavior under demanding conditions, when they must carry out an unrelated secondary task while trying to reorient themselves (Hermer-Vazquez, Spelke, & Katsnelson, 1999). It appears that common cognitive processes are at work in children's and adults' reorienting; in both cases, the use of geometric information is more robust than the use of featural information. Thus, the changes that lead to variability across development (as children progress from reorienting on the basis of geometric information alone to reorienting through featural information as well) are likely to be relevant to understanding the parallel variability that adults show in reorienting under different conditions.

Another example arises in children's and adults' perseveration, or the repeating of prior behaviors when they are no longer relevant. Children often perseverate in very obvious ways, repeating incorrect behaviors again and again. For example, after 3-year-olds sort cards according to one rule (e.g., by their shape), they perseverate with this rule even after they are asked repeatedly to switch to sorting the cards by a new rule (e.g., by their color) (Zelazo et al., 1996). Moreover, they perseverate despite being able to answer questions about the new rule correctly (e.g., about where blue cards should go in the color game). Again, adults seem to have no difficulty with such simple tasks, but they show similar patterns of behavior in more subtle ways. Specifically, adults are slowed in their responses under the same conditions in which children perseverate (e.g., when they must switch to a new rule; Diamond & Kirkham, 2005; Morton & Munakata, 2004). And, adults show this slowing despite being able to respond quickly to questions about the new rule (Morton & Munakata, 2004). Thus, it again appears that the processes contributing to variability across development (as children progress from perseverating despite answering questions correctly to flexibly switching) are likely relevant to understanding the parallel variability that adults show in their response times for tasks of flexibility. We will return to this example in the final section of the chapter, to consider implications for working memory processes.

Developmental Trajectory

An understanding of developmental trajectories could also inform debates about neural specializations in the mature system. For example, there is considerable debate about neural specializations for face processing (e.g., Haxby et al., 2001; Kanwisher, 2000; Tarr & Gauthier, 2000). If there are neural regions that are specialized for processing faces, does this reflect an inherent specialization tuned for faces per se? Or, does this reflect a more general system that gets tuned to frequently attended stimuli through learning? If children showed increasing use of these brain regions with the development of expertise for faces (or other kinds of stimuli), this might support the more domain-general account. In contrast, if infants showed high use of these brain regions with early exposures to faces, this might support the more domain-specific account.

We will discuss in the final section some initial attempts to understand the development of representations in PFC that can support systematic behavior in an "adult"-like model. In this case, the developmental process is critical because the adult system appears to be capable of "magical" powers of generalization—we can

almost instantly perform novel tasks without the kinds of extensive training procedures required by monkeys (and standard neural network models). We think these "magical" powers actually reflect the extended development of a large vocabulary of basic cognitive skills, which can then be flexibly deployed in the adult to rapidly solve novel tasks. Thus, studying the development of this vocabulary is critical for understanding the functioning of the adult system.

In these ways, we believe that variability across development provides an important window onto general cognitive processes, which can lead to the discovery of parallel, more subtle, indicators of these processes in adults and an understanding of how the mature system functions.

But Is Development Really Relevant?

Some investigators have expressed skepticism about the relevance of developmental variability for understanding variability in the mature system. The reasoning goes as follows: as children develop, they progress from not having a skill to having that skill; variability across development thus arises from the addition of new skills. In contrast, adults have all of the various candidate skills of interest; variability across adults thus must arise from factors other than the addition of new skills. Variability across development and across adults must come from different sources.

We believe this argument is flawed for many, if not most, cases of developmental variability. Children rarely progress from simply not having a skill to having that skill. Development is instead generally more graded and variable (e.g., Munakata et al., 1997; Siegler, 1996; Thelen & Smith, 1994), with children progressing from less automatic, robust, or frequently used skills to skills that are more advanced on these dimensions. For example, in the domain of arithmetic, a rough glance might suggest that children progress from simply not knowing how to add to knowing how to add (e.g., around 7 years of age). A more careful analysis, however, shows that children across an age span of several years possess a similar repertoire of adding strategies (e.g., counting on fingers, starting with the larger addend and counting up by the smaller addend, and retrieving the answer from memory). The developmental variation comes from differences in the weighting of these various strategies, rather than the addition of new strategies. This is not to say that children (or adults, for that matter) have all of the relevant cognitive skills, and change is always a matter of gradual changes in weighting. However, much of the variation across development can be understood in terms of such gradual changes.

As a result, in many cases like this it is inaccurate to view development in terms of a staircase model, with children cleanly progressing from one developmental stage with a particular set of skills to the next stage with a new set of skills. A more appropriate model may be one of overlapping waves, with children progressing through graded changes in a variety of skills (Siegler, 1996). The latter model highlights the potential relevance of developmental changes to understanding individual differences in the mature system. That is, graded differences in skills in their automaticity, robustness, and frequency of use likely contribute to variability across development and in the mature system.

Prefrontal–Basal Ganglia Working Memory Gating and Information-Updating Models

As discussed earlier, we believe that modeling work is essential for informing and advancing theory. We have described our models of active maintenance and how they may contribute to understanding variation in working memory. Here, we discuss how such active maintenance mechanisms may be modulated to support behaviors in more complex situations.

Active maintenance in PFC can be modulated by adaptive gating mechanisms that can dynamically switch between robust maintenance and rapid updating. As summarized earlier, we have identified neural mechanisms in the basal ganglia that are well suited for this adaptive gating role (Frank et al., 2001; O'Reilly & Frank, 2006). Specifically, the Go (direct-pathway) neurons in the dorsal striatum

can disinhibit the PFC, allowing it to rapidly update what it is maintaining. The indirect-pathway NoGo neurons compete with these Go neurons to prevent this updating, enabling robust maintenance of currently active PFC representations. These gating mechanisms raise a number of important questions, including two that we address in this section. The first is, what determines when these Go and NoGo neurons fire? Without a clear mechanistic explanation of this, the gating mechanism would amount to a homunculus. The second question is, what implications does the presence of an adaptive gating mechanism have for the development of PFC representations?

Learning to Gate in the Basal Ganglia

Our general answer to the first question regarding the firing of the Go and NoGo gating neurons in the basal ganglia is that powerful learning mechanisms shape the firing of these neurons in response to task demands. Specifically, our PBWM model uses a Pavlovian-style reinforcement learning mechanism called *perceived value and learned value* (PVLV) that represents a synergy between biological mechanisms and computational demands (O'Reilly & Frank, 2006). Biologically, such a mechanism is supported by the dopaminergic systems of the ventral basal ganglia in much the same way as the closely related temporal-differences learning mechanism (Contreras-Vidal & Schultz, 1999; Houk et al., 1995; Joel et al., 2002; Schultz et al., 1997; Suri & Schultz, 2001). Computationally, PVLV solves the *temporal credit assignment* problem, which is the critical problem in training an adaptive gating system.

The temporal credit assignment problem arises when the consequences of an action are delayed in time from the point when the action needs to be taken. For example, consider a simple working memory task like the spatial working memory task, where a spatial location must be encoded, maintained over a delay, and then a response to that location must be made. From the gating mechanism's perspective, this task requires a Go signal at the time of the stimulus to update working memory. However,

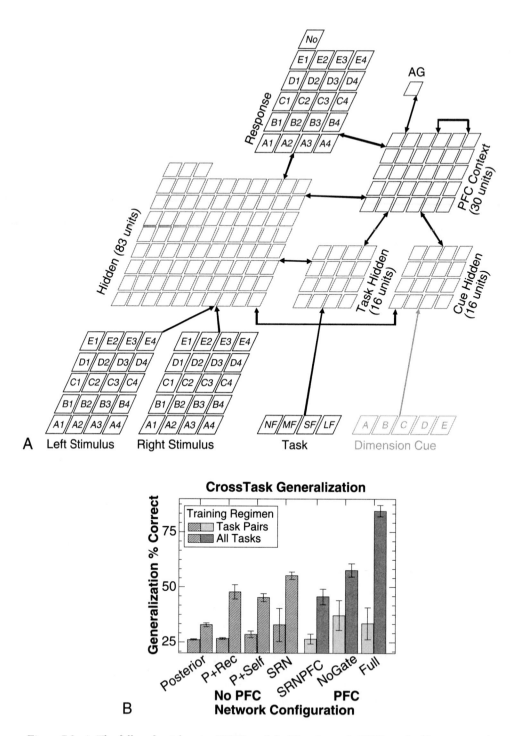

Figure 7.9. A: The full prefrontal cortex (PFC) model of Rougier et al. (2005, used with permission)
Stimuli are presented in two possible locations (left, right). Rows represent different dimensions,
labeled A–E, and columns represent different features (1–4). Other inputs include a task input
indicating current task to perform (NF, MF, SF, LF), and, optionally, a verbal cue as to the currently
relevant dimension (explicit cue conditions only). Output responses are generated over the verbal-
response layer. The AC unit is the adaptive critic, providing a temporal differences–based dynamic

the benefits of having correctly activated this Go signal do not come until after the delayed response based on the encoded stimulus. Therefore, the learning mechanism must somehow learn from these subsequent rewards to perform a Go gating action earlier in time. This is a challenging computational problem. The PVLV mechanism solves it by perceiving reward value (PV) associated with stimuli (maintained in PFC) that were previously associated with learned reward values (LV). So, by trial-and-error, the system maintains stimuli in PFC, and if these are associated with reward, then when these stimuli later appear again, the resulting PV signal reinforces Go firing to these stimuli. Biologically, the firing of dopamine neurons in the ventral tegmental area (VTA) and substantia nigra pars compacta (SNc) (heavily innervated by the basal ganglia) reflect the firing patterns of the PVLV model (O'Reilly & Frank, 2006; Schultz et al., 1997). These dopamine neurons then modulate learning in the striatum, producing appropriate patterns of reinforcement for Go and NoGo firing in our PBWM model.

One of the most important features of the PBWM model relative to earlier gating models is that it can provide selective gating signals to different regions of PFC, so that some PFC working memory representations can be maintained while others are updated. We refer to these separately updatable PFC regions (and associated parallel cite-loops through the basal ganglia) as *stripes*, in reference to the anatomically isolated patterns of connectivity characterized by Levitt et al. (1993). By virtue of having these separate stripes, the learning mechanism

must also solve a *structural credit assignment* problem in determining which stripes are responsible for maintaining different separable items of task-relevant information. This additional mechanism is based on inhibitory projections from the substantia nigra pars reticulata (SNr) to the dopamine neurons in the SNc, which produces a shunting inhibition that modulates dopamine firing in a stripe-specific manner. The resulting stripe-specific dopamine signals provide selective reinforcement for only those stripes that are responsible for the current perceived value (PV) reinforcement signals.

Development of Rule-like Prefrontal Cortex Representations

The presence of an adaptive gating mechanism can impose important constraints on the types of representations that form in the PFC system, which in turn can impact the overall behavior of the system in important ways. In particular, we have recently shown that a network having an adaptive gating mechanism developed abstract, rule-like representations in its simulated PFC, whereas models lacking this mechanism did not (Rougier et al., 2005). Furthermore, the presence of these rule-like representations resulted in greater flexibility of cognitive control, as measured by the ability to generalize knowledge learned in one task context to other tasks. These results may have important implications for understanding how PFC can contribute to tasks in ways that are not obviously related to working memory function (e.g., by supporting more regular, rule-like behavior).

---

gating signal to the PFC context layer. To evaluate the features of this architecture, many variants were tested, from a single 145 hidden-unit layer between inputs and verbal response (with and without recurrent connectivity) to a simple recurrent network (SRN), with a context layer that is a copy of the hidden layer on the prior step. B: Cross-task generalization results (% correct on test set) for the full PFC network and a variety of control networks, with either only two task (Task Pairs) or all four tasks (All Tasks) used during training. Overall, the full PFC model generalizes substantially better than the other models, and this interacts with the level of training such that performance on the all-tasks condition is substantially better than the task-pairs condition. With one feature left out of training for each of four dimensions, training represented only 31.6% (324) of the total possible stimulus inputs (1024); The roughly 85% generalization performance on the remaining test items therefore represents good productive abilities.

Rougier et al. (2005) trained a range of different models on a varying number of related tasks operating on simple visual stimuli (e.g., *name* a "feature" of the stimulus along a given "dimension" such as its color, shape, or size; *match* two stimuli along one of these dimensions; *compare* the relative size of two stimuli). The generalization test for the cognitive flexibility of the models involved training a given task on a small percentage (e.g., 30%) of all the stimuli, and then testing that task on stimuli that were trained in other tasks. To explore the impact of the adaptive gating mechanism and other architectural features, a range of models having varying numbers of these features were tested.

As shown in Figure 7.9, the model with the full set of prefrontal working memory mechanisms achieved significantly higher levels of generalization than those of otherwise comparable models that lacked these specialized mechanisms. Furthermore, this benefit of the prefrontal mechanisms interacted with the breadth of experience the network had across a range of different tasks. The network trained on all four tasks generalized significantly better than one trained on only pairs of tasks, but this was only true for the full PFC model. Thus, the model exhibited an interesting interaction between nature (the specialized prefrontal mechanisms) and nurture (the breadth of experience): both were required to achieve high levels of generalization. We consider the protracted period of development of the PFC (up through late adolescence; Casey et al., 2001; Diamond & Goldman-Rakic, 1986; Huttenlocher, 1990; Lewis, 1997; Morton & Munakata, 2002b) as the time frame over which prefrontal representations are shaped, and the huge breadth of experience during that time then leads to what systematic reasoning abilities we have as adults.

The main reason why the prefrontal mechanisms led to such good generalization in our simple task domain is that they enabled the network to develop discrete, abstract, rule-like representations of the stimulus dimensions (Fig. 7.10). Specifically, the network was trained such that a given stimulus dimension was relevant across a series of individual training trials. Furthermore, in some cases, the network had to "guess" what this relevant dimension was on the

basis of trial-and-error feedback, and maintain it over a sequence of trials in which the dimension was the same. Critically, the robust activation-based working memory functions of the prefrontal model enabled the network to maintain the same representation over time, and therefore these representations learned to abstract the dimensional information that was common across trials, while filtering out the irrelevant information that varied across these trials.

Other comparison networks that could maintain information over time, but lacked a dynamically gated working memory system (e.g., a simple recurrent network or SRN; Elman, 1990), ended up using a variable set of representations over a given dimension and thus did not develop the appropriate abstractions. We think this pattern of results reflects a general rationale for the PFC developing more abstract representations than posterior cortex, and thus facilitating flexible generalization to novel environments: abstraction derives from the maintenance of stable representations over time, interacting with learning mechanisms that extract commonalities over varying inputs. Supporting this view are data showing that damage to PFC impairs abstraction abilities (e.g., Dominey & Georgieff, 1997) and that PFC in monkeys develops more abstract category representations than those in posterior cortex (Freedman, Riesenhuber, Poggio, & Miller, 2002; Nieder, Freedman, & Miller, 2002; Wallis, Anderson, & Miller, 2001).

Importantly, the rule-like PFC representations that developed in the model differ from the symbolic representations typically assumed by traditional symbolic models of higher-level cognition (e.g., Anderson & Lebiere, 1998; Newell, 1990). Unlike symbolic models, these rule-like PFC representations do not support arbitrary symbol-binding operations, and are instead much more like standard neural-network representations, in that they obtain their meaning through gradually adapting synaptic connections with other representations in the system. Thus, they have considerably less intrinsic flexibility relative to arbitrary symbols. This is evident in that our model predicts moderate but far from perfect levels of generalization or transfer to new tasks (e.g., the 85% transfer

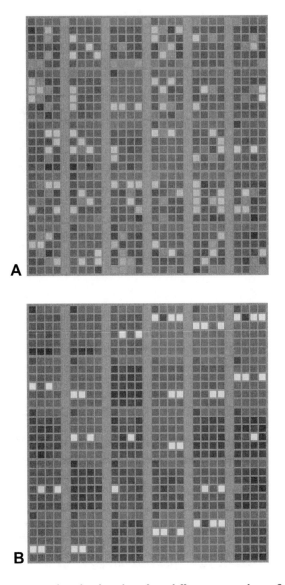

Figure 7.10. Representations that developed in four different network configurations tested by Rougier et al. (2005). A: No prefrontal cortex (PFC) (posterior cortex) trained on all tasks. B: PFC without the adaptive gating mechanism (all tasks). C: Full PFC (all tasks). D: Full PFC trained only on task pairs (NF & MF in this case). Each panel shows the weights from the hidden units (A) or PFC (B–D) to the verbal-response layer. Larger squares correspond to units (all 30 in the PFC, and a random and representative subset of 30 from the 145 hidden units in the posterior model), smaller squares designate strength of the connection (lighter = stronger) from that unit to each of the units in the verbal-response layer. Note that each row designates connections to verbal-response units representing features in the same stimulus dimension (see Fig. 7.1). It is evident, therefore, that each of the PFC units in the full model (D) represents a single dimension and, conversely, that each dimension is represented by a distinct subset of PFC units. This pattern is less evident in the model lacking an adaptive gating mechanism (B) and in the PFC model trained only on task pairs (D), and is almost entirely absent in the posterior model (A) in which the hidden units appear to encode arbitrary combinations of features across dimensions. Panel (E) shows the correlation of generalization performance in these cases with the extent to which the units distinctly and orthogonally encode stimulus dimensions in a rule-like manner.

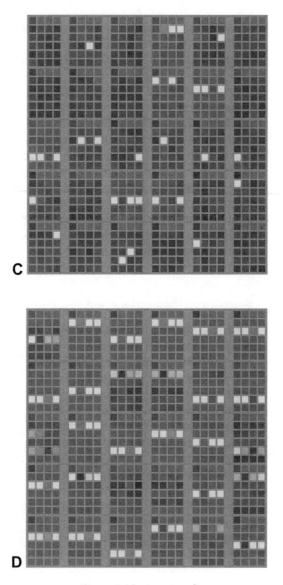

Figure 7.10. (*continued*)

shown in Fig. 7.9B), which is consistent with the empirical data (e.g., Gick & Holyoak, 1987). In contrast, purely symbolic models incorrectly predict perfect generalization performance, unless otherwise artificially handicapped. Nevertheless, the rule-like representations in our model can support flexible cognitive control through a combination of other properties. One is that the PFC representations are more abstract and discrete in nature than representations that develop in posterior cortical areas, which results in enhanced generalization in novel environments or task contexts. Another is that a large "vocabulary" of such representations can develop over sufficiently broad experience, which then enables novel tasks to be performed by flexibly combining existing representations (generativity). Finally, specialized neural mechanisms support both rapid updating and robust maintenance of PFC representations, as well as the ability of these representations to bias or influence processing

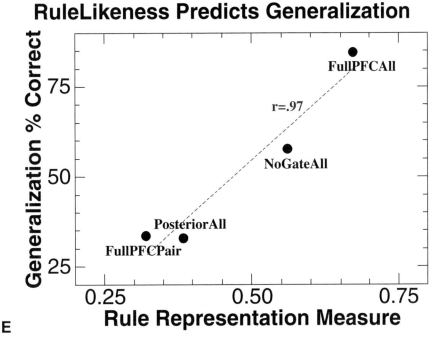

E

Figure 7.10. (*continued*)

in other cortical areas (Cohen, Dunbar, & McClelland, 1990).

For example, to support generalization in a novel environment, an appropriate abstract representation for the task at hand must be rapidly activated and then maintained in the face of novel distractions. This abstract representation then imposes rule-like, top-down constraints on processing in other cortical areas, resulting in more systematic, regular behavior. When demands change, the system must be able to rapidly update to a new, more appropriate representation. To support generativity, appropriate *novel combinations* of existing representations must be rapidly activated and maintained or updated as necessary. In short, we argue that flexible cognitive control emerges from mechanisms that control the *dynamics of activation of existing representations*, in contrast to traditional symbolic approaches where flexibility derives from arbitrary symbol binding, or other approaches suggesting that flexibility depends on rapidly learning entirely new representations (Duncan, 2001).

The extent to which development of these abstract, rule-like PFC representations support more flexible cognitive control could be a very important source of individual variability in working memory function. In the extreme case, we argue that the vastly greater levels of cognitive flexibility exhibited by people relative to that of other primate species may derive from the greatly extended time window over which human PFC representations develop (Casey et al., 2001; Diamond & Goldman-Rakic, 1986; Huttenlocher, 1990; Lewis, 1997; Morton & Munakata, 2002b), coupled, of course, with the expanded size of human PFC. In our model, the breadth of experience was a critical factor in shaping these PFC representations. Thus, we would predict that individual variability in exposure to a wide range of cognitive task demands would play an important role in determining subsequent cognitive flexibility. Increased levels of cognitive flexibility could potentially impact a wide range of working memory tasks. For example, an individual's ability to more flexibly and efficiently perform a novel task (few working memory tasks are routinely performed in everyday life) may result in a higher effective level of working memory span. Also, the correlations between working memory span and more direct measures of cognitive flexibility (e.g., Raven's progressive matrices) could be explained in terms of differences in basic working memory span capacity producing corresponding differences in the formation of abstract, rule-like PFC representations, which are tapped by these tasks.

CONSIDERATION OF OTHER SOURCES OF WORKING MEMORY VARIATION

There are likely many similarities between our theory of working memory variation and other sources proposed in this volume, as well as possible points of contrast. We view our framework as almost identical to that of Braver et al. (with whom we collaborate; see Chapter 4), and share much in common with those of Kane, Conway, Hambrick, and Engle (Chapter 2) and Friedman and Miyake (2004). For example, Braver et al. and Kane et al. emphasize the role of the PFC in providing a controlled attentional system for activating and supporting task-relevant information. This is also central to our approach, as discussed in the context of models of variation in strength of working memory representations. We go further, however, in that we also emphasize the dynamic interactions between PFC and hippocampus to support performance on complex span tasks (see O'Reilly, Braver, et al., 1999, for elaboration).

In general, we believe that a crucial step in identifying similarities and differences (between our theories and others, and among other theories) will be to clarify the precise meaning of central theoretical constructs such as "working memory," "activation," and "inhibition," and to more directly map them to underlying mechanisms. In what follows, we attempt to relate some of these constructs to the central mechanisms in our framework. We also discuss how domain-general and domain-specific individual differences can arise from these underlying mechanisms. Finally, we explore the roles of the PFC and posterior sensory areas in working memory within our framework.

Mapping Constructs and Mechanisms

To explore the issue of mapping theoretical constructs onto underlying neural mechanisms, we start with Chapter 9 (by Hasher, Lustig, and Zacks) in this volume, which contrasts contributions from "activation" processes with those from "inhibition" processes to working memory tasks. The authors find that priming or retrieval of semantic associates, tasks considered to tap activation processes, is unrelated to individual differences in working memory (e.g., across aging). In contrast, prevention of interference from stimuli presented on prior trials in order to respond correctly on the present trial, considered an inhibitory process, does correlate with working memory variation. They conclude that inhibition processes are central to working memory, and that variation in activation does not account for variation in working memory. As a result, inhibition might not reflect the flip side of activation, as others have argued (Cohen & Servan-Schreiber, 1992; Goldman-Rakic, 1987; Kimberg & Farah, 1993; Miller & Cohen, 2001; Munakata, 1998; O'Reilly, Braver, et al., 1999; Roberts, Hager, & Heron, 1994). The studies by Hasher and colleagues are very elegant, and we believe they point to important aspects of working memory function and variability. However, we believe that their data support somewhat different conclusions about working memory, given a consideration of the mechanisms that might underlie their constructs of activation and inhibition.

Specifically, their measures of activation (e.g., semantic retrieval and priming) do not tap sustained, prefrontally mediated activation of the sort that is crucial for working memory. Instead, the "activation" tasks likely tap the richly interconnected semantic networks of posterior cortex. In support of this interpretation, frontal lesions do not affect fluency tasks that require generation of instances of existing semantic categories (e.g., "name as many animals as you can in 1 minute"), but they do affect more arbitrary fluency tasks (e.g., the FAS task: "name as many words starting with the letters F, A, and S as you can in 1 minute"; Benton, 1968; Butler, Rorsman, Hill, & Tuma, 1993). From this perspective, we are not surprised that Hasher et al. did not find a strong link between their activation tasks and working memory. In contrast, an activation–working memory link might be revealed by activation tasks that tap the sustained activation of information across delays, in the face of interfering stimuli, and so on. The FAS task requires such sustained activation (and updating) because the existing semantic connectivity in posterior cortex is not organized along the dimensions required (i.e., initial letter of a word) such that controlled top-down activation of this information is required, and the participant must also avoid activating responses that were already given.

In addition, performance on the inhibition tasks need not tap inhibitory processes per se. The tasks are inhibitory only in the sense that success requires selection of items from the most recent trial instead of those from prior trials, but this does not mean that the mechanisms underlying this process are specifically inhibitory. Neural network models have demonstrated how active maintenance of correct options can lead indirectly to the inhibition of other options, and how changes in active maintenance abilities alone can lead to variation in working memory performance (e.g. Cohen & Servan-Schreiber, 1992; Munakata, 1998; O'Reilly, Braver, et al., 1999). Indeed, many directed-forgetting "inhibitory" tasks demonstrate that irrelevant items are not actually suppressed and can be easily recalled later on. It is more plausible to consider that top-down activation supports the activation of task-relevant information instead of suppressing task-irrelevant information. From a purely functional and computational perspective, the amount of task-relevant information is typically much smaller than the amount of task-irrelevant information, so it makes sense to focus on the few task-relevant items rather than imagine an inhibitory process that specifically suppresses the representations of the large number of task-irrelevant items. (The maintenance load for such a list of items can be huge in typical proactive interference experiments like those used by Hasher et al.)

To emphasize our central claims, we think that prefrontally mediated activation-based working memory is most important for maintaining information in the face of other sources of distraction or interference. In the prototypical case, this interference comes from distractor items presented during an interval when a stimulus item must be maintained in an active state (e.g., Miller et al., 1996). However, distracting information can also come from strong activation of task-irrelevant information even when the task-relevant information is fully visible, as in the Stroop task (Cohen et al., 1990) and a towel-pulling task described in the final section (Aguiar & Baillargeon, 2000; Stedron et al., 2005). In this case, top-down prefrontal activation is needed to support the weaker task-relevant representations in the face of interference from stronger representations. In the case of proactive interference as studied by Hasher et al. and a number of other investigators (Bunting, 2006; Friedman & Miyake, 2004; Chapter 2), the strength of task-irrelevant representations comes from immediately prior learning, instead of a lifetime of learning as in the Stroop task, but the underlying mechanistic principles are the same.

The above discussion provides one example of the general point that purely psychological constructs such as activation and inhibition may not have a clear mapping onto underlying neural mechanisms. Many researchers who have considered the underlying neural mechanisms conclude as we do that controlled inhibition emerges as a consequence of sustained activation in PFC. Activation and inhibition are thus directly related to one another, with activation serving as the primary mechanism. Given that individual variability is likely related to differences in underlying neural mechanisms, we think it is important that greater consideration be given to such mechanisms in assessing the potential role of psychological constructs in individual variability.

Domain Specificity vs. Domain Generality

Another major theme in this research is the domain generality versus specificity of working memory and related individual capacities. Caplan, Waters, and DeDe (Chapter 11) show an extreme case of domain specificity for syntax processing, while other researchers have shown varying levels of generality (e.g., accounting for performance on the Raven's progressive matrices or the antisaccade task; see for example Chapters 2 and 3). As we elaborate below, the neural network models central to our framework can exhibit both domain-specific and domain-general effects. Further, they may provide important insights into what kinds of mechanisms lead to these effects. For example, we describe below how a domain-specific effect can sometimes arise from a very general neural parameter, and vice-versa. Therefore, we reiterate our view that empirical findings of domain specificity or generality cannot be transparently mapped onto underlying neural mechanisms and that consideration of these mechanisms can lead to different interpretations of these kinds of results.

In general terms, neural-network models can explain domain specificity because all knowledge and processing in a network takes place across dedicated sets of neurons and synaptic connections. Thus, different domains of knowledge will tap different sets of neurons and synapses. The efficacy of one set of synapses depends on the complex history of experience that has entrained these connections, thus introducing a strong element of cross-task variability. These general properties of networks have been strongly confirmed in the striking context- and task-specificity of human performance and, consequently, moderate levels of generalization or transfer (Glick & Holyoak, 1987). Furthermore, the observed correlations between working memory and other cognitive functions rarely exceed .5.

Against this backdrop of domain specificity are a number of factors that can lead to some amount of shared variability across tasks. Obviously, the extent to which tasks share content and processing demands will determine their ability to tap the same sets of connections, and this can produce the observed shared variability within content domains, such as within verbal processing and spatial processing. Variability in global neural parameters can also give rise to shared variability across a range of tasks. For example, variability in the production or release of a global neuromodulator like dopamine, which broadly impacts neocortical processing and learning, could clearly lead to corresponding variability across a range of tasks.

Nevertheless, variability in global parameters such as dopamine need not affect *all* tasks equally. An interesting example comes from people with phenylketonuria (PKU), who have a disturbance in the production of dopamine (Diamond, 2002). Specifically, they cannot convert phenylalanine to tyrosine, the precursor to dopamine. Treatment takes the form of restricting dietary intake of phenylalanine, which allows ingested tyrosine more opportunity to compete with phenylalanine for transport into the brain. Without any dietary remediation severe mental retardation results, with impairments in performance across a broad range of cognitive tasks, presumably due to the broad effects of dopamine across the cortex. With moderate dietary remediation (which leads to blood phenylalanine levels three to five times the normal level), performance on tasks that do not depend on frontal cortex (e.g., spatial discrimination, visual paired comparison, line bisection) improves substantially (to normal levels), but frontal-like deficits remain. Diamond (2002) interpreted this pattern as reflecting the higher firing rate and higher rate of dopamine turnover in dopamine neurons projecting to PFC than in other dopamine neurons. As a result, residual deficits in producing dopamine with moderate dietary remediation affected dopamine levels more in PFC than in other areas. Thus, variability in the global parameter of dopamine production caused more variability in some tasks (those dependent on frontal cortex) than in others. More extreme dietary restrictions are required to avert such deficits in frontal function (Diamond, Prevor, Callender, & Druin, 1997).

Another study in which global dopamine efficacy was manipulated via dopamine receptor agonists also revealed an interesting and complex pattern of effects on frontal task performance (e.g., Kimberg, D'Esposito, & Farah, 1997; Kimberg & D'Esposito, 2003). The authors found that the effects of dopaminergic manipulations interacted with the working memory span of subjects, such that increased dopamine levels improved performance of low-span subjects, whereas it impaired performance of those with high spans. The implications here are that base rate levels of dopamine differ between the span groups and that there is an optimal level of dopamine, with the low spans being below this level (so that increases produce benefits) while the high spans are already at the optimal level, so that increases actually impair performance.

The patterns of results discussed above are what we would predict from our computational models of the PFC–basal ganglia system. Dopamine plays a critical role in our models, having both learning and performance effects on the PFC–basal ganglia gating system. For example, our most recent models include a role for dopamine in establishing the balance between Go working-memory updating signals and NoGo working-memory maintenance signals from the basal ganglia. This model predicts the optimal-level effects observed above by Kimberg and colleagues, and more generally suggests that this system is going to be more sensitive to dopamine levels than the posterior cortical system, where dopamine does not have such an important performance effect in our models. In addition to systematically exploring the effects of dopamine variability in our models, we plan to investigate a number of other more global parameters. For example, overall strength of connectivity among PFC neurons and factors affecting the disinhibitory dynamics in the basal ganglia could have similarly generalized effects on working memory performance. These global parameters are the most likely candidates for explaining correlations between complex span measures and such basic tasks as the antisaccade task.

The implications of the model used above for researchers conducting factor-analytic work is that it provides possible avenues for anchoring and independently measuring the sources of domain-general effects. Instead of focusing only on generalized speed of processing measures (which appears to be the only global parameter to have been given strong consideration to date), we advocate exploring other measures of underlying neural parameters (e.g., dopaminergic tone) as a

way of determining what underlies the shared variance across tasks for a given individual.

Complementing such empirical explorations, we plan to subject our computational models to factor analysis while manipulating a variety of plausible global parameters to determine the extent to which these factors globally impact performance on working memory tasks, compared to other non–working memory tasks. We expect such an exercise would be highly illuminating for both understanding the models and using them to make links with empirical factor-analytic work.

Co-opting of Sensory Areas for Working Memory

Reuter-Lorenz and Jonides (Chapter 10) emphasize the extent to which working memory functions can be supported by brain areas that are typically activated in sensory processing tasks, instead of requiring specialized brain areas dedicated solely to working memory functions. We endorse this view to some extent, but we also emphasize that the unique neural specializations of the PFC–basal ganglia system are essential for demanding working memory functions.

Specifically, our view is, given the interactive connectivity of the brain, anything maintained in an active state in PFC will tend to be reflected in activations in other relevant areas of the brain (e.g., maintaining object information will activate inferior temporal [IT] areas, and maintaining spatial information will activate parietal areas). Furthermore, because these other areas contain rich semantic information, these reverberatory activations will be beneficial for processing the maintained information and in supporting its maintenance to some extent.

However, activations in posterior systems may be more susceptible to spread (of the sort explored earlier in the simple simulations) and are less robust to interference. As discussed earlier, neurons in posterior (e.g., in IT) systems continued to represent a prior stimulus during a delay period, as long as there were no interfering inputs (Miller & Desimone, 1994; Miller et al., 1996; Steinmetz et al., 1994). Note that it remains possible that such transient maintenance in posterior areas is driven by more robust maintenance in PFC. In the face of interfering inputs, maintenance was uniquely supported by PFC neurons, not by posterior areas. Thus, when precise and robust representations are needed, as for working memory, the unique specializations of the PFC–basal ganglia system may become essential.

Summary

The main theme that we have emphasized here is that the grounding of constructs in neural mechanisms can provide important constraints on interpretations of behavioral findings of individual variability. What looks like variability in inhibitory function may actually reflect variability in active maintenance abilities. What looks like domain-specific behavior may actually reflect differential sensitivity to a global neural parameter. What looks like an undifferentiated cluster of brain areas supporting working memory may actually reflect the interactions among more clearly specialized neural systems.

CONCLUSIONS

So, how do we manage to find our keys as we search around the house for them? We believe that the developmental and computational approaches described in this chapter provide insights into two processes—active maintenance and information updating—that are central to working memory abilities for such tasks.

First, we must keep in mind the goal of searching for the keys as we wander around the house. This kind of active maintenance requires specialized mechanisms, because there is a computational trade-off between interactive representations (that can support semantic networks in posterior cortex) and isolated representations (that can support active maintenance abilities in prefrontal cortex). Further, we need to be able to revise our subgoals on the basis of where we have already searched for the keys and where we have yet to search. This kind of updating requires a gating mechanism that may be implemented through the specialized neural circuitry of the basal ganglia. Understanding these computa-

tional demands can help make sense of specialized brain regions being required for different functions. Further, individual variation can then be understood in terms of computational differences in the abilities of these brain regions, such as in the strength of active representations in PFC, or in the Go–NoGo dynamics of the basal ganglia.

As discussed throughout the chapter, we believe that developmental and computational approaches have been very important for understanding such working memory processes. The developmental work on perseveration provides a window into similar processes in adults. The computational work has been critical for exploring complex interactions (e.g., between the PFC and basal ganglia during development) and for demonstrating how basic mechanisms could subserve behaviors in nonintuitive ways (e.g., with variation in strength of working memory representations alone leading to knowledge–action dissociations, and perseveration in the face of visible solutions).

There are many other aspects of working memory that we have not considered here (e.g., Baddeley, 1986) that will be important to incorporate into complete accounts. We believe that it will be essential to map theoretical constructs onto underlying mechanisms in this process. Investigating the computational bases of different aspects of working memory should help to ground such theoretical constructs, which should in turn inform our understanding of how and why individuals vary in their working memory abilities.

Note

1. A more complete exploration of this idea would implement greater interactivity among related non-PFC units, but this has not yet been investigated.

Acknowledgments

The writing of this chapter was supported by NICHD Grant 1R29 HD37163 and ONR grant N00014-03-1-0428. We thank members of the Cognitive Development Center and Computational Cognitive Neuroscience Lab at the University of Colorado,

---

BOX 7.1.   SUMMARY ANSWERS TO BOOK QUESTIONS

1. THE OVERARCHING THEORY OF WORKING MEMORY

Our research focuses on the computational mechanisms underlying two components of working memory: active maintenance of information (e.g., maintaining driving directions such as "Turn left at the light") and updating of information (e.g., after turning left at the light, replacing those directions with the next step). We investigate the types of representations and learning mechanisms that allow different brain systems (particularly prefrontal cortex and basal ganglia) to specialize in these components of working memory. We believe that an understanding of such underlying mechanisms is essential for informing and advancing theorizing about working memory.

2. CRITICAL SOURCES OF VARIATION IN WORKING MEMORY

Possible sources of working memory variability include (1) differences in the strength of actively maintained representations (e.g., with representations becoming more robust across delays and in the face of interference with development), and (2) differences in the tendency to update or maintain information (e.g., with such differences contributing to variations observed in diseases and disorders such as Parkinson's disease and ADHD, as well as within the typical population). We focus on these types of sources of variability because they can be related to computational mechanisms contributing to working memory and seem to be plausible candidate sources of variability given biological, behavioral, and computational considerations.

3. OTHER SOURCES OF WORKING MEMORY VARIATION

We believe there are many other potential sources of working memory variability, such as those proposed in this volume. There are likely many similarities between our approach and others', as well as points of contrast. For example, we share with Braver et al. (Chapter 4) and Kane et al. (Chapter 2) the view of working memory representations providing a controlled attentional system for activating task-relevant information. We differ from Hasher et al. (Chapter 9) in how we map theoretical constructs onto underlying mechanisms; we believe that a consideration of underlying mechanisms leads to very different conclusions about constructs such as activation and inhibition.

4. CONTRIBUTIONS TO GENERAL WORKING MEMORY THEORY

Variability observed across development provides an important window into the basic components of working memory. For example, the same working memory tasks that children robustly fail give adults difficulty in more subtle ways (e.g., as evidenced in their reaction times). This continuity across the life span suggests that theories of working memory that can explain variability across children of different ages may also explain working memory in the mature system. For instance, a more robust ability to actively maintain information may explain developmental differences as well as individual differences across people of the same age, and serve as a critical component of working memory in general.

Boulder, and members of the Cognitive Development Centre at the University of Western Ontario for useful comments and discussion.

References

Aguiar, A., & Baillargeon, R. (2000). Perseveration and problem solving in infancy. In H. Reese (Ed.), *Advances in child development and behavior* (Vol. 27, pp. 135–180). New York: Academic Press.

Ahmed, A., & Ruffman, T. (1998). Why do infants make A-not-B errors in a search task, yet show memory for the location of hidden objects in a non-search task? *Developmental Psychology, 34,* 441–453.

Alexander, G. E., DeLong, M. R., & Strick, P. L. (1986). Parallel organization of functionally segregated circuits linking basal ganglia and cortex. *Annual Review of Neuroscience, 9,* 357–381.

Anderson, J. R., & Lebiere, C. (1998). *The atomic components of thought.* Mahwah, NJ: Lawrence Erlbaum Associates.

Baddeley, A. D. (1986). *Working memory.* New York: Oxford University Press.

Bell, M. A., & Fox, N. A. (1992). The relations between frontal brain electrical activity and cognitive development during infancy. *Child Development, 63,* 1142–1163.

Benton, A. L. (1968). Differential effects of frontal lobe disease. *Neuropsychologia, 6,* 53–60.

Braver, T. S., Cohen, J. D., Nystrom, L. E., Jonides, J., Smith, E. E., & Noll, D. C. (1997). A parametric study of frontal cortex involvement in human working memory. *NeuroImage, 5,* 49–62.

Brown, R. G., & Marsden, C. D. (1990). Cognitive function in Parkinson's disease: From description to theory. *Trends in Neurosciences, 13,* 21–29.

Bunting, M. F. (2006). Proactive interference and item similarity in working memory. *Journal of Experimental Psychology: Learning, Memory and Cognition, 32,* 183–196.

Butler, R. W., Rorsman, I., Hill, J. M., & Tuma, R. (1993). The effects of frontal brain impairment on fluency: Simple and complex paradigms. *Neuropsychology, 7,* 519–529.

Casey, B. J., Durston, S., & Fossella, J. A. (2001). Evidence for a mechanistic model of cognitive control. *Clinical Neuroscience Research, 1,* 267–282.

Cohen, J. D., Braver, T. S., & O'Reilly, R. C. (1996). A computational approach to prefrontal cortex, cognitive control, and schizophrenia: Recent developments and current challenges. *Philosophical Transactions of the Royal Society (London) B, 351,* 1515–1527.

Cohen, J. D., Dunbar, K., & McClelland, J. L. (1990). On the control of automatic processes: A parallel distributed processing model of the Stroop effect. *Psychological Review, 97,* 332–361.

Cohen, J. D., & Servan-Schreiber, D. (1992). Context, cortex, and dopamine: A connectionist approach to behavior and biology in schizophrenia. *Psychological Review, 99,* 45–77.

Contreras-Vidal, J. L., & Schultz, W. (1999). A predictive reinforcement model of dopamine neurons for learning approach behavior. *Journal of Computational Neuroscience, 6,* 191–214.

Dehaene, S., & Changeux, J. P. (1989). A simple model of prefrontal cortex function in delayed-response tasks. *Journal of Cognitive Neuroscience, 1,* 244–261.

Diamond, A. (1985). Development of the ability to use recall to guide action, as indicated by infants' performance on AB̄. *Child Development, 56,* 868–883.

Diamond, A. (2002). A model system for studying the role of dopamine in prefrontal cortex during early development in humans. In M. H. Johnson, Y. Munakata, & R. O. Gilmore (Eds.), *Brain development and cognition: A reader* (pp. 441–493). Oxford: Blackwell.

Diamond, A., & Goldman-Rakic, P. S. (1986). Comparative development in human infants and infant rhesus monkeys of cognitive functions that depend on prefrontal cortex. *Society for Neuroscience Abstracts, 12,* 742.

Diamond, A., & Kirkham, N. (2005). Not quite as grown-up as we like to think: Parallels between cognition in childhood and adulthood. *Psychological Science, 16,* 291–297.

Diamond, A., Prevor, M., Callender, G., & Druin, D. (1997). Prefrontal cortex cognitive deficits in children treated early and continuously for PKU. *Monographs of the Society for Research in Child Development, 62,* Monograph 252.

Dominey, P. F., & Georgieff, N. (1997). Schizophrenics learn surface but not abstract structure in a serial reaction time task. *Neuroreport, 8,* 2877.

Duncan, J. (2001). An adaptive coding model of neural function in prefrontal cortex. *Nature Reviews Neuroscience, 2,* 820–829.

Durstewitz, D., Kelc, M., & Gunturkun, O. (1999). A neurocomputational theory of the dopaminergic modulation of working memory functions. *Journal of Neuroscience, 19,* 2807.

Durstewitz, D., Seamans, J. K., & Sejnowski, T. J. (2000). Dopamine-mediated stabilization of delay-period activity in a network model of prefrontal cortex. *Journal of Neurophysiology, 83,* 1733–1750.

Elman, J. L. (1990). Finding structure in time. *Cognitive Science, 14*, 179–211.

Elman, J. L., Bates, E. A., Johnson, M. H., Karmiloff-Smith, A., Parisi, D., & Plunkett, K. (1996). *Rethinking innateness: A connectionist perspective on development.* Cambridge, MA: MIT Press.

Farah, M. J., Monheit, M. A., & Wallace, M. A. (1991). Unconscious perception of "extinguished" visual stimuli: Reassessing the evidence. *Neuropsychologia, 29*, 949–958.

Farah, M. J., O'Reilly, R. C., & Vecera, S. P. (1993). Dissociated overt and covert recognition as an emergent property of a lesioned neural network. *Psychological Review, 100*, 571–588.

Fellous, J. M., Wang, X. J., & Lisman, J. E. (1998). A role for NMDA-receptor channels in working memory. *Nature Neuroscience, 1*, 273–275.

Frank, M. J., Loughry, B., & O'Reilly, R. C. (2001). Interactions between the frontal cortex and basal ganglia in working memory: A computational model. *Cognitive, Affective, & Behavioral Neuroscience, 1*, 137–160.

Freedman, D. J., Riesenhuber, M., Poggio, T., & Miller, E. K. (2002). Visual categorization and the primate prefrontal cortex: Neurophysiology and behavior. *Journal of Neurophysiology, 88*, 929–941.

Friedman, N. P., & Miyake, A. (2004). The relations among inhibition and interference control functions: A latent variable analysis. *Journal of Experimental Psychology: General, 133*, 101–135.

Fuster, J. M. (1989). *The prefrontal cortex: Anatomy, physiology and neuropsychology of the frontal lobe.* New York: Raven Press.

Gick, M. L., & Holyoak, K. J. (1987). The cognitive basis of knowledge transfer. In S. M. Cormier & J. D. Hagman (Eds.), *Transfer of learning: Contemporary research and applications* (pp. 9–46). Orlando, FL: Academic Press.

Goldman, P. S., & Rosvold, H. E. (1972). Effects of selective caudate lesions in infant and juvenile rhesus monkeys. *Brain Research, 43*, 53.

Goldman-Rakic, P. S. (1987). Circuitry of primate prefrontal cortex and regulation of behavior by representational memory. In F. Plum & V. Mountcastle (Eds.), *Handbook of physiology: Vol. 5, The nervous system* (pp. 373–417). New York: Oxford University Press.

Haxby, J. V., Gobbini, M. I., Furey, M. L., Ishai, A., Schouten, J. L., & Pietrini, P. (2001). Distributed and overlapping representations of faces and objects in ventral temporal cortex. *Science, 293*, 2425–2429.

Hermer, L., & Spelke, E. S. (1994). A geometric process for spatial reorientation in young children. *Nature, 370*, 57–59.

Hermer-Vazquez, L., Spelke, E. S., & Katsnelson, A. S. (1999). Sources of flexibility in human cognition: Dual-task studies of space and language. *Cognitive Psychology, 39*, 3.

Hochreiter, S., & Schmidhuber, J. (1997). Long short-term memory. *Neural Computation, 9*, 1735–1780.

Hofstadter, M. C., & Reznick, J. S. (1996). Response modality affects human infant delayed-response performance. *Child Development, 67*, 646–658.

Houk, J. C., Adams, J. L., & Barto, A. G. (1995). A model of how the basal ganglia generate and use neural signals that predict reinforcement. In J. C. Houk, J. L. Davis, & D. G. Beiser (Eds.), *Models of information processing in the basal ganglia* (pp. 233–248). Cambridge, MA: MIT Press.

Huttenlocher, P. R. (1990). Morphometric study of human cerebral cortex development. *Neuropsychologia, 28*, 517–527.

Joanisse, M. F., & Seidenberg, M. S. (2003). Phonology and syntax in specific language impairment: Evidence from a connectionist model. *Brain and Language, 86*, 40–56.

Joel, D., Niv, Y., & Ruppin, E. (2002). Actor-critic models of the basal ganglia: New anatomical and computational perspectives. *Neural Networks, 15*, 535–547.

Kanwisher, N. (2000). Domain specificity in face perception. *Nature Neuroscience, 3*, 759–763.

Kimberg, D. Y., & D'Esposito, M. (2003). Cognitive effects of the dopamine receptor agonist pergolide. *Neuropsychologia, 41*, 1020–1027.

Kimberg, D. Y., D'Esposito, M., & Farah, M. J. (1997). Effects of bromocriptine on human subjects depend on working memory capacity. *Neuroreport, 8*, 3581–3585.

Kimberg, D. Y., & Farah, M. J. (1993). A unified account of cognitive impairments following frontal lobe damage: The role of working memory in complex, organized behavior. *Journal of Experimental Psychology: General, 122*, 411–428.

Lambon-Ralph, M. A., Patterson, K., Garrard, P., & Hodges, J. R. (2003). Semantic dementia with category specificity: A comparative case-series study. *Cognitive Neuropsychology, 20,* 307–326.

Levitt, J. B., Lewis, D. A., Yoshioka, T., & Lund, J. S. (1993). Topography of pyramidal neuron intrinsic connections in macaque monkey prefrontal cortex (areas 9 & 46). *Journal of Comparative Neurology, 338,* 360–376.

Lewis, D. A. (1997). Development of the prefrontal cortex during adolescence: Insights into vulnerable neural circuits in schizophrenia. *Neuropsychopharmacology, 16,* 385–398.

McClelland, J. L., & Rogers, T. T. (2003). The parallel distributed processing approach to semantic cognition. *Nature Reviews Neuroscience, 4,* 310–322.

Miller, E. K., & Cohen, J. D. (2001). An integrative theory of prefrontal cortex function. *Annual Review of Neuroscience, 24,* 167–202.

Miller, E. K., & Desimone, R. (1994). Parallel neuronal mechanisms for short-term memory. *Science, 263,* 520–522.

Miller, E. K., Erickson, C. A., & Desimone, R. (1996). Neural mechanisms of visual working memory in prefontal cortex of the macaque. *Journal of Neuroscience, 16,* 5154.

Miyake, A., & Shah, P. (Eds.). (1999). *Models of working memory: Mechanisms of active maintenance and executive control.* New York: Cambridge University Press.

Morton, J. B., & Munakata, Y. (2002a). Active versus latent representations: A neural network model of perseveration and dissociation in early childhood. *Developmental Psychobiology, 40,* 255–265.

Morton, J. B., & Munakata, Y. (2002b). Are you listening? Exploring a knowledge action dissociation in a speech interpretation task. *Developmental Science, 5,* 435–440.

Morton, J. B., & Munakata, Y. (2004). *The appearance (and disappearance) of knowledge-action dissociations in adults.* Unpublished manuscript.

Munakata, Y. (1998). Infant perseveration and implications for object permanence theories: A PDP model of the task. *Developmental Science, 1,* 161–184.

Munakata, Y. (2001). Graded representations in behavioral dissociations. *Trends in Cognitive Sciences, 5,* 309–315.

Munakata, Y., McClelland, J. L., Johnson, M. J., & Siegler, R. S. (1997). Rethinking infant knowledge: Toward an adaptive process account of successes and failures in object permanence tasks. *Psychological Review, 104,* 686–713.

Munakata, Y., & Yerys, B. E. (2001). All together now: When dissociations between knowledge and action disappear. *Psychological Science, 12,* 335–337.

Newell, A. (1990). *Unified theories of cognition.* Cambridge, MA: Harvard University Press.

Nieder, A., Freedman, D. J., & Miller, E. K. (2002). Representation of the quantity of visual items in the primate prefrontal cortex. *Science, 298,* 1708–1711.

O'Reilly, R. C., Braver, T. S., & Cohen, J. D. (1999). A biologically based computational model of working memory. In A. Miyake & P. Shah (Eds.), *Models of working memory: Mechanisms of active maintenance and executive control* (pp. 375–411). New York: Cambridge University Press.

O'Reilly, R. C., & Frank, M. J. (2006). Making working memory work: A computational model of learning in the frontal cortex and basal ganglia. *Neural Computation, 18,* 283–328.

O'Reilly, R. C., Mozer, M., Munakata, Y., & Miyake, A. (1999). Discrete representations in working memory: A hypothesis and computational investigations. *The Second International Conference on Cognitive Science* (pp. 183–188). Tokyo: Japanese Cognitive Science Society.

O'Reilly, R. C., & Munakata, Y. (2000). *Computational explorations in cognitive neuroscience: Understanding the mind by simulating the brain.* Cambridge, MA: MIT Press.

Petrides, M. (1994). Frontal lobes and working memory: Evidence from investigations of the effects of cortical excisions in nonhuman primates. In F. Boller, & J. Grafman (Eds.), *Handbook of neuropsychology* (Vol. 9, pp. 59–82). Amsterdam: Elsevier.

Piaget, J. (1954). *The construction of reality in the child.* New York: Basic Books.

Plaut, D. C., & Booth, J. R. (2000). Individual and developmental differences in semantic priming: Empirical and computational support for a single-mechanism account of lexical processing. *Psychological Review, 107,* 786–823.

Ragozzino, M. F., Ragozzino, K. E., Mizumori, S. J. Y., & Kesner, R. P. (2002). Role of the dorsomedial striatum in behavioral flexibility for response and visual cue discrimination learning. *Behavioral Neuroscience, 116,* 105–115.

Rao, S. G., Williams, G. V., & Goldman-Rakic, P. S. (1999). Isodirectional tuning of adjacent interneurons and pyramidal cells during working memory: Evidence for microcolumnar organization in PFC. *Journal of Neurophysiology, 81,* 1903.

Roberts, R. J., Hager, L. D., & Heron, C. (1994). Prefrontal cognitive processes: Working memory and inhibition in the antisaccade task. *Journal of Experimental Psychology: General, 123,* 374–393.

Rougier, N. P., Noelle, D., Braver, T. S., Cohen, J. D., & O'Reilly, R. C. (2005). Prefrontal cortex and the flexibility of cognitive control: Rules without symbols. *Proceedings of the National Academy of Sciences USA, 102,* 7338–7343.

Rumelhart, D. E., & McClelland, J. L. (1986). *Parallel distributed processing: Explorations in the microstructure of cognition,* Vols. 1 and 2. Cambridge, MA: MIT Press.

Schultz, W., Dayan, P., & Montague, P. R. (1997). A neural substrate of prediction and reward. *Science, 275,* 1593–1599.

Seidenberg, M. (1993). Connectionist models and cognitive theory. *Psychological Science, 4,* 228–235.

Siegler, R. (1996). *Emerging minds: The process of change in children's thinking.* New York: Oxford University Press.

Smith, E. E., & Jonides, J. (1998). Neuroimaging analyses of human working memory. *Proceedings of the National Academy of Sciences USA, 95,* 12061–12068.

Stedron, J., Sahni, S. D., & Munakata, Y. (2005). Common mechanisms for working memory and attention: The case of perseveration with visible solutions. *Journal of Cognitive Neuroscience, 17,* 623–631.

Steinmetz, M., Connor, C., Constantinidis, C., & McLaughlin, J. (1994). Covert attention suppresses neuronal responses in area 7a of the posterior parietal cortex. *Journal of Neurophysiology, 72,* 1020–1023.

Stuss, D., & Benson, D. (1984). Neuropsychological studies of the frontal lobes. *Psychological Bulletin, 95,* 3–28.

Suri, R. E., & Schultz, W. (2001). Temporal difference model reproduces anticipatory neural activity. *Neural Computation, 13,* 841–862.

Tarr, M. J., & Gauthier, I. (2000). FFA: a flexible fusiform area for subordinate-level visual processing automatized by expertise. *Nature Neuroscience, 3,* 764–770.

Thelen, E., & Smith, L. B. (1994). *A dynamic systems approach to the development of cognition and action.* Cambridge, MA: MIT Press.

Wallis, J. D., Anderson, K. C., & Miller, E. K. (2001). Single neurons in prefrontal cortex encode abstract rules. *Nature, 411,* 953–956.

Wang, X.-J. (1999). Synaptic basis of cortical persistent activity: The importance of NMDA receptors to working memory. *Journal of Neuroscience, 19,* 9587–9603.

Zelazo, P. D., Frye, D., & Rapus, T. (1996). An age-related dissociation between knowing rules and using them. *Cognitive Development, 11,* 37–63.

8

Variation in Working Memory across the Life Span

SANDRA HALE, JOEL MYERSON, LISA J. EMERY,
BONNIE M. LAWRENCE, and CAROLYN DUFAULT

Our interest in working memory evolved out of our research on life span changes in cognitive processing speed. Given the profound changes in response times (RTs) that are associated with cognitive development and aging (for a review, see Cerella & Hale, 1994), we wondered how age differences in speed might affect other aspects of cognitive function. With respect to working memory in particular, there seemed to be multiple ways in which it might be affected by changes in processing speed as well as multiple ways in which working memory might affect higher-order cognitive processes such as reasoning. For example, when the time available for processing is limited, slower processing of memory items might lead to poorer encoding, whereas slower processing of non-memory information might take time away from rehearsal, leading to more forgetting. The potential effects of speed on encoding are similar to those of Salthouse's (1996) limited-time mechanism, whereas the effects on forgetting are similar to those of Salthouse's simultaneity mechanism and to Towse and Hitch's (Chapter 5) task-switching account of the development of working memory. Both poorer encoding and more forgetting lead to weaker memory traces, which would provide a less adequate basis for reasoning. Therefore, we speculated that changes in cognitive processing speed might precipitate a cascade in which increases or decreases in speed would lead to changes in working memory function which, in turn, would directly affect higher levels of cognition (Fry & Hale, 1996, 2000; Kail & Salthouse, 1994). It should be noted that the account proposed by Salthouse and that proposed by Towse and Hitch both emphasize how the consequences of having to switch back and forth between tasks are affected by age-related changes in the time it takes to perform these tasks. These views should be distinguished from accounts of age-related changes in working memory that emphasize changes in the ability to switch itself, a putative executive function (to be discussed later).

When we began our research on working memory we were immediately drawn to the framework proposed by Baddeley (1986), largely because Baddeley hypothesized that the working memory system contains separate verbal and visuospatial subsystems. This hypothesis was consistent with our findings on age-related slowing of verbal and visuospatial processing, findings that also imply the existence of domain-specific processing systems. Specifically, older adults are generally slower to process all information, but they are slowed to a substantially greater degree in the visuospatial domain and to a much lesser degree in the verbal domain (e.g., Hale & Myerson, 1996; Lawrence, Myerson, & Hale, 1998; Lima, Hale & Myerson, 1991). Accordingly, we hypothesized (correctly, as it turns out) that working memory for visuospatial information would be more age sensitive than working memory for verbal information (Myerson, Emery, White, & Hale, 2003; Myerson, Hale, Rhee, & Jenkins, 1999).

The methodology that we adopted for studying age differences in working memory was influenced by Logie, Zucco, and Baddeley's (1990) elegant study of domain-specificity in the working memory function of young adults. The basic design of this study, which involved testing memory spans for verbal and visuospatial information while participants performed verbal and visuospatial secondary tasks, seemed ideally suited for examining age-related differences in working memory. Logie et al. found that memory for verbal and visuospatial information was selectively affected by secondary tasks, so that a secondary task from the same domain as that of the memory items produced much greater interference than a secondary task from the other domain. Nevertheless, in both cases a secondary task from one domain did produce some interference with memory for items from the other domain, and this cross-domain interference was interpreted as showing the role of the central executive. That is, performing any two tasks concurrently, in this case the primary memory task and the interfering secondary task, was assumed to require attentional resources, leaving less resources for control of the domain-specific slave systems directly responsible for maintaining the memory items. This would be true regardless of whether the primary and secondary tasks were from the same or different domains, but when they were from

the same domain, the secondary task also selectively interfered with the slave system for that domain, producing further interference with memory performance.

The experimental paradigm pioneered by Logie et al. (1990) seemed to provide an excellent tool for dissecting the effects of age-related changes in working memory. By developing verbal and visuospatial span tasks that produced equivalent performance in young adults when there was no secondary task (i.e., equivalent domain-specific simple span tasks), we could then administer these tasks to other groups and assess the relative rates of development or decline in the efficiency of the two domain-specific slave systems. Importantly, by going on to examine interference by a secondary task from a different domain than that of the primary memory span task we could assess age differences in executive function, and by measuring the extent to which a secondary task from the same domain produced additional interference, we could assess age differences in the sensitivity of the slave systems. Such sensitivity could reflect either decay of memory traces during performance of the secondary task, which presumably interrupts rehearsal, or the actual displacement or degradation of memory traces by interference from secondary task information.

This experimental paradigm, involving combining span tasks and secondary tasks from both verbal and visuospatial domains, also seemed well suited to evaluating the proposals of other developmental researchers. A dominant perspective in recent theorizing about changes in working memory across the life span has been one emphasizing changes in resistance to interference (e.g., Dempster & Brainerd, 1995; Richardson et al., 1996). Such changes have been described by a variety of terms, including attentional capacity, inhibitory function, and executive control, by researchers advocating different working memory models. Moreover, similar viewpoints have been adopted by those who study children (e.g., Bjorklund & Harnishfeger, 1990) and older adults (Hasher & Zacks; 1988), as well as by those who focus not on age differences but on individual differences among young adults (Conway & Engle, 1996). This perspective has considerable face validity, given the age-related changes that occur in the frontal lobes considered in the context of the effects of frontal lobe lesions (Dempster, 1992; Kane & Engle, 2002; Moscovitch & Winocur, 1995; West, 2000). Although differences in terms (e.g., attention, inhibition, capacity, resources, and control) may reflect different conceptualizations of the issue to some extent, there are nonetheless core similarities, and these similarities are sufficient to lead to similar predictions regarding the fundamental issue: resistance to interference.

Thus, using the Logie et al. (1990) paradigm we were prepared to assess a number of critical sources of working memory variation: potential differences in executive function and in the efficiency of the verbal and visuospatial slave systems, as well as in the sensitivity of these systems to interference. Of particular interest was whether measures of these functions would rise and fall in concert, or whether a particular measure would follow a unique trajectory, lagging or leading through development and/or aging. In addition, having established the often dramatic changes in processing speed that occur at both ends of the life span (e.g., Hale, 1990; Hale, Lima, & Myerson, 1991; for a review see Cerella & Hale, 1994), we wondered what role these changes had in other aspects of cognition (see also Kail & Salthouse, 1994). Our conjectures ultimately turned into the *developmental cascade model*, which posits that the changes in processing speed that occur with age lead to corresponding changes in working memory (i.e., faster processing leads to increases in working memory capacity and function, and slower processing leads to decreases in working memory capacity and function). The cascade model also posits that these speed-related changes in working memory have consequences for other, higher-order aspects of cognition, with reasoning ability, as measured by tests of fluid intelligence, being the paradigmatic example (Fry & Hale, 1996).

It has been said that individual differences represent a crucible in which to test general (nomothetic) psychological theory (Underwood, 1975), and the same argument can be applied

to age differences (e.g., Kotary & Hoyer, 1995). For example, if Baddeley's (1986) theoretical framework is correct, then given an age group known to have an executive deficit, this deficit should render the group's performance of a primary memory span task especially sensitive to interference by a secondary task from the same domain as the primary task. Similarly, if items are maintained in working memory through rehearsal, and faster rehearsal permits more items to be maintained, then given a group with a deficit in the speed of processing information from one specific domain, that group's memory span for items from that domain should be lower than their span for items from another domain.

Of course, observing age differences consistent with the predictions of a general theory provides support, but not proof, of the theory's validity. Moreover, when predictions are not supported, the fault may lie either with the theory or with the additional assumptions involved in the test. For example, a failure to observe enhanced sensitivity to interference by a cross-domain secondary task in a group with a putative executive deficit could occur because the theoretical assumptions are incorrect about executive involvement in performance of two concurrent tasks. Alternatively, the failure could occur because the group does not have the hypothesized deficit, and often only further research can resolve such questions. In either case, age differences can play a critical role in testing theoretical assumptions about the fundamental mechanisms underlying working memory performance as well as those about the nature of differences between age groups.

Over the past several years our research interests have expanded to include not only questions regarding age differences but also more basic questions, such as the nature of the differences between simple and complex span tasks, and how these differences play out in both normal and pathological development and aging. This focus on more basic issues arose naturally from our developmental research, in part because of the general theoretical implications of age differences in working memory. In this chapter, we will first describe what we have observed in experiments with young adults, who are assumed to be performing at peak efficiency relative to other groups. These findings will then be compared with what we have observed in experimental studies of children and adolescents, followed by a comparison with healthy, normally aging older adults. In the present context it is important to note that young adults are not just a control group for studying age differences. Rather, young adulthood is just another developmental stage, albeit one from which it is often easiest to recruit experimental subjects. Thus, in our view, findings from young adults are an important part of the life span developmental story. After describing the results of studies that focused directly on age differences, we will describe the results of two studies on individual differences in working memory and fluid intelligence, one at each end of the life span. Finally, we will review the implications of our findings for the four focal questions on working memory proposed by the editors of this volume.

WORKING MEMORY IN
YOUNG ADULTS

Baddeley (1986) proposed that the working memory system consists of at least three components. There are two domain-specific subsystems, the phonological loop for maintenance of verbal information and the visuospatial sketchpad for maintenance of visuospatial information, and a central executive that exercises attentional control and performs other executive functions. Following the approach used by Baddeley and colleagues (e.g., Logie et al., 1990), our initial goal was to develop a set of memory span tasks that would enable independent assessment of these three components in different age groups across the life span.

Accordingly, we developed two simple span procedures to serve as primary tasks, which we hypothesized would each engage one of the two domain-specific subsystems for temporally storing the memory items, and two secondary tasks, one verbal and one visuospatial, which we hypothesized would interfere with the maintenance

of verbal and visuospatial information, respectively (Hale, Myerson, Rhee, Weiss, & Abrams, 1996; for a review, see Jenkins, Myerson, Hale, & Fry, 1999). Of particular interest was the extent to which a secondary task from one domain would affect performance on memory span for items from the other domain (e.g., the effect of a visuospatial secondary task on verbal memory span), indicating executive involvement in the coordination of tasks from different domains (Hale et al., 1996; Hale, Bronik, & Fry, 1997; Myerson et al., 1999).

For the primary memory span tasks, a series of items (either digits or letters in the verbal tasks or locations in a grid in the visuospatial tasks) were displayed one by one on a computer monitor, followed by a signal to recall the items that were just presented. For the verbal secondary task, participants had to say aloud the color of each item as it appeared. For the visuospatial secondary task, participants had to indicate the color of each item by touching the matching color in a palette located to the right of the primary span stimuli. A schematic drawing depicting these procedures is shown in Figure 8.1. Although our early studies required vocal recall of digits and manual recall of locations (using marks made directly on the computer monitor), our more recent studies have used a touch screen (with letters rather than digits for recall of verbal items) or a computer mouse to indicate recall responses (e.g., Jenkins, Myerson, Joerding, & Hale, 2000; Lawrence, Myerson, Oonk, & Abrams, 2001).

Several features of these procedures should be noted. First, to better isolate the mechanisms that cause verbal and visuospatial secondary tasks to have different effects on working memory, we designed these tasks using an approach pioneered by Brooks (1968). That is, our verbal and visuospatial secondary tasks both depend on the same simple color discriminations, and differ primarily in terms of how those discriminations are reported (i.e., by naming the color aloud in the verbal secondary task, and by pointing to a matching color in the visuospatial secondary task). Thus, it is the response requirement that makes the secondary tasks either verbal or visuospatial in nature.

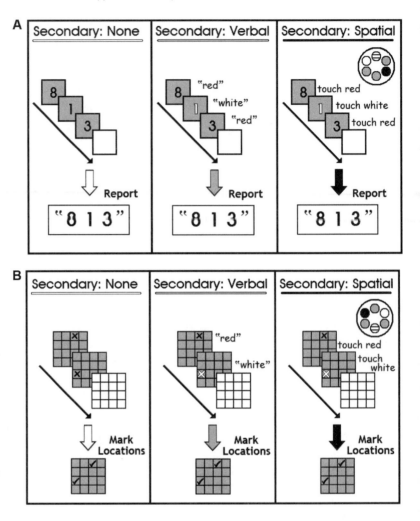

Figure 8.1. Schematic drawings of the procedures used in the three working-memory task conditions for the verbal (A) and spatial (B) domains. Note that the color palette represents red as black and blue as horizontal stripes, and that red memory items are shown as black. (Although memory items could be blue, no blue items are shown.) Also, the color palette, which is shown once in this illustration, actually appeared adjacent to each memory item; the positions of the colors in the palette varied randomly from item to item.

Second, we chose to interleave the primary and secondary tasks, rather than requiring participants to perform them concurrently. That is, participants were not performing the secondary task when a memory item was presented and presumably processed by the participant. Only after the item had been presented could the participant perform the secondary task. This procedure was intended to minimize the possibility that our secondary tasks would compete with the encoding of memory items, although the secondary tasks might compete with rehearsal of the items.

In addition, the interleaving of primary and secondary tasks was intended to make our complex span procedures formally analogous to other working memory procedures such as the reading span and computation span tasks (Babcock & Salthouse, 1990; Daneman & Carpenter, 1980). Note, for example, that in the prototypical reading span task, participants read a series of sentences and then try to recall, in order, the last word of each sentence. That is, participants are presented with multi-attribute stimuli (i.e., strings of words, each of which may be thought of as an attribute of the whole sentence) to be processed, although only one attribute (i.e., the last word of each sentence) of these stimuli is relevant to the primary memory task.

Similarly, the verbal and visuospatial items used in these procedures can be thought of as stimuli with multiple attributes (e.g., color, identity, and location), at least two of which must be processed (color and identity in the verbal task and color and location in the visuospatial task), although only one attribute (identity or location) must be recalled later. In the reading span task, performance of the secondary task (correctly reading a sentence) implies that the memory item (the last word) has been encoded. Similarly, Hale et al. (1996) argued that successful performance of the secondary task (correctly reporting the color of the item) in these procedures implies that the memory item has been encoded, allowing us to focus on why and how the secondary tasks interfere with the maintenance of these items in memory.

Third, and finally, we measured memory span as the length of the series of memory items that can be correctly recalled, because use of this metric facilitates comparison of performance on different memory span tasks. The advantage of measuring span in terms of series length may be illustrated by comparing this approach with performance measures based on the number or proportion of correct trials. With such measures, scores depend on both the range of series lengths tested and the number of trials at each length. In the case of the working memory measures included in the Wechsler Adult Intelligence Scale–third edition (WAIS-III) and Wechsler Memory Scale–third edition (WMS-III; Psychological Corporation, 1997), for example, it is difficult to compare scores on the Digit Span, Spatial Span, and Letter-Number Sequencing subtests, because all three subtests differ in terms of the total number of correct trials that are possible. One may get around this problem, at least in part, by using z scores (e.g., Myerson, Emery, et al., 2003). However, such an approach sacrifices information on the absolute level of performance, and thus may obscure the practical implications of any age differences observed. In designing Web sites that are friendly to users of all ages, for instance, it is not helpful to know that there are significant age differences if one does not also know how many items, on average, young and older adults can hold in working memory.

In our first working memory study, the experimental procedures depicted in Figure 8.1 were administered to a group of undergraduates. We observed that a secondary task requiring a response in the same domain as the primary memory span task led to a decrease in

span of approximately 1.5 items or more, relative to when the primary memory task was performed without a secondary task (Hale et al., 1996, Experiment 1). Moreover, this was true for both verbal and visuospatial spans (i.e., both for digit span combined with naming the color of the memory items and for location span combined with touching the matching colors). In contrast, memory spans were surprisingly unaffected by a secondary task when it required a response in the other domain (i.e., location span combined with naming the color of the memory items and digit span combined with touching the matching colors). These results represent a classic double dissociation and are strongly supportive of Baddeley's (1986) model of a working memory system with separate verbal and visuospatial subsystems.

The interference with memory span produced by a same-domain secondary task appears to reflect the additional demands that the secondary task places on the specific subsystem engaged in maintaining memory items. For example, naming colors aloud may interfere with subvocal rehearsal of verbal items. Nevertheless, the failure of secondary tasks from one domain to cause at least a small decrement in memory span for items from the other domain is puzzling (e.g., the lack of effect of pointing to a matching color on digit span). It suggests that task switching, which is generally thought to be an executive function, does not always lead to a decrease in the efficiency of the verbal and visuospatial memory subsystems. Or put another way, the attentional control involved in coordinating performance of the primary and secondary tasks in this study does not appear to use the same resources as those used in the maintenance of memory information.

Our interest in understanding the way in which the visuospatial secondary task engaged the visuospatial memory subsystem was piqued by these data. The effect of the verbal secondary task on verbal memory span was explainable in terms of the idea that the verbal secondary task interrupted covert articulatory rehearsal of verbal memory items (e.g., Baddeley, Lewis, & Vallar, 1984; Gathercole & Baddeley, 1993; cf., Nairne, 2002). The mechanism underlying the effect of the visuospatial secondary task on visuospatial span was less apparent, in part because the visuospatial sketchpad (and in particular, the nature of visuospatial rehearsal) has received far less investigation than the phonological loop, and in part because the very existence, let alonethe nature, of visuospatial rehearsal is controversial (e.g., Postle, Awh, Jonides, Smith, & D'Esposito, 2004; Washburn & Astur, 1998; see Chapter 10, this volume).

Accordingly, we were interested in evaluating two of Baddeley's (1986) suggestions regarding the types of processes that might be engaged during the maintenance of visuospatial memory items: mental imagery and covert eye movements. We found that, contrary to the hypothesis of imagery-based rehearsal, a secondary task requiring mental rotation did not affect memory span for spatial locations (Hale et al., 1996, Experiment 2). However, simply requiring an eye movement away from the grid in which the memory items were presented did lead to a reduction in memory span, and requiring a visually guided pointing movement in addition to the eye movement significantly added to the interference (Hale et al., 1996, Experiment 3). Taken together, these findings suggest that the shifts in spatial attention that accompany eye movements and direct limb movements disrupt the mechanism(s) used to temporarily maintain location information.

Lawrence et al. (2001) explored this issue further by using sophisticated eye-monitoring equipment to ensure that participants actually made accurate saccades in the eye-movement conditions and maintained fixation in the other conditions, including those involving shifts of spatial attention. Again, visuospatial and verbal memory span tasks were interleaved with secondary tasks by means of an experimental paradigm similar to that described above and shown in Figure 8.1. In Lawrence et al.'s first experiment, the secondary task required participants to saccade to a sudden-onset peripheral target presented following each memory item. The saccade target was randomly located to the right or the left of where the memory items appeared. As can be seen in the upper left panel of Figure 8.2, having to execute saccades caused a decrease in memory for locations of approximately

2.5 items but had relatively little effect on memory span for letters.

Lawrence et al.'s (2001) second experiment used the same two types of primary memory tasks (verbal and visuospatial) and three types of secondary eye-movement tasks: "reflexive" saccades (using the same procedure as in Experiment 1), antisaccades, and prosaccades. The antisaccade task required participants to execute a saccade *away* from the peripheral target rather than towards the target as in the reflexive saccade condition. The prosaccade task required participants to execute an eye movement in the direction indicated by a central cue (an arrow pointing right or left). As shown in the upper right panel of Figure 8.2, all three types of saccades produced decreases of approximately the same size in visuospatial memory span. This finding is surprising from theoretical perspectives that emphasize the role of inhibition, controlled attention, or frontal lobe functions in working memory, because such perspectives predict a special status for antisaccades, as these are assumed to require inhibition and controlled attention, functions that have been attributed to the frontal lobes (e.g., Kane, Bleckley, Conway, & Engle, 2001).

In a third experiment, Lawrence et al. (2001) demonstrated that directional limb movements also led to a decrease in visuospatial memory span approximately equivalent to that produced by saccadic eye movements. Importantly, the limb movements were executed in the absence of eye movements and without visual feedback. These findings suggest that the interference produced by eye movements is not the result of their visual consequences (i.e., visual transients, saccadic suppression, or the resetting of retinal coordinates), because the limb movements had no visual consequences. Rather, interference from eye movements is a property of both directed limb and eye movements, perhaps because they both are accompanied by shifts in spatial attention. It should be noted that these results do not show that attention shifts are used to rehearse visuospatial memory items. They do suggest, however, that such shifts disrupt the processes involved in active maintenance of location information.

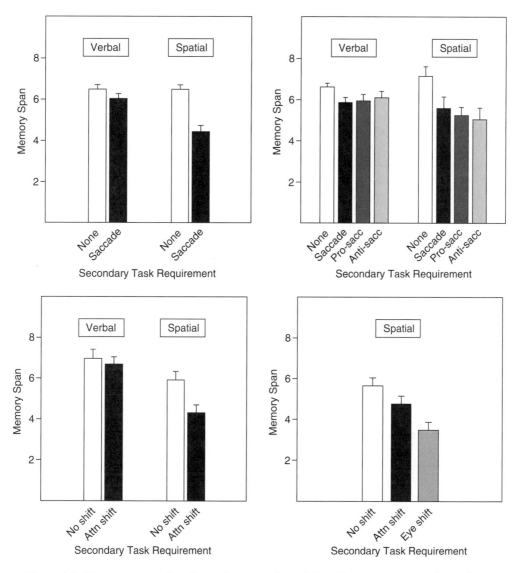

Figure 8.2. Memory spans plotted as a function of condition. Data in upper panels are from Lawrence et al. (2001); data from lower panels are from Lawrence et al. (2004). The spans for the None conditions in the upper panels represent the average of two no-eye-movement control conditions.

In a follow-up study, Lawrence, Myerson, and Abrams (2004) conducted two experiments designed to more directly determine whether covert shifts of spatial attention differentially disrupt working memory function in the verbal and visuospatial domains. In Experiment 1, which again using the interleaved secondary-task paradigm, participants were required to make a same–different discrimination about two successive stimuli (two **X**s, two +s, or one **X** and one +) that were both presented either centrally or peripherally. For the peripheral stimuli, one stimulus was presented approximately 10 degrees to the left of fixation and the other was presented approximately 10 degrees to the right of fixation. Importantly, participants maintained a central fixation (i.e., no eye movements were allowed) while making this same–different discrimination, so that covert attention shifts were required to identify the peripheral stimuli. As shown in the lower left panel of Figure 8.2, visuospatial memory span was much lower (approximately 1.5 items) when the secondary task stimuli were presented in the periphery (and shifts of spatial attention were required) than when the stimuli were presented centrally, and this decrease in memory span due to spatial attention shifts was observed only in the visuospatial domain.

Experiment 2 of Lawrence et al. (2004) addressed the question of whether overt and covert attention shifts differentially affect visuospatial working memory. Three different secondary tasks involving discrimination of a target (an **X** or a +) were interleaved with a primary memory span task. One of these secondary tasks required that the participant maintain fixation (as in Experiment 1) while discriminating centrally presented targets, and another required them to maintain fixation while discriminating targets that appeared either to the right or left of the fixation point. In the third condition, the target also appeared to the right or the left of fixation, but participants were required to make an eye movement to the target.

Relative to the condition in which participants discriminated central targets, the secondary tasks requiring attention shifts and eye movements caused a decrease in visuospatial memory span. The decrease, however, was much greater (nearly twice as large) for the eye-movement condition than for the attention-shift condition (see lower right panel of Fig. 8.2), even though both conditions involved exactly the same stimuli. Whether actual eye movements simply involve more spatial attention than covert shifts of attention or whether there are actual differences in the quality of the attention involved is still unclear. On the basis of this series of experiments, however, we would stress that the highly selective consequences of both eye movements and shifts of spatial attention (which exclusively affect memory spans for location information) argue against the idea that spatial attention involves a general (i.e., domain-independent) resource.

Recently, we turned back to Baddeley's original concept of the working memory system, which he described in terms of the temporary holding *and manipulation* of information (Baddeley, 1986). Although a large number of working memory experiments have been conducted using both interleaved and concurrent secondary tasks that require processing information irrelevant to the primary memory task, far fewer studies have been conducted with working memory tasks that actually require manipulation of the memory items.

For example, consider the reading span task, which is perhaps the paradigmatic working memory task and the one that provided the model for the interleaved secondary task procedures used in all of our studies described thus far. The secondary task in reading span (i.e., reading sentences) involves processing information, most of which (except for the final words) is irrelevant to the memory task. Although such procedures are clearly appropriate for investigating attentional aspects of working memory, they may be less appropriate for investigating certain aspects of working memory that underlie performance on higher-order cognitive tasks. Specifically, reasoning and problem solving often require that some subset of information be held for a short period of time while it is manipulated or combined with other information to produce an acceptable solution to the problem being solved. Mental arithmetic problems, for example, clearly require use of this aspect of working memory.

Emery, Myerson, and Hale (2002) have suggested that this aspect of working memory function (i.e., the temporary storage of items in order to manipulate them) may be better studied using what may be termed *manipulation span tasks* than by pairing primary span tasks with interleaved or concurrent secondary tasks. Letter-number sequencing, a working memory task that has been added to the most recent version of the Wechsler Memory Scale (WMS-III; Psychological Corporation, 1997), is an example of a manipulation span task. In letter-number sequencing, a series of alternating letters and numbers (e.g., "K 2 G 8") are presented, and individuals being tested are required to sequence and then recall these items; numbers must be recalled first in ascending order followed by letters in alphabetical order ("2 8, G K"). Unlike backward span tasks, which appear to involve off-line manipulation of memory items (i.e., rearrangement occurs after the whole series has been presented), letter-number sequencing, at least in the form that we have adapted for computer administration, appears to involve on-line manipulation of the items, and this manipulation may actually facilitate recall.

Our interest in letter-number sequencing was stimulated by the unexpected results of our first experiment using this procedure (Emery et al., 2002, Experiment 1). This experiment was designed specifically to compare manipulation span procedures with those combining primary and secondary tasks. As in many of our previous experiments, participants performed two different primary memory span tasks, one from the visuospatial domain (i.e., memory for locations in a grid) and one from the verbal domain (i.e., memory for letters and numbers). For each of these span tasks, there were three conditions: (1) a simple span condition involving forward recall, (2) a complex span condition that combined the primary span task with an (interleaved) secondary task from the same domain, and (3) a manipulation span condition requiring participants to reorganize the memory items prior to recall (see Fig. 8.3). Participants recalled verbal memory items by touching the appropriate boxes in two grids, one containing digits and the other containing letters, and they recalled visuospatial memory items by touching the appropriate boxes in an empty grid. In all conditions, memory items were presented at a rate of one every 3 s to allow time for secondary task responses or on-line manipulation of the memory items, depending on the condition.

In the complex-span conditions, the secondary tasks involved color judgments (reported either by saying the color of each memory item or by pointing to a matching color, depending on the domain of the primary task) and were similar to those used in Hale et al.'s (1996) study. For the manipulation span condition in the visuospatial domain, participants were told to imagine each memory item shifted one column to the right and to recall these new locations (n.b., if shifting an item resulted in a location that was off the grid, participants were

instructed to wrap it around to the leftmost column of the grid). For the manipulation span condition in the verbal domain, we used a computerized version of the letter-number sequencing task described previously. Letters and digits were presented alternately, and participants were required to sort and sequence the items, recalling the digits first (in numerical order) and the letters second (in alphabetical order).

The question of interest in this experiment was whether secondary tasks and manipulation tasks would have similar negative effects on working memory, relative to the corresponding simple, forward span tasks in each domain. The results revealed that both types of procedures (performing a visuospatial secondary task and spatially manipulating the memory items) caused approximately equivalent amounts of interference with visuospatial memory span. The results for the verbal conditions, however, revealed a very different pattern: requiring a verbal secondary task caused verbal memory span to decrease significantly (replicating our previous studies), but requiring participants to reorganize the memory items actually resulted in better performance than simple forward recall of letters and numbers!

This puzzling finding may be best understood in the context of two follow-up experiments by Emery et al. (2002) that focused exclusively on letter-number sequencing. In the first follow-up study, we found that the beneficial effect of sequencing letters and numbers depends on the rate at which they are presented. When the presentation rate was 2.25 s per item, participants' spans were approximately 1.0 item larger when they had to sequence the items than when they had to recall them in the order presented. When the rate was 1.25 s per item, however, memory spans in the forward and sequenced recall conditions were approximately equal. The fact that the benefit from sequencing the items depends on the presentation rate (whereas simple, forward spans are relatively unaffected by rate) suggests that sequencing occurs on-line, contingent on the amount of time available, and not just off-line, after all the items have been presented.

In the second follow-up study, Emery et al. (2002) added a condition in which the stimuli

Letter-Number Span Tasks

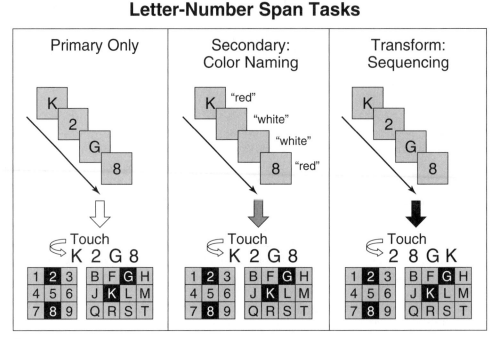

A

Location Span Tasks

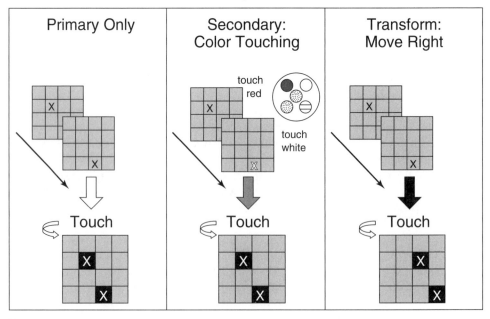

B

Figure 8.3. Schematic drawings of the procedures used in the three conditions of the letter-number span tasks (A) and the three conditions of the location span tasks (B). As in Figure 8.1, red memory items are depicted as black, and no blue items are shown.

were presented in a presorted order (i.e., ascending numbers first, alphabetically ordered letters second), rather than being sequenced by the participants. Memory span for items presented in order was higher than forward recall of alternately presented (and randomly ordered) letters and numbers. When participants had to sequence the items themselves, memory spans were intermediate between those for the other two conditions. Thus, there appear to be both costs and benefits associated with manipulating memory items: ordered items can be recalled more readily than unordered items, but memory items may be lost during the reorganization process that produces an ordered list.

The costs and benefits observed with letter-numbering sequencing stands in contrast to the results for backward spans (e.g., Myerson, Emery, et al., 2003), in which only the costs of manipulation are seen. The sources of these costs are probably not hard to explain: rearranging memory items not only takes time, it may result in proactive interference from the original sequence. As Emery et al. (2002) have shown, however, the costs of reorganization may sometimes be outweighed by the benefits, and analysis of the difference between backward span and letter-number sequencing procedures may shed light on the source of these benefits.

Span tasks deliberately test participants at the limits of their abilities, which implies that the representations of at least some memory items will be degraded by the time participants must attempt to recall them. Reorganization of items into a more familiar, predictable series, as in letter-number sequencing, may facilitate the reconstruction of such degraded representations (a process sometimes termed *redintegration*; Schweickert, 1993). In contrast, rearranging memory items in reverse order probably fails to benefit recall because the backward version of the list is typically no more familiar or predictable than the original, forward version of the list.

Of course, degradation of memory representations (whether through decay or interference) occurs continuously, and the sooner that items can be organized the less likely it is that their representations will become too degraded to be recoverable. This would explain why slower presentation rates, which permit more

on-line reorganization, result in greater benefits to recall performance. Interestingly, the processes involved in reorganizing memory items on-line, like those involved in their active maintenance, appear to be highly domain specific. This is evidenced by the fact that, as Emery et al. (2002) observed in a final experiment, an interleaved visuospatial secondary task had relatively little effect on letter-number sequencing performance, whereas an interleaved verbal secondary task completely eliminated the benefits of sequencing. These results suggest that sequencing uses relatively little in the way of general attentional resources.

Taken together, the series of memory span experiments with young adult participants described above provides strong support for Baddeley's (1986) hypothesis of separate subsystems for the temporary maintenance of verbal and visuospatial information. A particularly robust finding, observed in a number of experiments and with a variety of procedures, is that interleaved secondary tasks produce predominantly domain-specific interference with performance on primary memory span tasks. For example, color and shape discriminations only interfere with memory for numbers and letters if the response is vocal rather than manual. In contrast, verbal memory spans are relatively unaffected by having to point to colors that match those of the memory items, by eye movements or directed limb movements (regardless of whether they are or are not visually guided), or by spatial-attention shifts, all of which do affect visuospatial spans. Importantly, the antisaccade task produces no more interference with visuospatial working memory than other eye-movement tasks.

These findings suggest that the executive functions involved in inhibiting responses, controlling attention, and switching back and forth between primary and secondary tasks produce relatively little interference with the temporary maintenance of information in working memory. Indeed, the presence or absence of an additional processing requirement consistently played a much smaller role in determining the number of items that could be recalled than when the additional processing and the information to be maintained involved the same domain (i.e., verbal vs. visuospatial). Manipulation span experiments suggest that the processes involved in manipulating the contents of working memory may also be relatively domain specific. Taken together, these insights into what does and does not affect memory span in young adults have helped guide the design and interpretation of our studies of age-related differences in working memory across the life span.

WORKING MEMORY ACROSS THE LIFE SPAN

A major difficulty in comparing the effects of experimental manipulations on the performance of different age groups is the lack of equivalent baseline performance. Perhaps the most familiar examples of this come from studies of age differences in RTs, and the problem of comparing semantic priming effects is typical (e.g., Chapman, Chapman, Curran, & Miller, 1994; Hale & Myerson, 1995; Myerson, Ferraro, Hale, & Lima, 1992). Children and older adults both show larger semantic priming effects than young adults. That is, their RTs decrease more than those of young adults when a lexical decision is primed by the preceding semantic context. The difficulty in interpreting this reliable finding, which on the face of it would seem to imply that children and older adults are better at using context, is that children and older adults have longer RTs than those of young adults to begin with (i.e., in the absence of any relevant context). Thus, children and older adults may benefit more from context simply because they find decisions more difficult in the absence of context, and not because they use context more effectively.

Various analytical tools (e.g., regression analyses based on Brinley plots and state-trace graphs) have been developed to deal with the problem of unequal baselines with respect to RTs (e.g., Myerson, Adams, Hale, & Jenkins, 2003; Verhaeghen & Cerella, 2002). The problem of unequal baselines also occurs, however, with respect to memory spans (e.g., Jenkins et al., 1999), for which graphical and regression approaches similar to those used with RTs are ar-

guably less appropriate (Oberauer & Süß, 2000; cf., Myerson, Jenkins, Hale, & Sliwinski, 2000). One approach to dealing with this problem in the case of memory span data is to do what amounts to an "end run" around it. If two tasks are matched in difficulty for one of the groups being compared, then any difference in performance of the two tasks by another group clearly indicates that the latter group is more (dis)advantaged with respect to one of the tasks. More specifically, if a verbal and a visuospatial span task are equally difficult for young adults, then if older adults have lower visuospatial spans than verbal spans (and they do), clearly age affects visuospatial working memory more than it affects verbal working memory. In this case, interpretation of the result is straightforward even though older adults may have lower spans than those of young adults on both verbal and visuospatial tasks.

How does one create verbal and visuospatial tasks of equal difficulty? One approach takes advantage of the fact that memory spans are larger for items drawn from a smaller set. Thus, digit span is larger than letter span, which is larger than word span. Similarly, the number of locations in a matrix that can be remembered decreases as the size of the matrix increases. As it turns out, young adults' digit spans are approximately the same size as their visuospatial spans when they are required to remember locations in a 4×4 grid (e.g., Hale et al., 1996; see Fig. 8.1 above), thereby facilitating comparisons with other age groups on these tasks. Alternatively, one can match spans in a child or older-adult group and then compare spans on the same tasks in young adults (Jenkins et al., 2000). Other approaches are possible as well, but for the most part we have relied on matching young adults' verbal and visuospatial spans, and this strategy has been relatively successful, as we will show in the following sections on children and older adults.

Children

To examine how development affects working memory, we tested children with the same basic experimental paradigm that we had previously used with young adults (Hale et al., 1996), but with two of the task parameters modified so as to simplify the procedure slightly and allow more time. On the basis of pilot testing of children, we decided to use only three colors (red, white, and blue, rather than the six colors used originally with young adults) and to slow the presentation of memory items (to one item every 3.0 s rather than one item every 1.5 s). Data obtained from a small group of young adults suggested that the pattern of results for this age group would be unaffected by these modifications.

Using these parameter values, Hale et al. (1997) compared performance of two groups of children (mean ages, 8 and 10 years) and a young-adult comparison group (mean age, 19 years) on the six working memory conditions examined previously in Hale et al.'s (1996) study. Memory span improved as a function of age in all conditions. The data also suggest developmental changes in task switching, a putative executive function, as indicated by age differences in the pattern of effects of secondary tasks on the primary memory span tasks. As can be seen in Figure 8.4, only the 8-year-olds showed evidence that secondary tasks from one domain interfered with primary tasks from the other domain, although in both cases the size of the interference effect was much smaller than that caused by same-domain secondary tasks. That is, unlike the other groups, 8-year-olds' verbal

memory spans were lower when they had to perform a visuospatial secondary task than on the primary task alone. Similarly, 8-year-olds' visuospatial memory spans were lower when they had to perform a verbal secondary task than on the primary task alone. In contrast, 10-year-olds and 19-year-olds only showed evidence of domain-specific interference.

From the perspective of Baddeley's (1986) model, these findings might be interpreted as showing that the central executive is still immature in 8-year-olds, as reflected in the decrease in their memory spans when they had to switch back and forth between primary and secondary tasks from different domains. That is, although switching back and forth between primary and secondary tasks appears to make minimal demands on the central executive (or requires relatively little in the way of attentional resources) from age 10 onwards, at younger ages task switching may make more than minimal demands on the central executive.

Consistent with previous developmental research (for a review, see Gathercole, 1999), the results of the Hale et al. (1997) study reveal that, in general, memory span increases with age. However, the data also suggest that there may be differences between the rates at which verbal and visuospatial working memory develop. Such differences are also apparent in the data from a study by Fry and Hale (1996) that examined verbal and visuospatial memory spans

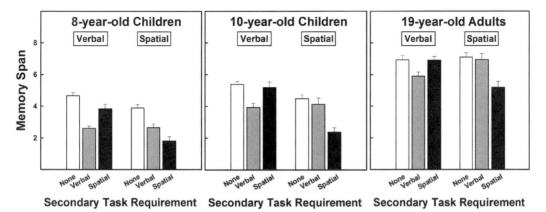

Figure 8.4. Memory span plotted as a function of secondary task requirement for each of the three age groups. Data are from Hale, Bronik, and Fry (1997).

in 8-, 10-, 12-, and 19-year-olds. (Importantly, Fry and Hale also administered processing-speed and fluid-intelligence tests, the results for which will be considered below in the section Individual Differences.) In both studies, simple verbal and visuospatial memory spans were roughly equivalent in young adults, but in children, verbal spans were higher than visuospatial spans, with the difference between the two domains decreasing with the age of the child group (see Fig. 8.5). The finding that visuospatial memory span approaches adult levels more slowly than verbal memory span is an intriguing one, and may be related to the finding that visuospatial memory spans decline more rapidly in old age, as discussed in the following section.

Older Adults

To understand how normal aging affects working memory, we tested healthy younger and older adults (mean ages, 20 and 67 years, respectively) using the experimental paradigm introduced by Hale et al. (1996), with the same two modifications (fewer colors and slower presentation rates) used by Hale et al. (1997) in testing children. As reported by Myerson et al. (1999), and shown here in Figure 8.6, the pattern of the data from both the young- and older-adult groups conformed to the double

dissociation observed in our original study of younger adults (Hale et al., 1996). That is, for both groups, only same-domain secondary tasks negatively affected memory span performance. As can be seen, however, there was a striking difference between the two age groups: on the visuospatial tasks, older adults showed deficits that were considerably larger (i.e., nearly 2.5 items) than those on the three verbal tasks (i.e., approximately 1 item).

From several theoretical perspectives, including Baddeley's (1986) working memory model, frontal-lobe aging theories (Moscovitch & Winocur, 1995; West, 2000), and the inhibition-deficit framework (Hasher & Zacks, 1988; Zacks, Radvansky, & Hasher, 1996), it is interesting to note that normal aging does not appear to be associated with a decline in executive functions, at least as measured in terms of the effects of having to switch back and forth between tasks. That is, different-domain secondary tasks had little or no effect on memory span in older adults, and although same-domain secondary tasks did interfere with performance of primary memory span tasks, the observed interference effects were no larger than those observed in young adults. In contrast to this preservation of function, the marked decrease in visuospatial memory spans with age appears to be part of a more general decline in the efficiency of visuospatial processing, as evidenced by greater visuospatial than verbal slowing and greater age-related deficits in visuospatial than verbal learning (Jenkins et al., 2000).

This decline in visuospatial processing efficiency without an accompanying breakdown in the independence of the two domain-specific working memory subsystems may be contrasted with the results obtained in children. Recall that, like older adults, children show lower visuospatial than verbal spans (see Fig. 8.4 above), but whereas secondary tasks from one domain produce interference with memory spans in the other domain in children (at least before 10 years of age), older adults' spans are relatively unaffected by such procedures (Hale et al., 1997; Myerson et al., 1999). These findings suggest that differences in verbal and visuospatial working memory on the one hand, and

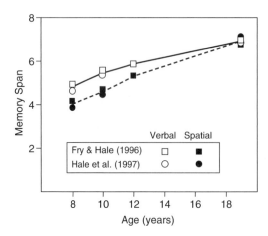

Figure 8.5. Verbal and spatial memory span plotted as a function of age. Data are from Fry and Hale (1996) and Hale, Bronik, and Fry (1997).

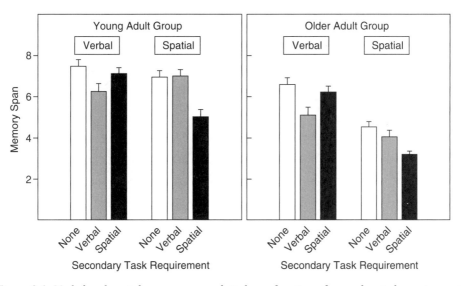

Figure 8.6. Verbal and spatial memory span plotted as a function of secondary task requirement for the young-adult group (left panel) and the older-adult group (right panel). Data are from Myerson, Hale, Rhee, and Jenkins (1999).

differences in the functional independence of the two domains on the other may reflect two separate developmental phenomena.

As documented by Jenkins et al. (1999), the differential decline in older adults' verbal and visuospatial working memory has been replicated in our laboratory several times. Although this finding has been somewhat controversial, its robustness is evidenced by the results of our analysis of the normative data from the most recent Wechsler Memory Scale (WMS-III). In particular, our analyses revealed more rapid adult age-related decline in visuospatial span than in digit (i.e., verbal) span (Myerson, Emery, et al., 2003). Confidence in this finding stems not only from its consistency with previous results in our laboratory, but more importantly from the fact that the verbal–visuospatial difference in the WMS-III data is based on a normative sample of more than 1000 participants between the ages of 20 and 90 years.

The WMS-III data also reveal two other significant findings. Perhaps surprisingly, the difference between forward and backward spans is not affected by age in either domain. The effect of age on the difference between forward and backward spans, like the difference between verbal and visuospatial spans, has been controversial; indeed, the WAIS-III technical manual specifically states that backward digit span is more affected by aging than forward digit span. Nevertheless, as depicted in the left panel of Figure 8.7, the normative sample data clearly show that the difference between forward and backward spans remains constant as people age (Myerson, Emery, et al., 2003).

The second important observation based on the WMS-III data is that performance on the letter-number sequencing subtest shows a unique curvilinear pattern of decline (see Fig. 8.7, right panel), decreasing relatively slowly until around age 65, after which the decline is more precipitous. In contrast, digit and spatial spans (both forward and backward) showed relatively more linear declines (Myerson, Emery, et al., 2003). These findings, taken together with the results of our previous study of letter-number sequencing in young adults (Emery et al., 2002), suggest that the distinction between off-line and on-line manipulation may be important for understanding age differences on these working memory tasks.

Two recent experiments by Emery, Myerson, and Hale (2003) addressed the question of the

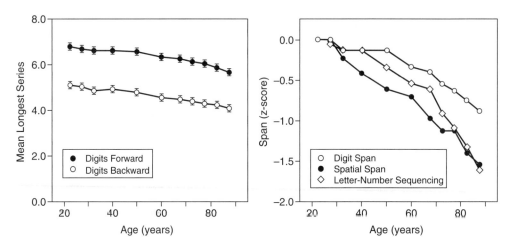

Figure 8.7. Performance on memory span tests plotted as a function of age. Mean longest series of digits forward and backward are shown in the left panel. Z scores for digit span, spatial span, and letter-number sequencing are shown in the right panel. Data are from Myerson, Emery, White, and Hale (2003).

role of on-line manipulation of memory items in the effects of age on letter-number sequencing. In Experiment 1, Emery et al. (2003) tested younger and older adults (mean ages of 20 and 76 years) on the letter-number sequencing tasks described earlier along with an additional condition in which the series of memory items was followed by a cue indicating the order in which the items were to be recalled (see Fig. 8.8). Focusing first on the three conditions previously studied by Emery et al. (2002), the results for young adults replicated those of the earlier study (see the three right-most bars in the left panel of Fig. 8.9): Memory spans were lowest for forward recall of alternating letters and numbers and highest for forward recall of presorted memory

items, whereas sequenced recall produced intermediate-sized spans. As shown in the right panel of Figure 8.9, although the memory spans of older adults in these three conditions were not as large as those of young adults, they otherwise had a similar pattern.

Of particular interest in this experiment was the condition with the sequencing cue. This condition encouraged off-line processing because participants had to maintain the memory items in the order of presentation (alternating letters and numbers) until the end of the series, at which time the cue informed them whether or not to sequence the memory items (ascending digits followed by ascending letters). Memory spans on off-line processing trials (repre-

Figure 8.8. Schematic drawings of the procedures for the letter-number span tasks used in Emery, Myerson, and Hale (2003).

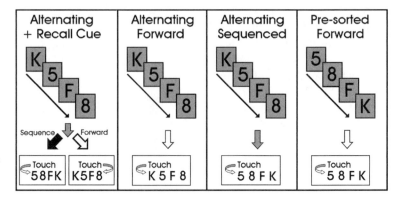

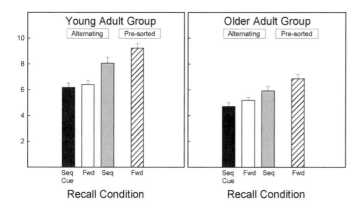

Figure 8.9. Memory span plotted as a function of recall condition for young- and older-adult groups. Data are from Emery, Myerson, and Hale (2003).

sented by the left-most bar in each of the two panels of Fig. 8.9) were lower than spans in the sequencing condition (third bar from the left in each panel), in which participants could rearrange the items on-line (i.e., during presentation of the items). Although both groups benefited from the opportunity to rearrange items on-line (as compared with off-line), the younger adults benefited to a greater extent than the older adults.

One possible explanation for this greater benefit from on-line sequencing observed in the younger adults is that age-related slowing may have made it more difficult for the older adults to manipulate memory items on-line. In Experiment 2, Emery et al. (2003) directly tested this hypothesis by presenting memory items (alternating letters and numbers) at three different rates (1.5 s per item, 2.5 s per item, and 3.5 s per item), including one faster and one slower than that in the preceding experiment. Presentation rate was crossed with recall order

(forward vs. sequenced) to yield six conditions. The data, shown in Figure 8.10, show that presentation rate did not affect performance by either young or older adults (mean ages of 20 and 77 years) in the forward span conditions. In the sequenced conditions, however, presentation rate did affect memory spans. Rather than eliminating age differences, slower presentation rates actually caused them to increase. Presumably, young adults' faster processing speed means that they can reorder more memory items than older adults given the same amount of time, and thus young adults benefit more than older adults from increases in the amount of time available for on-line sequencing.

Overall, our studies of working memory in younger and older adults have led us to the following conclusions. Regardless of the task, older adults show smaller memory spans than those of younger adults, and this is particularly true for visuospatial working memory tasks, which show reliably larger age differences than

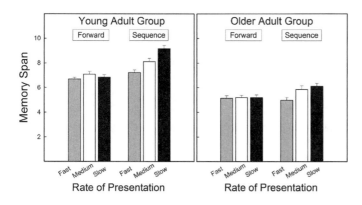

Figure 8.10. Memory span plotted as a function of rate of item presentation for the young-adult and older-adult groups in the forward and sequenced recall conditions. Data are from Emery, Myerson, and Hale 2003).

verbal working memory tasks. Within the verbal and visuospatial domains, however, the patterns of memory spans on different tasks are remarkably similar in the two groups and appear to provide little evidence that executive deficits underlie age differences in working memory. Recently, research in our lab has focused on manipulation span tasks and revealed an important distinction between tasks that involve on-line and off-line reorganization of memory items. On the one hand, the effects of requiring off-line manipulation, as reflected in the difference between forward and backward spans, appear to be relatively age invariant, contrary to common belief. On the other hand, the effects of on-line manipulation, as evidenced by the difference between forward spans and letter-number sequencing spans, appear to depend on both the amount of time allowed to accomplish the reordering and the difference in processing speed between the groups being compared.

INDIVIDUAL DIFFERENCES IN WORKING MEMORY

In addition to studying age-related differences in working memory through an experimental approach, we have also conducted research using an individual-differences approach. The advantage of this approach is that it permits one to test causal models by means of multiple variables and to evaluate all of the hypothesized relationships simultaneously. Importantly, the individual-differences approach allows us to test hypotheses about the linkage between age, working memory, and higher cognitive processes, such as the processes measured by tests of fluid intelligence. In particular, we have examined age and individual differences in cognitive abilities during childhood (Fry & Hale, 1996) as well as during middle and late adulthood (Hale, 2003). Thus, our models focus on the relationship between age and fluid intelligence, and evaluate the role of potential mediating, hypothetical constructs (and the connections among these constructs).

We first used the individual-differences approach in a cross-sectional study of children,

adolescents, and young adults (Fry & Hale, 1996). This study was designed to determine the extent to which age-related improvements in fluid ability (as measured by the Raven's matrices) are the result of age-related improvement in working memory ability that are, in turn, the result of age-related improvement in cognitive processing speed. We termed this hypothetical causal account the *developmental cascade model*. We contrasted the developmental cascade model with a full developmental model (shown in the upper panel of Fig. 8.11) in which age, cognitive processing speed, and working memory function are all potential predictors of fluid ability (paths 1, 2, and 3, respectively). In the full model, speed is also a potential predictor of working memory function (path 4), and age serves as a predictor of both speed and working memory (paths 5 and 6, respectively). According to the developmental cascade hypothesis, only paths 5, 4, and 3 should be significant. (Note that the use of path analysis in lieu of a structural-equation model was dictated by the low number of variables associated with the each of the constructs.)

To test the developmental cascade model, Fry and Hale (1996) assessed 219 participants between the ages of 7 and 19 years using a battery of tests that included four measures of cognitive processing speed similar to those used previously in our laboratory (Hale, 1990; Hale, Fry, & Jessie, 1993). Four working memory tests, selected from the six original tasks (shown in Fig. 8.1, above), were also included in the battery: verbal without a secondary task, verbal plus a verbal secondary task, spatial without a secondary task, and spatial plus a visuospatial secondary task. Fluid ability was measured using Raven's Standard Progressive Matrices.

The results of the Fry and Hale (1996) study provide considerable support for the developmental cascade hypothesis in terms of how age affects speed and working memory, and how these variables in turn affect fluid ability. As seen in the lower panel of Figure 8.11, the relationship between age and working memory was, as predicted, mediated by processing speed, and the relationship between speed and fluid ability was mediated by working memory. Counter to

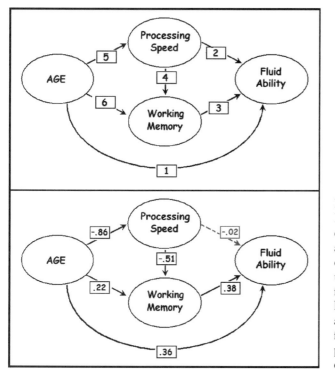

Figure 8.11. Path analysis of data from Fry and Hale (1996). The full developmental model of relations among age, processing speed, working memory, and fluid ability is shown in the upper panel, and the path coefficients for the full model are shown in the lower panel. The path between speed and fluid ability (shown by broken line) failed the Wald test. Retesting with that path omitted resulted in negligible changes in the path coefficients.

the developmental cascade hypothesis, however, paths 1 and 6 were statistically significant. That is, age had a direct effect on working memory, even with speed statistically controlled, and age also had a direct effect on fluid ability, even with both speed and working memory statistically controlled.

Recently, we revisited the Fry and Hale (1996) data set to examine the unique and shared variances among age, speed, working memory, and fluid ability (Fry & Hale, 2000). Two separate hierarchical multiple-regression analyses revealed that nearly all of the variance (i.e., 97%) in working memory that could be accounted for by age was shared variance, and most of the variance (i.e., 80%) in fluid ability that could be accounted for by age was also shared variance. That is, all but 3% of the total age contribution to working memory was mediated by speed, and all but 20% of the total age contribution to fluid ability was mediated by working memory. Thus, although the developmental cascade model did not provide a

perfect fit to the data, it does tell much of the story. Given that chronological age is only a proxy for various maturational changes and environmental events, future research is needed to determine what can account for the remaining 20% of the age-related variance in fluid ability.

It may be noted that our analyses used a single working memory construct based on verbal and visuospatial tests of simple and complex memory spans. In contrast, Jarrold and Bayliss (Chapter 6) distinguished two working memory constructs, simple span (or storage) and complex span, in their analysis of the determinants of working memory in children between the ages of 6 and 11. Jarrold and Bayliss reported that although both speed and simple span contributed to complex memory span, speed did not contribute to simple span. From the perspective of the developmental cascade hypothesis, this latter finding is somewhat surprising, and appears to contradict the results of previous studies (e.g., Kail, 1992; Kail

& Park, 1994). This apparent inconsistency led us to revisit the developmental data collected by Fry and Hale (1996).

To facilitate comparison of our data set and the one obtained by Jarrold and Bayliss (Chapter 6), we used age, rather than the logarithm of age (Fry & Hale, 1996, 2000), as a predictor, and initially restricted our analysis to the data from the 165 children who were between the ages of 7.0 and 13.2 years. We constructed composite indices for speed (four tasks), simple span (two tasks), and complex span (two tasks) by summing each individual's z scores on the relevant tasks. As shown in Figure 8.12, our analysis revealed a pattern generally consistent with a developmental cascade: processing speed made a direct contribution to simple memory span, which in turn contributed to complex span. In addition to the indirect effect via simple span, speed also had a direct effect on complex span. Although the contributions of speed and simple span to complex span are consistent with Jarrold and Bayliss's findings, our findings are in contrast to theirs in at least two respects. In the Fry and Hale data, processing speed and storage do not completely explain all of the age-related variance in children's complex memory span, and, more importantly, processing speed has a direct effect on simple span.

Multiple-regression analyses revealed that together, processing speed and simple memory span accounted for more than 97% of the age-related variance in children's complex span. In addition, processing speed accounted for more than 90% of the age-related variance in simple span. An analogous path analysis including high school and college students (a total of 214 participants) showed a similar pattern, in which processing speed and simple span accounted for 100% of the age-related variance in working memory, and processing speed accounted for 87% of the age-related variance in simple span. Although the results of our analysis and those reported by Jarrold and Bayliss (Chapter 6) differ with respect to the relation between speed and simple span, what seems more important is the finding on which both analyses clearly agree: together, speed and simple span explain the large majority, if not all, of the age-related variance in complex span. Moreover, this conclusion holds not only for elementary school children, as Jarrold and Bayliss showed, but also for the whole developmental period from the age at which children start elementary school through to young adulthood.

Turning to the other end of the life span, we recently completed a latent-variable analysis of data collected from healthy older adults between the ages of 60 and 96 years. These individuals were recruited from the pool of volunteers maintained by the Alzheimer's Disease Research Center at the Washington University School of Medicine in St. Louis, Missouri. All members of this pool were evaluated annually by trained clinicians using the Clinical Dementia Rating (CDR) scale. Importantly, the 72 older adults (mean age, approximately 76 years) whose data are reported here all received a CDR rating of 0 representing no dementia, all had no signs of depression at the time of

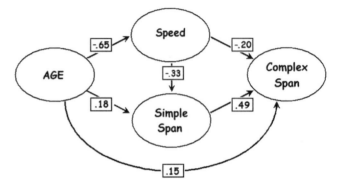

Figure 8.12. Path coefficients from analysis of the relations among age, processing speed, simple memory span, and complex memory span. Data are from Fry and Hale (1996). To facilitate comparison of this analysis with that of Jarrold and Bayliss (Chapter 6), this analysis is based on the data for 165 children and excludes the data from the high school and college students.

testing, and all had visual acuity corrected to 20/40 or better.

The participants were administered a battery of three verbal and three visuospatial working memory tasks similar to those used in our previous studies but adapted for the touch screen (two of the visuospatial conditions are shown in the first two conditions depicted in the lower panel of Fig. 8.3), and two tests of fluid ability, Raven's Progressive Matrices and the Woodcock Johnson Concept Formation subtest. The Woodcock Johnson Concept Formation subtest consists of a series of simple shapes shown in a variety of colors and one of two sizes (small or large). In each problem, a subset of adjacent objects appears inside a rectangle, and participants are instructed to state the rule that governs which shapes are inside the rectangle and which are outside. For example, if a small red triangle and a large yellow square were inside the rectangle, and a large blue triangle, a large red circle, and a large blue square were outside the rectangle, then the correct response would be "small or yellow."

Examination of the zero-order correlations between the working memory measures and the fluid-ability tests revealed that the single best predictor of both the Raven's test and Woodcock Johnson subtest was the simple visuospatial working memory measure (i.e., visuospatial memory span when there was no secondary task requirement). The correlations between simple visuospatial span and the Raven's test and Woodcock Johnson subtest were .63 and .55, respectively. With regard to the verbal span tasks, the complex verbal working-memory measure (verbal span with a verbal secondary task) was the best predictor of the two fluid measures, with rs of .38 and .40, respectively. Nevertheless, it should be noted that all three of the visuospatial working memory tasks had higher correlations with the fluid-ability measures than the best verbal predictor.

Our finding of a high correlation of simple visuospatial span with fluid ability in older adults is consistent with recent findings in young adults (see Chapters 2 and 3). The high correlations observed among the visuospatial span tasks, and between both the simple and complex spans and the tests of fluid ability, are also consistent with the finding that simple visuospatial span predicts performance tests of visuospatial abilities as well as complex visuospatial span and that the two types of visuospatial span tasks are not easily differentiated psychometrically (Miyake, Friedman, Rettinger, Shah, & Hegarty, 2001; Shah & Miyake, 1996).

Next, the data from these working memory tasks and tests of fluid ability were subjected to confirmatory factor analysis. We hypothesized that our working memory tasks would load on two factors, one visuospatial and one verbal, and that the fluid-ability tests would load on a third factor. This model provided an extraordinarily good fit to the data ($\chi^2 = 9.80$, $p = .912$, RMSEA $< .0001$; see Fig. 8.13, left panel). It should be noted that two of the constructs (spatial working memory and fluid ability) were themselves highly correlated ($r = .99$), an issue we will return to later. We also conducted a confirmatory factor analysis of data from the working memory tasks in which there were two hypothesized factors based on the distinction between simple and complex span tasks, as suggested by Engle, Tuholski, Laughlin, and Conway (1999). This analysis, which contrasted span tasks with and without secondary tasks, revealed that a model based on the simple–complex distinction provided an inadequate fit to the data, although it is important to recall that our sample consisted of older adults whereas Engle et al.'s sample consisted of young adults.

Given that our hypothesized three-factor structure (consisting of verbal working memory, spatial working memory, and fluid ability) was confirmed, we proceeded to use structural equation modeling to address the following question: are age-related deficits in visuospatial (but not verbal) working memory the cause of age-related deficits in fluid ability? Our structural equation model (see Fig. 8.13, right panel) provided an excellent fit to the data, $\chi^2 = 23.91$, $p = .409$, RMSEA $= .024$. The only statistically significant predictor of fluid ability was visuospatial (not verbal) working memory, so the effect of age on fluid ability was entirely indirect, via the influence of age on

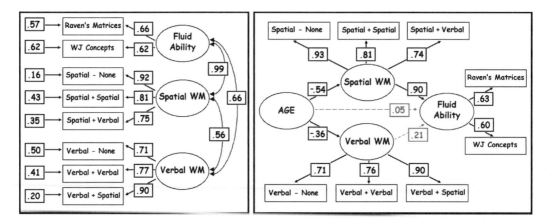

Figure 8.13. Results of confirmatory factor analysis (left panel) and structural equations modeling (right panel) of data from Hale (2003). Note that for the model shown in the right panel, neither the path between age and fluid ability nor the path between verbal working memory (WM) and fluid ability reached statistical significance. WJ = Woodcock Johnson subtest.

visuospatial working memory. Although age also affected verbal working memory, this effect was not nearly as pronounced as the effect of age on visuospatial working memory. Age explained more than twice as much of the variance in older adults' visuospatial working memory, compared with their verbal working memory.

Finally, the high correlation between the spatial working-memory and fluid-ability factors observed in our first confirmatory factor analysis suggested that a two-factor (rather than three-factor) solution might provide a good fit to the data. Therefore, we conducted another confirmatory analysis to test a factor model consisting of a verbal-ability (or verbal working memory) factor and a visuospatial-ability factor (based on both visuospatial working memory and fluid ability). The results of this analysis showed that the fit to the data was slightly improved ($\chi^2 = 10.46, p = .941$, RMSEA < .0001). This small improvement aside, application of Ockham's razor would suggest a preference for the simpler (two-factor) model given that both provide adequate fits. This finding implies that, at least for older adults, visuospatial working memory (including both simple and complex spans) and fluid ability represent facets of a unitary visuospatial factor (namely, visuospatial ability) that shows a general decline throughout late adulthood.

DISCUSSION OF THE FOUR QUESTIONS

Overarching Theory of Working Memory

Baddeley's (1986) model has served as a framework for much of our research on working memory. From our perspective, the attraction of Baddeley's model is that it includes separate, content-specific subsystems. As we noted previously, a model of working memory with separate verbal and visuospatial subsystems was particularly appealing because our work on cognitive aging has shown that older adults are less efficient at processing visuospatial information than verbal information (e.g., Hale & Myerson, 1996; Lawrence et al., 1998; Lima et al., 1991). Moreover, it seemed to us that data from different age groups (from childhood to late adulthood) might prove to be a fertile testing ground for Baddeley's model. For the most part, our results have been consistent with this model, although our findings suggest that secondary tasks interfere with memory span when they engage the same domain-specific systems as the primary memory task, rather than when they engage domain-independent executive functions.

Many studies of working memory (including our own) have examined the effect of requiring people to maintain information while performing secondary tasks that require additional processing. However, the additional processing typically involves information irrelevant to the primary memory task (e.g., Daneman & Carpenter, 1980; Engle et al., 1999; Hale et al., 1996; Lawrence et al., 2001). Most recently, we have been motivated by Baddeley's (1986) original definition of the working memory system to explore tasks such as letter-number sequencing that explicitly involve manipulating memory items (Emery et al., 2002, 2003; Myerson, Emery, et al., 2003). We believe that such tasks are in some ways closer to the original concept of working memory and provide a necessary supplement to studies using primary and secondary tasks.

Critical Sources of Working Memory Variation

The major source of variation in working memory ability among the participants in our studies is age. Of course, chronological age is not itself a causal variable. Rather, age is a proxy for at least two distinct sets of neurobiological processes, with the term *maturation* used to distinguish the neurobiological changes that occur during childhood from the changes during this period that are due to learning, and the term *senescence* used to refer to neurobiological changes during adulthood. The specific physiological and anatomical changes that occur with age are presently not well understood, but with changes in the number of cortical neurons now ruled out, researchers have increasingly focused their attention on changes in white matter. The nature of these changes appears to differ qualitatively at the two ends of the life span (for reviews, see Paus et al., 2001; Peters, 2002). In school-age children and adolescents, increases in white-matter volume are accompanied by decreases in gray-matter volume, whereas both white- and gray-matter volumes decrease throughout adulthood and there is an increase in the incidence of white-matter lesions. The route by which these neurobiological changes affect working memory is not yet clear, but the fact that white-matter changes are involved is consistent with the hypothesis that changes in processing speed contribute to changes in working memory at both ends of the life span.

The maturation of the working memory system from 8 to 20 years is itself a complex process, involving both increased myelination and synaptic pruning, which differentially affects executive, verbal, and visuospatial functions. Perhaps surprisingly, the ability to switch back and forth between tasks, an executive function, appears to mature most quickly—at least when switching involves alternating between a primary memory task and a simple secondary task (Hale et al., 1997)—with visuospatial memory function being the last to reach adult levels (Fry & Hale, 1996; Hale et al., 1997).

As might be expected from the neurobiological evidence, the process of senescent decline in working memory function in individuals 20 to 80 years of age is not a simple mirror image of the system's maturation during childhood. That is, although visuospatial working memory appears to decline at a faster rate than verbal working memory during adulthood (e.g., Cornoldi & Vecchi, 2003; Myerson et al., 1999; Myerson, Emery, et al., 2003), there appears to be no decline in the ability to switch between tasks, at least as measured by its effects on memory span. The substantial decline in memory for locations appears to be a specific instance of a more general age-related decline that affects a variety of visuospatial functions, including processing speed and learning ability as well as working memory (e.g., Hale & Myerson, 1996; Jenkins et al., 2000; Lawrence et al., 1998). This differential visuospatial decline may itself be an instance of a more general principle in which the later a function is acquired, the more sensitive it is to disruption, including disruption by age-related declines in basic neural processes.

The kind of information to be remembered also plays an important role in individual differences in working memory ability, just as it does in age differences. That is, the functional distinction between verbal and visuospatial working memory observed in experimental studies (e.g., Hale et al., 1996; Lawrence et al., 2001; Logie et al., 1990) appears to be important in studies of individual differences in ability as well (e.g., Hale, 2003; Shah & Miyake, 1996). Interestingly, working memory for numerical items appears to be highly related to that for verbal items (e.g., Oberauer, Süß, Schulze, Wilhelm, & Wittman, 2000), a finding suggesting that people remember the names of numbers rather than remembering more abstract concepts of quantities. The finding that working memory for syntactic information is distinct from that for verbal items (Caplan & Waters, 1999; DeDe, Caplan, Kemtes, & Waters, 2004; see Chapter 11) provides further evidence of the important role played by content in the structure of working memory.

Consideration of Other Sources of Variation in Working Memory

In addition to age and domain, processing speed is another important source of variation in working memory. Indeed, age-related variation in speed underlies much of the age-related variation in working memory. Correlations between speed and working memory factors are particularly strong in cross-sectional data from samples representing a large age range (e.g., Fry & Hale, 1996; Salthouse, 1996). The correlations observed in same-age samples are typically not quite as strong (e.g., Ackerman, Beier, & Boyle, 2002), although the difference may be due to restriction of range. The marked attenuation of correlations between age and working memory when speed is statistically controlled is consistent with developmental cascade models in which age-related changes in speed lead directly to changes in working memory capacity (Fry & Hale, 1996; Salthouse, 1996). Jarrold and Bayliss (Chapter 6) found that speed was related to complex but not simple spans in elementary-school children, but our data from a similar age group indicate that speed accounts for age differences in both types of spans. Importantly, there is general agreement that together, speed and simple span explain much of the age-related variance in complex span, and this conclusion appears to hold for the whole developmental period from the age at which children start elementary school through to young adulthood.

As Fry and Hale (1996) showed, however, age-related differences in speed do not completely explain age-related differences in work-

ing memory in school-age children and young adults. Similarly, the gradual slowing with age of cognitive processing in adults does not completely explain the age-related decline in adults' working memory (Verhaeghen & Salthouse, 1997). Similar views are expressed by Towse and Hitch (Chapter 5), who also found strong contributions of processing time on working memory spans, but acknowledged that they do not completely explain either age or individual differences in memory span.

In general, our findings on the effects of same-domain and different-domain secondary tasks provide little support for the hypothesis that executive processes draw on a general (i.e., domain-independent) attentional resource (e.g., Baddeley, 1986; Kane & Engle, 2002; Chapter 2). Indeed, Oberauer et al. (Chapter 3) argue that different executive processes share little common variance. Moreover, neither of the executive processes that have arguably the most face validity (i.e., switching between tasks and the ability to resist interference) is strongly related to working memory capacity (Oberauer, Lange, & Engle, 2004; Chapter 3). Rather than supporting the role of executive processes, our findings are more consistent with the hypothesis that interference results when primary and secondary tasks engage the same neural systems, as when secondary tasks requiring visual orienting are paired with visuospatial span tasks (Corbetta, Kincade, & Shulman, 2002; Smith & Jonides, 1999). This is not to say that when interference is observed, the neural systems engaged by the primary and secondary tasks overlap completely, merely that there is some overlap, and that it is this overlap that produces the interference.

Another possible explanation couched in more cognitive terms that might account for our results is that, as Nairne (2002) has suggested, interference results from overwriting due to similarity between primary and secondary task cues, rather than from decay of memory traces during performance of the secondary task or from depletion of domain-independent resources by having to coordinate primary- and secondary-task operations. As Baddeley (1996) has suggested, however, what is termed the central executive may not be a single, unified system but a set of separate, interacting control functions, and thus it may be premature to draw conclusions about executive functions in general.

Contributions to General Working Memory Theory

Our developmental research has taught us is to be wary of assuming that one has a good understanding of how young adults perform any task or battery of tasks, and this is true even when, at first blush, the nature of young-adult performance seems obvious. When we examined our first data from young adults performing two different types of primary memory span tasks (verbal and visuospatial) under three different secondary-task requirement conditions (i.e., none, same-domain, different-domain), we were delighted to obtain clear evidence of domain-specific interference. The fact that we did not obtain any different-domain interference (i.e., verbal interference with visuospatial span, or visuospatial interference with verbal span) seemed fortuitous, because it meant that if we did observe different-domain interference in other groups (e.g., older adults), we would be able to clearly interpret the findings as reflecting executive deficits.

Over the years, with systematic replication after replication in which not only young adults but also most school-age children and healthy older adults have failed to show different-domain interference, we have come to believe that the domain-specificity of secondary-task interference has a deeper meaning. Rather than making it possible to find central executive deficits easily, the relative lack of different-domain interference in healthy individuals between 10 and 80 years of age indicates that truly general (i.e., domain-independent) executive functions such as task switching simply may not play a major role in determining memory span. Thus, although task switching and attention switching may take time (e.g., Garavan, 1998; Rogers & Monsell, 1995), they do not necessarily interfere with working memory, unless the shifts are within a domain. For example, shifts of spatial attention affect memory for locations, but not memory for letters (Lawrence et al., 2004).

Inhibition is another putatively general-executive function that appears to play little role in determining memory span, at least with our procedures. Antisaccades (often assumed to be a good index of central-executive function because they require the inhibition of a pre-potent response) lead primarily to domain-specific interference. That is, such saccades appear to interfere primarily with the performance of visuospatial tasks, and the interference they generate is no greater than the interference produced by other types of eye movements (Lawrence et al., 2001). Again, however, it is important to note that central-executive functions may not be a single, unified system but a set of independent, interacting control functions (Baddeley, 1996). Caution may be especially warranted in the case of inhibition, where empirical studies have shown that putative measures of inhibition are often poorly correlated (Kramer, Humphrey, Larish, & Logan, 1994; Shilling, Chetwynd, & Rabbitt, 2002). Thus our findings on the antisaccade task may not necessarily be generalized to other situations involving inhibition.

There is one final implication that may be drawn from our findings on the domain-specificity of interference by secondary tasks that applies particularly to cognitive neuroscience, although as our knowledge in this area advances it will obviously have implications for general cognitive theory (e.g., Kane & Engle, 2002). If we are correct in thinking that interference results when primary and secondary tasks engage the same neural systems, then determining the overlap in activation in neural imaging studies may be as important as determining which areas are uniquely activated by specific tasks (e.g., Awh & Jonides, 2001; Corbetta et al., 2002; Smith & Jonides, 1999). The same implication applies to neurophysiologic research on neural activity at the single-unit level, where studying the neurons in a particular brain area whose activity is modulated by the same stimulus characteristics as those in other areas may be as important as studying those neurons whose activity is modulated by unique stimulus characteristics (e.g., Snyder, Batista, & Andersen, 2000). Indeed, Oberauer et al. (2004) have pointed to the need for theories of interference that indicate more precisely the conditions under which task similarity affects working memory. The present suggestion regarding overlap in neural activation answers their call. Of particular interest for both cognitive neuroscience and general cognitive theory will be whether the degree of overlap in activation by different tasks predicts the extent to which these tasks will interfere with each other, and whether age and individual differences in the degree of overlap can predict age and individual differences in interference.

BOX 8.1. SUMMARY ANSWERS TO BOOK QUESTIONS

1. THE OVERARCHING THEORY OF WORKING MEMORY

Baddeley's (1986) model of working memory with separate verbal and visuospatial subsystems has served us well in our research. Generally, our results have been consistent with this model, although we find that secondary tasks interfere with memory span only when they engage the same domain-specific subsystem as that of the primary memory task, rather than whenever they engage domain-independent executive functions. Recently, we have used procedures that explicitly involve manipulating memory items, consistent with Baddeley's original definition of working memory. These procedures (e.g., letter-number sequencing) provide an important complement to procedures in which secondary tasks require processing irrelevant information (e.g., operation span).

2. CRITICAL SOURCES OF WORKING MEMORY VARIATION

We have observed primarily quantitative differences across the life span from age 10 years onwards. Prior to age 10, the verbal and visuospatial subsystems are not yet completely independent. Following general improvements in late childhood and adolescence, older adults show a general decline that is exacerbated in the visuospatial domain. Chronological age is only a proxy, however, for neurobiological changes, especially those involving white matter because of its role in processing speed. Changes in processing speed affect working memory function at both ends of the life span, but the changes during senescence do not appear to be a simple mirror image of those during maturation.

3. OTHER SOURCES OF WORKING MEMORY VARIATION

Processing speed is an important source of variation that appears to underlie much of the age-related variation in working memory. We have shown, however, that processing speed and storage do not completely explain all of the age-related variance in children's complex memory span. We have considered, but rejected, roles for two important executive processes: the ability to inhibit irrelevant information and the ability to switch back and forth between tasks. Instead, our findings are more consistent with the hypothesis that, across most of the life span, interference results when primary and secondary tasks engage the same domain-specific neural systems.

4. CONTRIBUTIONS TO GENERAL WORKING MEMORY THEORY

Perhaps our strongest contribution to general working memory theory stems from a finding that we first observed in young adults: Only secondary tasks involving the same domain interfere with performance of a primary memory task. The relative lack of different-domain interference in cognitively healthy individuals between 10 and 80 years of age indicates that truly general (i.e., domain-independent) executive functions such as task switching do not play a major role in determining memory span. Thus, although task switching and attention switching take up processing time, they do not necessarily interfere with working memory except when the shifts are within a domain.

References

Ackerman, P. L., Beier, M. E., & Boyle, M. O. (2002). Individual differences in working memory within a nomological network of cognitive and perceptual speed abilities. *Journal of Experimental Psychology: General, 131*, 567–589.

Awh, E., & Jonides, J. (2001). Overlapping mechanisms of attention and spatial working memory. *Trends in Cognitive Sciences, 5*, 119–126.

Babcock, R. L., & Salthouse, T. A. (1990). Effects of increased processing demands on age differences in working memory. *Psychology and Aging, 5*, 421–428.

Baddeley, A. D. (1986). *Working memory*. New York: Oxford University Press.

Baddeley, A. D. (1996). Exploring the central executive. *Quarterly Journal of Experimental Psychology, 49A*, 5–28.

Baddeley, A. D., Lewis, V., & Vallar, G. (1984). Exploring the articulatory loop. *Quarterly Journal of Experimental Psychology: Human Experimental Psychology, 36A*, 233–252.

Bjorklund, D. F., & Harnishfeger, K. K. (1990). The resources construct in cognitive development: Diverse sources of evidence and a theory of inefficient inhibition. *Developmental Review, 10*, 48–71.

Brooks, L. R. (1968). Spatial and verbal components of the act of recall. *Canadian Journal of Psychology, 22*, 349–368.

Caplan, D., & Waters, G. S. (1999). Verbal working memory and sentence comprehension. *Behavioral and Brain Sciences, 22*, 77–126.

Cerella, J., & Hale, S. (1994). The rise and fall in information-processing rates over the life span. *Acta Psychologica, 86*, 109–197.

Chapman, L. J., Chapman, J. P., Curran, T. E., & Miller, M. B. (1994). Do children and the elderly show heightened semantic priming? How to answer the question. *Developmental Review, 14*, 159–185.

Conway, A. R. A., & Engle, R. W. (1996). Individual differences in working memory capacity: More evidence for a general capacity theory. *Memory, 4*, 577–590.

Corbetta, M., Kincade, J. M., & Shulman, G. L. (2002). Neural systems for visual orienting and their relationships to spatial working memory. *Journal of Cognitive Neuroscience, 14*, 508–523.

Cornoldi, C., & Vecchi, T. (2003). *Visuo-spatial working memory and individual differences*. New York: Psychology Press.

Daneman, M., & Carpenter, P. A. (1980). Individual differences in working memory and reading. *Journal of Verbal Learning & Verbal Behavior, 19*, 450–466.

DeDe, G., Caplan, D., Kemtes, K., & Waters, G. (2004). The relationship between age, verbal working memory, and language comprehension. *Psychology and Aging, 19*, 601–616.

Dempster, F. N. (1992). The rise and fall of the inhibitory mechanism: Toward a unified theory of cognitive development and aging. *Developmental Review, 12*, 45–75.

Dempster, F. N., & Brainerd, E. J. (1995). *Interference and inhibition in cognition*. San Diego: Academic Press.

Emery, L., Myerson, J., & Hale, S. (2002). *Letter-number sequencing: Costs and benefits of reorganizing items in working memory*. Presented at Psychonomic Society, Kansas City, MO, November.

Emery, L., Myerson, J., & Hale, S. (2003). *Adult age differences in transformation span measures of working memory*. Presented at the American Psychological Society, Atlanta, GA, May.

Engle, R. W., Tuholski, S. W., Laughlin, J. E., & Conway, A. R. A. (1999). Working memory, short-term memory, and general fluid intelligence: A latent variable approach. *Journal of Experimental Psychology: General, 128*, 309–331.

Fry, A. F., & Hale, S. (1996). Processing speed, working memory, and fluid intelligence: Evidence for a developmental cascade. *Psychological Science, 7*, 237–241.

Fry, A. F., & Hale, S. (2000). Relationships among processing speed, working memory, and fluid intelligence in children. *Biological Psychology, 54*, 1–34.

Garavan, H. (1998). Serial attention within working memory. *Memory & Cognition, 26*, 263–276.

Gathercole, S. E. (1999). Cognitive approaches to the development of short-term memory. *Trends in Cognitive Sciences, 3*, 410–419.

Gathercole, S. E., & Baddeley, A. D. (1993). *Working memory and language*. Hillsdale, NJ: Lawrence Erlbaum Associates.

Hale, S. (1990). A global developmental trend in cognitive processing speed. *Child Development, 61*, 653–663.

Hale, S. (May 2003). *Short-term memory, working memory, and fluid intelligence in older adults.* Presented at the American Psychological Society, Atlanta, GA.

Hale, S., Bronik, M. D., & Fry, A. F. (1997). Verbal and spatial working memory in school-age children: Developmental differences in susceptibility to interference. *Developmental Psychology, 33*, 364–371.

Hale, S., Fry, A. F., & Jessie, K. A. (1993). Effects of practice on speed of information processing in children and adults: Age-sensitivity and age-invariance. *Developmental Psychology, 29*, 880–892.

Hale, S., Lima, S. D., & Myerson, J. (1991). General cognitive slowing in the nonlexical domain: An experimental validation. *Psychology and Aging, 6*, 512–521.

Hale, S., & Myerson, J. (1995). Fifty years older, fifty percent slower? Meta-analytic regression models and semantic context effects. *Aging and Cognition, 2*, 132–145.

Hale, S., & Myerson, J. (1996). Experimental evidence for differential slowing in the lexical and nonlexical domains. *Aging, Neuropsychology, and Cognition, 3*, 154–165.

Hale, S., Myerson, J., Rhee, S. H., Weiss, C. S., & Abrams, R. A. (1996). Selective interference with the maintenance of location information in working memory. *Neuropsychology, 10*, 228–240.

Hasher, L., & Zacks, R. T. (1988). Working memory, comprehension, and aging: A review and a new view. In G. H. Bower (Ed.), *The psychology of learning and motivation: Advances in research and theory* (Vol. 22, pp. 193–225). San Diego: Academic Press.

Jenkins, L., Myerson, J., Hale, S., & Fry, A. F. (1999). Individual and developmental differences in working memory across the life span. *Psychonomic Bulletin & Review, 6*, 28–40.

Jenkins, L., Myerson, J., Joerding, J. A., & Hale, S. (2000). Converging evidence that visuospatial cognition is more age-sensitive than verbal cognition. *Psychology and Aging, 15*, 157–175.

Kail, R. (1992). Processing speed, speech rate, and memory. *Developmental Psychology, 28*, 899–904.

Kail, R., & Park, Y.-S. (1994). Processing time, articulation time, and memory span. *Journal of Experimental Child Psychology, 57*, 281–291.

Kail, R., & Salthouse, T. A. (1994). Processing speed as a mental capacity. *Acta Psychologica, 86*, 199–225.

Kane, M. J., Bleckley, M. K., Conway, A. R. A., & Engle, R. W. (2001). A controlled-attention view of working-memory capacity. *Journal of Experimental Psychology: General, 130*, 169–183.

Kane, M. J., & Engle, R. W. (2002). The role of prefrontal cortex in working-memory capacity, executive attention, and general fluid intelligence: An individual differences perspective. *Psychonomic Bulletin & Review, 9*, 637–671.

Kotary, L., & Hoyer, W. J. (1995). Age and the ability to inhibit distractor information in visual selective attention. *Experimental Aging Research, 21*, 159–171.

Kramer, A. F., Humphrey, D. G., Larish, J. F., & Logan, G. D. (1994). Aging and inhibition: Beyond a unitary view of inhibitory processing in attention. *Psychology and Aging, 9*, 491–512.

Lawrence, B., Myerson, J., & Hale, S. (1998). Differential decline of verbal and visuospatial processing speed across the adult life span. *Aging, Neuropsychology, and Cognition, 5*, 129–146.

Lawrence, B. M., Myerson, J., & Abrams, R. A. (2004). Interference with spatial working memory: An eye movement is more than a shift of attention. *Psychonomic Bulletin & Review, 11*, 488–494.

Lawrence, B. M., Myerson, J., Oonk, H. M., & Abrams, R. A. (2001). The effects of eye and limb movements on working memory. *Memory, 9*, 433–444.

Lima, S. D., Hale, S., & Myerson, J. (1991). How general is general slowing? Evidence from the lexical domain. *Psychology and Aging, 6*, 416–425.

Logie, R. H., Zucco, G. M., & Baddeley, A. D. (1990). Interference with visual short-term memory. *Acta Psychologica, 75*, 55–74.

Miyake, A., Friedman, N. P., Rettinger, D. A., Shah, P., & Hegarty, M. (2001). How are visuospatial working memory, executive function, and spatial abilities related? A latent-variable analysis. *Journal of Experimental Psychology: General, 130*, 621–640.

Moscovitch, M., & Winocur, G. (1995). Frontal lobes, memory, and aging. In J. Grafman, K. J. Holyoak, & F. Boller (Eds.), *Structure and functions of the human prefrontal cortex* (pp. 119–150). New York: New York Academy of Sciences.

Myerson, J., Adams, D. R., Hale, S., & Jenkins, L. (2003). Analysis of group differences in processing speed: Brinley plots, Q-Q plots, and other conspiracies. *Psychonomic Bulletin & Review, 10*, 224–237.

Myerson, J., Emery, L., White, D. A., & Hale, S. (2003). Effects of age, domain, and processing demands on memory span: Evidence for differential decline. *Aging, Neuropsychology, and Cognition, 10*, 20–27.

Myerson, J., Ferraro, F. R., Hale, S., & Lima, S. D. (1992). General slowing in semantic priming and word recognition. *Psychology and Aging, 7*, 257–270.

Myerson, J., Hale, S., Rhee, S. H., & Jenkins, L. (1999). Selective interference with verbal and spatial working memory in young and older adults. *Journal of Gerontology: Psychological Sciences and Social Sciences, 54B*, P161–P164.

Myerson, J., Jenkins, L., Hale, S., & Sliwinski, M. (2000). Stocks and losses, items and interference: A reply to Oberauer and Süß (2000). *Psychonomic Bulletin & Review, 7*, 734–740.

Nairne, J. S. (2002). Remembering over the short-term: The case against the standard model. *Annual Review of Psychology, 53*, 53–81.

Oberauer, K., Lange, E., & Engle, R. W. (2004). Working memory capacity and resistance to interference. *Journal of Memory and Language, 51*, 80–96.

Oberauer, K., & Süß, H. M. (2000). Working memory and interference: a comment on Jenkins, Myerson, Hale, and Fry (1999). *Psychonomic Bulletin & Review, 7*, 727–733.

Oberauer, K., Süß, H. M., Schulze, R., Wilhelm, O., & Wittman, W. W. (2000). Working memory capacity—facets of a cognitive ability construct. *Personality and Individual Differences, 29*, 1017–1045.

Paus, T., Collins, D. L., Evans, A. C., Leonard, G., Pike, B., & Zijdenbos, A. (2001). Maturation of white matter in the human brain: A review of magnetic resonance studies. *Brain Research Bulletin, 54*, 255–266.

Peters, A. (2002). The effects of normal aging on myelin and nerve fibers: A review. *Journal of Neurocytology, 31*, 581–593.

Postle, B. R., Awh, E., Jonides, J., Smith, E. E., & D'Esposito, M. (2004). The where and how of attention-based rehearsal in spatial working memory. *Cognitive Brain Research, 20*, 194–205.

Psychological Corporation (1997). *WMS-III administration and scoring manual.* San Antonio, TX: Harcourt Brace & Company.

Richardson, J. T., Engle, R. W., Hasher, L., Logie, R. H., Stolzfus, E. R., & Zacks, R. T. (1996). *Working memory and human cognition.* New York: Oxford University Press.

Rogers, R. D., & Monsell, S. (1995). Costs of a predictable switch between simple cognitive tasks. *Journal of Experimental Psychology: General, 124*, 207–231.

Salthouse, T. A. (1996). The processing-speed theory of adult age differences in cognition. *Psychological Review, 103*, 403–428.

Schweickert, R. (1993). A multinomial processing tree model for degradation and reintegration in immediate recall. *Memory & Cognition, 21*, 168–175.

Shah, P., & Miyake, A. (1996). The separability of working memory resources for spatial thinking and language processing: An individual differences approach. *Journal of Experimental Psychology: General, 125*, 4–27.

Shilling, V. M., Chetwynd, A., Rabbitt, P. M. A. (2002). Individual inconsistency across measures of inhibition: An investigation of the construct validity of inhibition in older adults. *Neuropsychologia, 40*, 605–619.

Smith, E. E., & Jonides, J. (1999). Storage and executive processes in the frontal lobes. *Science, 283*, 1657–1661.

Snyder, L. H., Batista, A. P., & Andersen, R. A. (2000). Intention-related activity in the posterior parietal cortex: A review. *Vision Research, 40*, 1433–1441.

Underwood, W. D. (1975). Individual differences as a crucible in theory construction. *American Psychologist, 30*, 128–134.

Verhaeghen, P., & Cerella, J. (2002). Aging, executive control, and attention: A review of meta-analyses. *Neuroscience and Biobehavioral Reviews, 26*, 849–857.

Verhaeghen, P., & Salthouse, T. A. (1997). Meta-analyses of age-cognition relations in adulthood: Estimates of linear and nonlinear age effects and structural models. *Psychological Bulletin, 122,* 231–249.

Washburn, D. A., & Astur, R. S. (1998). Nonverbal working memory of humans and monkeys: Rehearsal in the sketchpad? *Memory & Cognition, 26,* 277–286.

West, R. (2000). In defense of the frontal lobe hypothesis of cognitive aging. *Journal of the International Neuropsychological Society, 6,* 727–729.

Zacks, R. T., Radvansky, G., & Hasher, L. (1996). Studies of directed forgetting in older adults. *Journal of Experimental Psychology: Learning, Memory, and Cognition, 22,* 143–156.

III

Working Memory Variation Due
to Normal and Pathological Aging

9

Inhibitory Mechanisms and the Control of Attention

LYNN HASHER, CINDY LUSTIG, and ROSE ZACKS

"Bigger is better." So goes the message of many theoretical perspectives on working memory, views that emphasize working memory as a "mental workspace" which houses the representations and processes that, at any given moment, are in the focus of attention. The intuition of such views is that the larger this workspace, or the more representations one can have active at any given time, the better performance will be on most cognitive and social tasks.[1] Virtually all views of working memory share this perspective, including Baddeley's (1986, 1992, 2000) and Just and Carpenter's (1992). We describe an alternative view, one that could be described as "good things come in small packages." Our work as well as that of our collaborators focuses on the executive control processes that keep the mental representation "packages" small and goal relevant. This, we have argued, enables a maximally efficient information-processing system (e.g., Hasher & Zacks, 1988; Hasher, Zacks, & May, 1999).

Our focus is on a set of attentional or executive control processes, all inhibitory, that operate

in the service of an individual's goals to narrow and constrain the contents of consciousness to be goal relevant. An uncluttered or narrowly focused "working memory," rather than a large one, is the ideal processing system: it will be faster to achieve a goal than will a more broadly dispersed system because it will not be slowed by irrelevant stimuli that occur in the task context, or by environmentally triggered thoughts, or by self-generated distraction. The narrow focus maximizes the speed and accuracy of on-line processing because it reduces the likelihood of switching attention to goal-irrelevant representations such as those connected to a previous task, an upcoming task, environmental distraction, or subsidiary goals.

A narrowly focused processing system is also ideal because it has the downstream benefit of ensuring accurate and rapid retrieval of the information it once focused on (Anderson & Bower, 1973). This claim follows from a rich literature pointing to substantial costs for retrieval of having entertained irrelevant information during encoding. Sometimes the irrelevant information is explicitly part of the task environment, as is the case, for example, when highly similar or overlapping information is learned (Anderson & Bower, 1973; Watkins & Watkins, 1976), when encoding takes places under divided-attention conditions (Craik, Govoni, Naveh-Benjamin, & Anderson, 1996; Fernandes & Moscovitch, 2000), or when actually presented information triggers activation of related information (e.g., Deese, 1959; Roediger & McDermott, 1995; Underwood, 1965). Whatever the source, any additional information activated during encoding "enriches" the memory representation of presented items and forms the basis from which intrusions are drawn and memory lapses occur, the latter due to fundamental interference processes. We note that all tasks which depend on rapid and accurate retrieval of information that was once attended to will suffer to the degree to which the processing system was initially broadly, rather than narrowly, tuned at encoding.

The detrimental effects of an "embarrassment of riches"—i.e., of having *too much* information activated and in the focus of attention—have been the primary interest of our research program, rather than working memory per se. To that end, we have explored the nature of the inhibitory attentional-control processes that limit the momentary consideration of irrelevant information. We have also explored the importance of these attentional-regulation processes to a wide variety of cognitive tasks, including (a) traditional working memory tasks (e.g., simple span, verbal and visuospatial working memory span; Lustig & Hasher, 2002; Lustig, May, & Hasher, 2001; May, Hasher, & Kane, 1999; Rowe, Turcotte & Hasher, 2006); (b) basic-level perceptual speed tasks used in the intelligence, developmental, and aging literatures (Lustig, Hasher, & Tonev, in press); (c) more conceptual tasks such as reading speed and reading comprehension (Carlson, Hasher, Connelly, & Zacks, 1995; Connelly, Hasher, & Zacks, 1991; Li, Hasher, Jonas, Rahhal, & May, 1998), problem solving and decision making (May, 1999; Tentori, Osherson, Hasher, & May, 2001); (d) attentional regulation (May, Kane, & Hasher, 1995) and control of primed or prepotent (but task-irrelevant) responses (Butler, Zacks, & Henderson, 1999; May & Hasher,

1998); and (e) long-term explicit and implicit memory (Gerard, Zacks, Hasher, & Radvansky, 1991; Kim, Hasher & Zacks, in press; Lustig & Hasher, 2001; Rowe, Valderrama, Lenartowicz & Hasher, in press; Zacks, Radvansky, & Hasher, 1996).

Our particular focus on these *inhibitory-based* executive control processes differs from much of the early work on working memory, which centered on capacity for simultaneous mental operations and storage. Our emphasis on executive processes fits well, however, with the recent explosion of work on "executive control" across the cognitive and cognitive neuroscience literatures, including evidence that the control processes involved in attention, working memory, and long-term memory share common neural substrates (Cabeza et al., 2003; Ranganath, Johnson, & D'Esposito, 2003). Recent work by Engle and colleagues has a similar perspective to our own, as their emphasis has shifted toward working memory as an executive attention system rather than as a "memory" system (e.g., Engle, 2002; Kane, Bleckley, Conway, & Engle, 2001; see also Chapter 2, this volume). Finally, our work also fits well with the general effort to understand the processes involved in Baddeley's construct of the "central executive" (e.g., Baddeley, 2003).

In sum, our work is similar to that of many other investigators in its focus on executive processes as a critical source of working memory variation as well as variation in many cognitive domains. There is broad agreement that for individuals sharing common goals, it is the efficiency of executive processes that is a major source of variation in the contents of consciousness and in many of the mental and physical processes (e.g., memory and motor control) that are subsequently determined by the initial breadth of focus (e.g., see Chapters 2 and 4, but see Chapter 10 for a somewhat different view).

Our work differs from many others' in that we emphasize the role of *inhibitory* processes, or those processes that keep consciousness free of irrelevant information that can impede the successful and efficient completion of a current goal. Our assumption is that the initial stage of activating representations is largely automatic and is driven by environmental and social contexts, by specific perceptual cues, by instructions in the context of an experiment, and to some degree by an individual's momentary and long-term goals and values.[2] It is immediately after activation that goal-driven attentional or executive processes come into play, and we assume that these include both excitatory mechanisms that increase the activation of goal-relevant information and inhibitory processes that decrease the activation of irrelevant information.

We focus on inhibitory processes on the assumption that the initial stages of activation are largely automatic and so do not differ much among individuals within the same contexts and with the same goals. For example, semantic priming effects, or the facilitated recognition of one word (e.g., "nurse") after exposure to a related word (e.g., "doctor"), often do not differ across populations such as younger and older adults with different working memory abilities; or, if they do, the differences actually favor older adults (e.g., Cameli & Phillips, 2000; Giffard, Desgranges, Kerrouche, Piolino, & Eustache, 2003; Laver, 2000). Our reading of such results is that groups differing in age or working memory span or reading ability differ less in their abilities to activate relevant concepts than they do in their abilities to keep activation and attention restricted to what is relevant.

In our own work, the need to focus on the processes involved in restricting attention to goal-relevant information was initially stimulated by age differences found in an inference generation task, differences that could not be accounted for by those in working memory capacity, since estimates of the latter did not differ with age (Hamm & Hasher, 1992). The study tested for the inferences people generated while reading. When the context of a passage requiring an inference was slightly ambiguous, young adults generated one inference and older adults tended to generate two. When subsequent information made it clear that the initial inference drawn by young adults and one of the two inferences drawn by older adults was incorrect, young adults generated the correct inference and abandoned the no-longer correct one. Although older adults initially generated the correct inference, they did not abandon their

original, but no-longer correct, inference. These two findings from garden path passages, a larger range of inferences generated and a lengthier consideration of rejected inferences by older than by younger adults (see Hamm & Hasher, 1992, for details), led us to posit (Hasher & Zacks, 1988) the existence of inhibitory functions that in young adults limit the range of ideas entering the focus of attention and quickly suppress ideas that prove unhelpful. These mechanisms were clearly less efficient in older adults than in young adults.

These observations about inference generation and control, along with the failure of working memory to explain them, led us to build a theoretical framework in which variation in *inhibitory efficiency* accounts for much of the variation in cognitive performance. In fact, we take the strong position that inhibition is a fundamental determinant of the apparent differences in what many investigators term "working memory capacity."

Although much of our empirical work has used age-comparative studies rather than individual-differences methods per se, our theoretical work has always emphasized the general importance of inhibitory variation across groups and among individuals and more recently within the same individual across different physiological and psychological states (Hasher & Zacks, 1988, Hasher et al., 1999). Work on individual differences is generally supportive of the idea that inhibitory processes play a large role in cognition (Chiappe, Hasher, & Siegel, 2000; Chiappe, Siegel, & Hasher, 2002; Gernsbacher & Faust, 1991; Harnishfeger & Bjorklund, 1994; Kane et al., 2001; Lustig et al., 2001; Miyake, Friedman, Emerson, Witzki, & Howerter, 2000; Nigg, 2001; Persad, 2001; Persad, Abeles, Zacks & Denberg, 2002; Wenzlaff & Wegner, 2000; but see Park et al., 1996; Salthouse, 1996, for alternative interpretations). We note that the potential correspondence between individual-differences work and group-comparative work has tended to be overlooked (to judge from cross-citations), a situation we hope this volume will begin to redress.

Our major empirical efforts to understand inhibitory control over the contents of consciousness and implications of failures of control have taken two approaches: (1) the study of age-related inhibitory control deficits (i.e., group differences), and (2) the study of inhibitory control across the day (i.e., intra-individual differences). The latter line of work is quite unusual in mainstream cognition, but, as will be seen, it leads nicely to the conclusion that inhibitory control can vary not just among groups and individuals within a group but *within individuals themselves.*

Because the intra-individual-differences approach we take is an unusual one, we describe it briefly before returning to elaborate on inhibition. Our studies typically compare participants with a particular type of circadian arousal pattern (Evening types and Morning types; Horne & Ostberg, 1976) who are tested early in the morning and late in the afternoon to provide a snapshot of fundamental cognitive processes functioning across the day (see Winocur & Hasher, 2002, for a brief review of related animal model evidence). Despite the folk nomenclature of these two "types," they are well substantiated in physiology (e.g., Kerkhof & Lancel, 1991), including recent evidence of genetic contributions to extremes in arousal patterns (e.g., Cermakian & Boivin, 2003; Hur, Bouchard, & Lykken, 1998; see also the final section of this chapter). We also note that there are life span differences in overall arousal patterns, with more than 70% of older adults (and many young children) more likely to be at a peak in the morning than later in the day. This same time is likely a trough for many young adults, under 10% of whom have Morning-type arousal patterns (Kim, Dueker, Hasher, & Goldstein, 2002; Yoon, May, & Hasher, 2000; Yoon, May, Goldstein & Hasher, in press).[3]

Of particular importance for present purposes, the data suggest that regardless of whether one is a Morning- or Evening-type person, it is *inhibitory* processes that differ most across the circadian cycle; excitatory-based processes seem to show little variation across the day (e.g., Yoon et al., 2000). Our evidence suggests that inhibitory efficiency follows the arousal cycle and our assumption is that studying groups and individuals with varying degrees of inhibitory function (or single individuals at different points in their circadian arousal function) will help il-

luminate inhibitory processes and the roles they play in cognition, including in determining apparent differences in working memory capacity.

The decision to highlight inhibitory processes as critical determinants of both on-line and downstream efficiency places us within a small group of investigators who early on and quite independently looked at cognition from a similar point of view and across many different groups and individuals (initially, Gernsbacher & Faust, 1991, and Dempster, 1991). Many investigators subsequently arrived at similar or partially overlapping views (see Duchek, Balota, & Thessing, 1998; Harnishfeger & Bjorklund, 1994; Nigg, 2001; Wenzlaff & Wegner, 2000; Chapters 2, 3, 4, and 10, this volume). By focusing specifically on the role of inhibitory processes, we differ somewhat from other investigators who deal with executive or controlled attention processes in a generalized fashion, or who tie them to particular tasks such as set switching.

As more researchers focus on executive control processes, it has become increasingly clear that "executive control" is not a unitary construct and that the nature of the specific processes remains to be understood (e.g., Friedman & Miyake, 2004; Miyake et al., 2000; Sylvester et al., 2003). Although in its early stages, recent work suggests that different aspects of executive control (which we view largely as different aspects of inhibitory function) may be dissociable across individuals, brain regions, and times of day (e.g., Friedman & Miyake, 2004; Lustig & Meck, 2001; May, Hasher, & Foong, 2005; Sylvester et al., 2003; West, Murphy, Armilio, Craik, & Stuss, 2002).

Our own attempts to understand the nature of inhibitory processes and their contributions to performance led us to a framework that draws distinctions between three separate functions of inhibition, all of which serve to keep working memory (i.e., the focus of attention) free of irrelevant information (e.g., Hasher et al., 1999; Zacks & Hasher, 1994). Inhibitory processes act in the service of goals to (1) prevent irrelevant information from gaining *access* to the focus of attention, (2) *delete* no-longer relevant items from consideration, and (3) *restrain* prepotent responses so that other, initially weaker response candidates can be evaluated and influence behavior as appropriate for current goals.

In the next section of the chapter, we briefly describe inhibitory functions and the effects that variations in their efficiency can have on performance on a number of tasks with an emphasis on speed of processing and working memory. We suggest that a view of executive control that focuses on inhibitory processes can offer a competing account for group, individual, and intra-individual differences in speed and working memory (among other cognitive phenomenon) without appealing to notions of "capacity" that in the attention literature have been sharply criticized (e.g., Navon, 1984). Indeed, our evidence raises the possibility that what most working memory span tasks measure is inhibitory control, not something like the size of operating capacity (e.g., Just & Carpenter, 1992). In the final section, we discuss the potential neurobiological underpinnings of the age and circadian changes that have profound behavioral effects on inhibitory regulation.

INHIBITORY PROCESSES

We have posited three inhibitory functions: access, deletion, and restraint (Hasher et al., 1999; Hasher, Tonev, Lustig, & Zacks, 2001; Hasher & Zacks, 1988; Zacks & Hasher, 1994). Each is a powerful player in determining the speed and success of on-line processing. Two of them (access and deletion) are also major determinants of the speed and success of explicit retrieval while the third (restraint) can influence successes, for example, when strong or prepotent responses are correct (e.g., stopping at a traffic signal when it is red), and failures, when strong responses are wrong (cf. Radvansky & Curiel, 1998). Over the past 20 years our work has focused on exploring the nature of these inhibitory functions and showing that they (a) operate across a wide range of tasks, (b) diminish with age over adulthood, and (c) vary across the day with an individual's circadian arousal pattern. It is important to note that although our work takes a group- and intra-individual-differences approach, the theory be-

hind the work is a general theory of cognition and, as such, applies to individual differences.

Access

The initial activation of representations is presumed to be broad and virtually automatic. The *access* function of inhibition is engaged in the service of goals to determine which activated representations enter the focus of attention (e.g., Cowan, 1993). When efficient, all irrelevant representations are suppressed and the contents of consciousness will be narrowly tied to goals. A dramatic example of narrow focus of attention is the "inattentional blindness" effect, in which unattended items in the center of the visual field are literally not "seen" (Mack & Rock, 1998; Most et al., 2001). Another is the state of "flow" by which intense concentration enables individuals to ignore the external world and passing of time (e.g., Csikszentmihalyi, Rathunde, & Whalen, 1993).

Our original work on the inferences generated while reading suggested age differences in the amount of information that gains access to the focus of attention; as noted above, in an ambiguous context in which young adults generated only one interpretation, older adults generated more (Hasher & Zacks, 1988, Hamm & Hasher, 1992, Kim, Hasher, & Zacks, in press). Our recent work on the access function has focused on its role in determining the speed with which tasks can be performed. To this end, we manipulated the extent and nature of extraneous information present in a task environment.

For example, for older adults, the speed at which a decision is made about two letter strings (e.g., XPFGN and XPFCN) being the same or different is at least partially determined by whether there are other letter strings simultaneously present and competing for access to attention (Lustig et al., in press). For young adults, the presence of other letter-string problems has no effect on the speed at which problems are solved. These findings are critical, because letter comparison is one of a number of tasks used to assess the notion of "perceptual speed," a concept that in the life-span and intelligence literatures is thought of as a cognitive primitive that establishes limits to an individual's performance across a range of high-level cognitive tasks, including reasoning (Kail, 1993; Salthouse, 1996). As it happens, most tasks that assess "perceptual speed" use highly cluttered displays (with many similar problems on a page), an arrangement likely to disrupt the performance of some participants (those with reduced inhibitory function), but not others. Our work suggests that the source of disruption (and the underlying cognitive primitive) is the access function which determines the ability to constrain task focus to just the momentarily relevant item.

Inefficient control over access can also slow even highly practiced skills such as reading. For example, interspersing irrelevant words (in a distinctive font) amidst target text differentially slows reading for older adults (Carlson et al., 1995; Connelly et al., 1991; Duchek, et al., 1998; Dywan & Murphy, 1996; Li et al., 1998; Phillips & Lesperance, 2003). There are comparable data showing age differences in disruption effects when the distraction is in the auditory rather than visual mode (Tun, O'Kane, & Wingfield, 2002). The selective-attention literature shows a similar phenomenon: under many circumstances, older adults are differentially slowed to find a target amidst distraction (e.g., Plude & Hoyer, 1986; Zacks & Zacks, 1993). From our perspective, all of these effects are consistent with the idea that the access function of inhibition is not as efficient for older adults as it is for younger adults. These findings, and particularly those using simple perceptual-speed tasks, pose a challenge to views of processing speed as a cognitive primitive that underlies intelligence and the developmental trajectory of cognition across the life span (e.g., Kail, 1993; Salthouse, 1996). Such findings suggest that attentional regulation and particularly the access function of inhibition are part of the underlying mechanisms critical to cognition.

We note that the efficiency of the access function also varies across the day in patterns consistent with morning vs. evening arousal schedules. In one relevant study (May, 1999), participants were given a variant of the classic Remote Associates Task in which three very loosely related words (e.g., *rat*, *blue*, and *cot-*

tage) were presented and the task was to generate a word (*cheese*) that connects them. The target words were presented alone on control trials and with distraction on experimental trials; participants were warned to ignore the distraction that had been normed to either lead toward the solution word or away from it.

Evening-type younger and Morning-type older adults were tested early in the morning or late in the afternoon. Performance on the control (or distraction-free) sets did not differ with age or time of testing; however, the impact of distraction differed for both ages and times of testing. Young adults were completely able to ignore the distraction when tested in the afternoon, an effect similar to that seen in the inattentional blindness phenomenon (Mack & Rock, 1998; Most et al., 2001) and in perceptual speed tasks completed in the presence or absence of distraction (Lustig et al., in press). In the morning, however, young adults showed reliable costs and benefits as the distraction "leaked" in to influence performance. Thus, for young adults, control over the access function is more efficient in the afternoon than in the morning, a pattern consistent with their Evening-arousal typology.

For older adults, distraction is not ignored, it helps or hurts performance at both testing times, but more so in the afternoon than in the morning. The results for the older adults (and for young adults tested in the morning) cannot easily be written off as "general performance deficits," since baselines were equivalent when no distraction was present. Instead, the extraneous information sometimes led to greater costs but also to greater *benefits*, depending on the type of distraction that was present. What remained constant was the older adults' relative failure to restrict attention away from the distractor items, consistent with the assumption that control over the access function diminishes with age. This failure also held for everyone tested at suboptimal times of day.

More recent work shows that the consequences of a failure to control distraction are not just immediate, but can also impact on "downstream" performance 15 or 20 minutes after initial exposure to the distraction

(Kim et al., in press; Rowe, Valderrama, Le-nartowicz & Hasher, in press). Furthermore, these experiments show "far transfer" effects, such that distraction in the context of one task can influence performance on very different subsequent tasks. Indeed, in these two unique circumstances, the data show greater benefits for older as compared to younger adults, rather than the typically seen greater costs. As well, the benefits are greater at nonoptimal times than at optimal times (Rowe et al., in press).

As an aside, what the data also show is that failing to attend to the time at which younger and older adults are tested is probably a major mistake, since more than 70% of older adults are Morning types and a third or more of young adults in university settings are Evening types (see, e.g., May, Hasher, & Stoltzfus, 1993; Yoon et al., 2000; Yoon et al., in press). If early-morning testing times are not used, and most participants are tested later in the day (see May et al., 1993), age differences in access control will be exaggerated. As subsequent data show, this argument can likely be extended to the two other inhibitory functions (deletion and re-straint) and, critically, the argument can also be extended to other cognitive tasks that have inhibitory components.

In sum, our work and that of others suggests that across many situations, the ability to keep attention focused away from irrelevant infor-mation aids the fast and accurate processing of goal-relevant information. The access control function influences performance on tests of processing speed, a construct often used along or in competition with working memory capac-ity as an explanation for performance variation across the life span (Park et al., 1996; Salthouse, 1996), and on tests of reading and problem solv-ing, tasks often used as outcome measures in studies examining the predictive power of work-ing memory tasks (see review by Daneman & Merikle, 1996). From a theoretical perspective, efficient inhibitory function is critical for con-trolling which pieces of information gain ac-cess to attention and, on the assumption that co-occurrence is a major determinant of asso-ciation formation, how large the initial mem-ory bundles are. This in turn determines how

fast and accurate subsequent retrieval can be (Anderson & Bower, 1973). The impact of clut-tered or large memory bundles will be discussed following the next section.

Deletion

Inhibition also serves to *delete* irrelevant infor-mation from the focus of attention. Irrelevant information may be active in the first instance because of the failure of the access function to control "leakage" tied to subsidiary goals or to a mismatch between the goals of an individual and those set by an experimenter or situation. Deletion is critical for removing irrelevant representations from the focus of attention so as to enable efficient processing of goal-driven representations. Deletion also removes once-relevant information that has become irrelevant because of a change in goals, context, task, or situational demands, as can occur in a conver-sation when a topic changes, or in a task (whe-ther attention, memory, or problem solving) when one set of materials (or procedures) ends and another begins.

As noted earlier, the stimulus for this aspect of our theoretical framework comes from the ob-servation that older adults not only allow alter-native interpretations of a passage to gain *access* to their attention but also fail to *delete* those al-ternatives from consideration, even when it be-comes clear that they were incorrect (Hamm & Hasher, 1992; Hasher & Zacks, 1988). To es-tablish the generality of these initial findings, we created garden path sentences that ended with a highly predictable but missing word that the participant generated and that was replaced, a few seconds later, by a less predictable word pro-vided by the experimenter. We then used an implicit task to measure the accessibility of the initially generated word (the highly predictable ending)—a word that became irrelevant in the context of the task as soon as the experimenter provided an alternative ending to the sentence. We measured access to the no-longer relevant words (and for other control items) for both older and younger adults.

Across a series of studies, the ability to delete a no-longer relevant inference from memory varied as a function of adult age and time of testing (e.g., Hartman & Hasher, 1991; May & Hasher, 1998; May, Zacks, Hasher, & Multhaup, 1999). For Evening-type young adults tested in the afternoon (see May & Hasher, 1998), deletion actually *suppressed* the no-longer relevant word to such a degree that subsequent use of those words to end new sentences was actually *below* baseline levels. Early in the morning, however, the availability of the no-longer relevant term was reliably *above* baseline levels, showing time-of-day differences in the efficiency of the deletion function for young adults that are consistent with their arousal pattern. Older adults also showed time-of-day differences in deletion regulation, with worse performance in the afternoon, consistent with their circadian arousal type. Overall, there were profound age and time-of-day differences in inhibitory control over deletion.

Vulnerability to the effects of no-longer relevant information has been shown to vary across groups and individuals who differ in reading ability, in span scores, and on intelligence tests (e.g., Chiappe et al., 2000, 2002; Dempster, 1991; Gernsbacher & Faust, 1991; Kane & Engle, 2000). Note that if deletion is inefficient, the memory bundle representing a given event or moment will consist of (at least) both relevant information and irrelevant information that remained active in consciousness, thus enabling an "enriched" or cluttered memory bundle during encoding. These larger bundles in turn result in differentially poor retrieval (e.g., Anderson & Bower, 1973). In the next section, we consider the impact of the deletion function on tasks intended to measure working memory.

Deletion and Working Memory Span

Working memory span tasks, including the by-now classic reading span task of Daneman and Carpenter (1980), typically present the participant with a series of "study" and recall test trials, each of which consists of a set of sentences to understand while preparing to recall the final word of each, followed by an immediate recall of those final words. These sets vary in size (e.g., from two to six sentences), and by convention (i.e., at least since the earliest IQ tests developed

by Binet) they are presented in an "ascending" order so that the smallest sets are presented first. The largest set-size that a participant can reliably understand and for which all items in the set can be recalled is a commonly used index of working memory capacity.

The ascending administration requires deletion to be efficient so that at any point in the series of study trials consideration is narrowly focused on only the currently relevant set. If deletion is inefficient, items from prior sets will "enrich" the memory representations of the current set, reducing the ability of participants to recall the current set accurately. The failure to suppress no-longer relevant words enables proactive interference (PI) to build up across trials and to have its most detrimental effects on the large set-size trials that are last in the series yet critical to attaining a high working memory score.

On the basis of these observations of the typical operations involved in assessing working memory span, May, Hasher & Kane (1999) reversed the order of administration so that the largest trials occurred first, before PI had a chance to accumulate. This simple manipulation should have no effect on the measurement of working memory capacity per se, at least if capacity simply reflects the amount of information an individual can store and process in their "mental workspace." However, if deletion (and attendant PI) is involved in standard span tasks, the sequence manipulation should affect how much irrelevant information is available to that workspace from previous trials when participants are attempting to recall the current items. Indeed, the reversed administration dramatically improved the performance of older adults on the reading span task, so that, rather startlingly, their performance no longer differed from that of young adults. (A more extreme manipulation designed to reduce PI also improved the scores of young adults.) These findings suggest that variation in deletion function (or, inversely, in proactive interference caused by failures of the deletion function) plays a major role in producing variation in working memory span (see also Bowles & Salthouse, 2003).

Recent work suggests that this conclusion extends beyond the limits of the various versions of Daneman and Carpenter's reading and listening span tasks. The reversed-order manipulation also increased the span scores of older adults on a Corsi-block version of a visuospatial working memory span task (Rowe et al., 2006). Bunting (2006) has shown that the operation span task introduced by Engle and colleagues (e.g., Engle, Cantor, & Carullo, 1992), which is based on verifying the accuracy of equations while remembering words, is also vulnerable to PI (see also Rowe et al., 2006). We have also found that circadian influences can affect PI-heavy measures of working memory span (Hasher et al., 2005; Yoon et al., 2000), consistent with the conclusion that the efficiency of the deletion function varies across the day. Taken together, these data suggest that several of the most widely used versions of working memory span are likely measuring something other than capacity. We think it likely that they index the efficiency of inhibitory aspects of attention regulation.

Deletion may play a critical role not only in variability on working memory span tasks per se, but also in those tasks' ability to predict performance on other measures. Lustig et al. (2001) replicated the May, Hasher & Kane (1999) results by showing that delivering a span task in reverse order (so reducing PI) eliminated age differences in working memory span performance, and further showed that the deletion-demanding aspects of the span task were critical for its ability to predict performance on prose recall (a standard outcome measure in the individual difference tradition). For both younger and older adults, manipulations that reduced PI and improved span scores also reduced the ability of individual differences in span scores to predict individual differences in prose recall. By broad generalization, these data raise the possibility that whenever span tasks are used to select participants to perform on other tasks and whenever reliable correlations are obtained, the mediating variable may well be inhibitory control over nonrelevant information, not working memory capacity.

Further evidence that working memory span tasks do not measure capacity but instead something like interference proneness comes from a study demonstrating that prior experience with

other memory tasks can reduce estimates of the size of an individual's working memory span (Lustig & Hasher, 2002). Performance on other retrieval tasks (e.g., paired associates and serial learning) has long been known to be disrupted by prior laboratory experience (Greenberg & Underwood, 1950; Keppel, Postman, & Zavortink, 1968; Underwood, 1957; Zechmeister & Nyberg, 1982). As with these classic memory tasks, the Lustig and Hasher (2002) finding suggests that working memory span tasks may also be influenced by across-task proactive interference. Indeed, recent neuroimaging work suggests that the same brain areas may mediate both short- and long-term interference effects (Brush & Postle, 2003; Postle, Berger, Goldstein, Curtis, & D'Esposito, 2001), a finding consistent with the behavioral data.

The deletion function is critical not just for immediate performance and working memory tasks (with their immediate recall trials), it is also critical for longer-term retrieval, since a broad focus at encoding results in poorer retrieval (Anderson & Bower, 1973; Watkins & Watkins, 1976).[4] It is not surprising, then, that older adults typically show differentially poor retrieval relative to that of younger adults (see Kane & Hasher, 1995; Zacks, Hasher, & Li, 2000, for reviews). Consistent with this pattern of findings is evidence that retrieval is better, for both younger and older adults, at peak than at off-peak times of day. This conclusion stems from a series of studies using materials ranging from prose to word lists and test tasks ranging from free recall to recognition (see Winocur & Hasher, 2002; Yoon et al., 2000, in press, for reviews).

Restraint

Restraint is the inhibitory mechanism that controls strong responses. It is probably also the most widely studied inhibitory mechanism and is actually the mechanism that many simply refer to as "inhibition" (e.g., Miyake et al., 2000, among others). Restraint has been studied using a variety of tasks, including inhibition of return, Stroop tasks of various sorts, and the stop-signal task. It can also be studied by looking at slips of thought and action as well as at schema-driven errors at retrieval, on the assumption that schemas are strong responses to memory cues and so need to be restrained for more detailed memories to be retrieved (see Alba & Hasher, 1983).

Direct evidence showing age and time-of-day effects on control over strong responses comes from a variant of the stop-signal task, in which an occasional signal occurs informing people of the need to withhold a response that they otherwise make quickly and accurately. A critical dependent measure is the proportion of stop trials on which errors are made (i.e., a "go" response is made). In one study, older adults made more errors overall than young adults and everyone made more errors at a nonoptimal time of day (afternoon for older adults and morning for young adults) than at an optimal time (morning for older adults and afternoon for young adults). The ability to withhold a strong response is reduced with age as well as with performance at an off-peak time of day (May & Hasher, 1998).

Comparable evidence with respect to age differences comes from the antisaccade task, in which people are instructed to respond to a peripheral stimulus (a brief onset) by looking in the *opposite* direction to detect a limited-duration discrimination target. Because a peripheral onset elicits a reflex response of looking *toward* the cue, restraint is required to look in the correct direction (away from the onset location), and older adults have greater difficulty than younger adults deploying the required restraint. In particular, older adults make more looking-direction errors in the antisaccade task (Butler et al., 1999). Given the role inhibition plays in determining span size, it is not surprising that young adults show a relationship between span and performance on the antisaccade task (Kane et al., 2001).

The ability to control strong responses can also play a role in tasks requiring retrieval of detailed information when a strong response is triggered by a cue or context. A classic example of such errors occurs in the "Moses illusion" effect (Reder & Kusbit, 1991). Here people are asked to answer general-knowledge questions such as, "Who did Clark Kent turn into when he went into a telephone booth?" Embedded in the midst of sensible questions are some that are nonsense, such as "How many animals of each type did Moses take on the ark?" Yoon et al. (2000) reported that errors driven by strong responses (e.g., to the biblical theme in the sentence) are more likely to occur at nonpeak times of day, and are more likely to occur for older than for younger adults.

Other work shows that at nonoptimal times, people are more likely to use easily accessible stereotypes to judge individuals than they are at optimal times (Bodenhausen, 1990). These errors of thought can be termed "slips" of thought, relating them to the "slips" of action literature. This literature shows that strong motor responses are less controllable at nonoptimal times (Manley, Lewis, Robertson, Watson, & Datta, 2002; May & Hasher, 1998), just as thoughts are.

Attentional regulation of strong responses, like attentional regulation over distraction or access and deletion, appears to vary with circadian arousal, and those variations are also seen in old rats. Winocur and Hasher (1999) found a similar pattern for old rats tested in a classic Go–NoGo task at the beginning and at the end of their activity cycle (Winocur & Hasher, 1999). Go responses did not change across the day, although the ability to withhold a strong response was diminished at the end of the day for the old rats. Old rats also had more difficulty performing a delayed matching-to-sample test (on which they have to reverse a previous response) at the end of their activity cycle (Winocur & Hasher, 2004).

From a view emphasizing inhibitory function, restraint processes are likely involved in situations conceived of by others as tapping "task set" or "goal maintenance." For example, a series of Stroop experiments by Kane and Engle (2003) manipulated the ratio of congruent (so that the ink color matched the color named by the word) to incongruent (so that the ink color conflicted with the color named by the word) trials. When there were many congruent trials, participants with low working memory spans were error-prone on those few trials that were incongruent, and they were faster on congruent trials. This was the case even though low-span participants understood the goals of the task, and even when they received feedback after every trial. These data can be seen as reflecting a failure of "task set" or "goal maintenance," at least at the level of having a goal control behavior (e.g., Kane & Engle, 2003).

An inhibitory-based alternative explanation is at least equally possible. Like others (e.g., Arbuckle & Gold, 1993), we consider the Stroop task to be an inhibitory control task that requires control over strong responses (naming the word) in order to carry out a less dominant response (naming the color), thus primarily tapping into the restraint function. Since working memory tasks have an inhibitory component that includes control over deletion and, very likely, given deletion failures, control over strong responses from previous sets, it would not be surprising that control lapses in the Stroop task would be associated with poor performance on a span task. This might particularly be the case when the need to control the nondominant response is not regularly reinforced.

Thus strong responses can seize control of both action and thought, and both patterns can be seen for older adults and participants tested at nonoptimal times of day. These effects can be seen across a range of tasks, including attention, memory, and language comprehension. It is important to note that when strong responses are correct, no time-of-day differences are expected, since it is inhibition, not excitation, that varies with the arousal cycle and other important individual differences. As an example, the time it takes to classify a word (e.g., *chair*) as a member of a familiar category (furniture) does not differ across the day (e.g., May & Hasher, 1998; see Yoon et al., 2000).

WORKING MEMORY THEORY, CAPACITY, AND INHIBITION

In the previous sections we outlined our current understanding and some of the relevant evidence for the inhibitory control processes that in our view are responsible for much of the variation in working memory and cognition more generally. The relations between our views and those of other authors in this volume, and working memory theory in general, have been touched on throughout this discussion, but here we focus more specifically on them.

The working memory model of Baddeley and colleagues (Baddeley, 1986, 1992, 2000, 2003; Baddeley & Hitch, 1974) provides a common heritage for most of the chapters in this volume and for the vast majority of the working memory literature more generally. Our own work can be seen as focusing on the central executive component of Baddeley's system. Like Baddeley, we were initially influenced by Allport's (1989) and Shallice's (Shallice & Burgess, 1993) conceptions of control. Furthermore, we consider the executive processes important for "working memory" to be domain general, and important across many areas of cognition, particularly attention and memory, in close agreement with most of the contributors to this volume (see Chapters 2, 3, 4, 5, and 10). Finally, we note that several contributors address the potential relations between group-level variation and individual differences–level variation (see Chapters 2, 4, 8, 10, and 11). Like several other contributors (Chapters 8, 10, and 11), we are especially concerned with variation due to aging.

Our approach differs from most other views in emphasizing inhibitory processes as sources of attentional regulation and thus of working memory variation. Although inhibitory processes are included in other views (see especially Chapters 2, 3, and 10), we differ somewhat from these views by giving inhibition primary importance, and in so doing turning away from notions of capacity. We have avoided using this term in a loose sense, as we find it too easily confused with the idea that the ability to have more information activated and at the focus of attention is always beneficial. Thus, we also turn away from the metaphor of a large desk or workspace as the best working memory, and consider something more similar to a (truly effective) spam blocker, allowing into the system only information that is relevant to one's goals and concerns. As we have argued throughout this chapter, a mental workspace narrowly focused on current concerns will be fast and accurate at on-line processing, in part because it is only doing one task. Such a workspace is not cluttered with previous tasks, upcoming tasks, social obligations, and short- and long-term personal concerns; it is simply doing the current task. Simply doing the current task also happens to result subsequently in fast and accurate retrieval of the information within that task. What a narrow focus probably does not do is foster creativity (Carson, Peterson, & Higgins, 2003).

Where we differ from others in the life-span developmental literature and in the intelligence literature is in the notion that aspects of inhibitory regulation are central to determining individual and time-of-day differences in both perceptual speed and apparent working memory capacity. In our view, the cognitive primitives upon which higher-order tasks build are neither speed nor capacity, but instead are inhibitory regulation that occurs in the service of goals. It is important to note that individuals differ in their long-term goals (e.g., Kahneman, 1973) and values (e.g., Rokeach, 1976). When researchers are doing work across the adult life span (and probably with all non-university students), it is particularly important to recognize that younger and older adults differ on these important dimensions (e.g., Carstensen & Löckenhoff, 2003). If information matches goals and values, the use of inhibitory processes should be maximally efficient. Encoding will then be narrow and retention levels high. Indeed, recent evidence suggests that age differences in memory can be entirely eliminated when the materials to be remembered match the goals, values and interests of older adults (May, Rahhal, Berry, & Leighton, 2005; Rahhal, Hasher, & Colcombe, 2001; Rahhal, May, & Hasher, 2002).

BIOLOGICAL BASES FOR INHIBITORY VARIATION

The effects of age and time of day on inhibitory function described above strongly suggest that biological influences play a major role in variations in inhibitory efficiency. The field is in near-unanimous agreement that individual and group differences in frontal lobe structure and function contribute to individual and group differences in executive processes such as in-

hibition (e.g., Engle, Tuholski, Laughlin, & Conway, 1999; Miyake et al., 2000; Moscovitch & Winocur, 1995; Park, Polk, Mikels, Taylor, & Marschuetz, 2001; Persad et al., 2002; West, 1996, 2000). The evidence for frontal lobe involvement in individual and group differences in inhibition and other executive attention processes has been reviewed extensively elsewhere and is covered in more depth in other chapters in this volume (see especially Chapters 2, 4, 7, 10, and 11). Here we focus specifically on biological evidence for variability in inhibitory function, especially that due to age and circadian arousal.

Adult age differences in the structure and function of the frontal lobe structures most often associated with working memory and inhibition are a major focus of work in the cognitive neuroscience of aging (see reviews by Cabeza, 2002; Grady & Craik, 2000; Raz, 2000; Reuter-Lorenz, 2002; Reuter-Lorenz et al., 2001). The relevant neuroimaging findings are discussed in more detail in Chapter 10; we will summarize some of the more ubiquitous patterns here. Prefrontal cortex structures, including those most often associated with working memory and inhibition, typically show the largest effects of age in structural brain studies (Raz, 2000). In functional imaging studies, older adults often differ from young adults in showing either less activation in the brain regions typically associated with task performance in young adults or showing more activation, often in regions not associated with task performance in young adults (Cabeza, 2002; Grady & Craik, 2000; Reuter-Lorenz, 2002; Reuter-Lorenz et al., 2001). This additional activation is frequently interpreted as a form of compensation for age-related increases in task difficulty or damage to structures more typically associated with the task. Other investigators have raised the possibility that it may represent a failure to create distinct representations or a lack of functional inhibition (e.g., Logan, Sanders, Snyder, Morris, & Buckner, 2002; see Reuter-Lorenz & Lustig, 2005, for discussion of the functional implications of additional activations).

Although the neuroimaging literature most often focuses on changes in prefrontal cortex, there are also large changes in the subcortical structures and neurotransmitter systems that interact with prefrontal cortex to modulate its function. The size of age effects on the caudate and putamen, basal ganglia structures involved in dopamine function, and on the locus coeruleus, a brain structure involved in norepinephrine function, is a close second to the amount found for prefrontal cortex (Raz, 2000). These two catecholamine neurotransmitters, dopamine and norepinephrine, play important roles in attention and working memory. Changes in these systems may play an important but underrated role in age changes in cognition (see discussions by Braver & Barch, 2002; Li & Sikström, 2002; Rubin, 1999).

Of particular interest to the current discussion is that dopamine and norepinephrine function appears to be essential to the "gating" of information—that is, maintaining target information and preventing irrelevant, nontarget information from becoming activated (see reviews by Arnsten, 1998; Aston-Jones, Rajkowski, & Cohen, 1999; Berridge, Arnsten, & Foote, 1993; Braver & Barch, 2002; see Chapter 4, this volume). For example, neural-recording studies in rodents and primates show that the phasic (stimulus-related) firing of certain basal ganglia and locus coeruleus neurons is largely target specific under normal conditions, with little or no firing to distractors (see review by Arnsten, 1998). However, disruptions in the tonic (state-related) levels of either dopamine or norepinephrine lead to a loss of discriminability; both phasic firing to distractors and behavioral false alarms increase (Arnsten, 1998; Aston-Jones et al., 1999). In humans and other mammals, dopamine and norepinephrine function shows variation with both age (Arnsten, 1998; Volkow et al., 1998) and circadian cycle (Aston-Jones, Chen, Zhu, & Oshinksy, 2001; Karlsson, Farde, & Halldin; 2000; Wirz-Justice, 1984, 1987). Further, there is an interaction such that increased age is associated with shorter, flatter, and often more irregular circadian cycles (Edgar, 1994; Hofman, 2000; Monk & Kupfer, 2000; Weinert, 2000). These systems are thus prime candidates for the source of age- and circadian-related variation.

Event-related potentials (ERPs) also provide evidence for age- and circadian-related changes in the brain functions associated with working memory. In particular, P300, an ERP component strongly associated with the detection of target or unusual stimuli against a background of distractors, shows significant variation in both amplitude and latency over the course of the day (Geisler & Polich, 1990, 1992; Higuchi, Lui, Yuasa, Maeda, & Motohashi, 2000; Polich & Kok, 1995). P300 also shows differences as a result of aging (see review by Polich, 1996), and animal studies provide compelling evidence for its link to locus coeruleus activity (Foote, Berridge, Adams, & Pineda, 1991; Swick, Pineda, Schacher, & Foote, 1994). Thus far there has been very little functional neuroimaging (PET or fMRI) evidence of the influence of circadian or age–circadian interactions on brain function. However, the evidence from neurotransmitter and ERP studies suggests that these interactions are very promising areas for future investigation.

With regard to the possible relationships among different functions of inhibition, we note a recent fMRI study that compared the brain regions involved in switching with those involved in the restraint of a prepotent response (Sylvester et al., 2003; see Nelson, Reuter-Lorenz, Sylvester, Jonides, & Smith, 2003, for a similar study by this group). On each trial, participants were presented with an arrow facing either the right or left. For the switching task, participants had to count the number of times each type of arrow (right or left) appeared during a block of trials; the arrow's direction switched unpredictably during the block. For the restraint task, participants had to press a button either corresponding to the direction in which the arrow was pointing (i.e., press the right button if the arrow is pointing right; low-restraint condition) or one opposite this direction (i.e., press the left button if the arrow is pointing right; high-restraint condition).

Although each task undoubtedly tapped multiple processes, the switching task might be thought of as preferentially requiring the *deletion* of one task set from working memory (e.g., count right arrows) to allow concentration on another (e.g., count left arrows). In contrast, the restraint task likely preferentially required the restraint or *suppression* of a natural inclination to press the button corresponding to the direction in which the arrow was pointing. An intriguing question is the degree to which these two tasks elicited the same patterns of brain activity, thus suggesting a general executive function involved in both, or distinct patterns specific to each task, implying different functions of executive control or inhibition.

There was a good deal of overlap in the brain regions activated by the two tasks: regions in superior parietal cortex, medial frontal cortex, and left dorsolateral prefrontal cortex. There were also several interesting differences. The switching task activated several posterior regions more than the restraint task did—that is, switching differentially activated bilateral extrastriate cortex and left posterior parietal cortex. The restraint task preferentially activated regions in right parietal cortex, premotor cortex, frontopolar cortex, and bilateral basal ganglia regions including caudate and putamen. These results on young-adult participants provide intriguing evidence for the possibility that different functions of inhibition (or executive control more generally) may be mediated by different brain structures (Sylvester et al., 2003). These different structures may vary in their sensitivity to factors such as age and time of day, and this difference should manifest itself behaviorally.

In short, there is extensive evidence that the brain structures associated with working memory show a great deal of change with age, and that the functioning of those structures may show further variation across different times of day. In addition, recent brain imaging data support the idea of a distinction between different functions of inhibition or executive control, by suggesting that different functions may be distinguished by the regions of the brain most involved in their implementation (Sylvester et al., 2003). Behavioral evidence (e.g., Friedman & Miyake, 2004) is also suggestive in this regard. Attempts to make direct connections between age-, circadian-, and function-related variations in working memory performance are relatively new, but represent a rich and exciting area for future research.

Our central view is that working memory capacity is not the main issue for understanding higher-order cognition (nor is speed, as has been argued in the literature on aging), rather, been argued in the literature on aging), rather,

inhibition and possibly other executive functions are. The contents of consciousness, or working memory, are controlled by executive functions operating in the service of goals. These executive functions are largely inhibitory in nature. There is a good deal of evidence to support this view, both in the present volume and elsewhere. Indeed, many views in this book have some overlap with those we propose here, the ideas of Kane and colleagues (Chapter 2) being the closest. For example, Kane et al. now describe executive attention as the critical resource that determines both working memory capacity and inhibition. Of course, approaches favoring inhibitory processes have not gone uncriticized (e.g., MacLeod, Dodd, Sheard, Wilson, & Bibi, 2003: Miller & Cohen, 2002). The aging and time-of-day differences reviewed here, however, will ultimately require some accommodation by these alternative views.

CONCLUSIONS

Our emphasis on inhibitory processes, rather than on constructs such as capacity or resources, may be the characteristic that most differentiates our view from that of others. We have consistently maintained that inhibitory *control* processes are the most likely sources of individual, group, and intra-individual variation in measures of working memory. We have proposed the existence of three inhibitory processes, access, deletion, and restraint (e.g., Hasher et al., 1999), that together and possibly independently operate to regulate the contents of consciousness. Our age and time-of-day work with individuals at different points in their arousal cycle suggests that all three processes change with age and across the day, such that regulation is better at peak times of day than at off-peak times. The findings from animal models overlap, albeit not precisely, both the age and time-of-day effects we have seen for people (Winocur & Hasher, 1999, 2002, 2004), suggesting a biological basis for these mechanisms. We have also reported evidence that inhibitory processes underlie age differences in speed of processing and underlie most tasks that measure working memory capacity, as well as

BOX 9.1. SUMMARY ANSWERS TO BOOK QUESTIONS

1. THE OVERARCHING THEORY OF WORKING MEMORY

We proposed a general theory of cognition whose central view is that the best performance on a variety of tasks occurs when the contents of consciousness are narrowly focused on goal-relevant information (e.g., Hasher et al., 1999). Narrowing occurs in the face of an individual's internal and external context—a world in which there is massive activation triggered by the environment, the recent past, near-future tasks, and subsidiary goals. To tune this massive activation, we suggest that inhibitory control is required, through at least three control processes: access, deletion, and restraint. Together with goals, these processes determine the contents of consciousness, or working memory. Our hypothesized attentional mechanisms can be thought of as at least partially fulfilling the functions of the executive system of Baddeley's working memory model (1986, 1992, 2003).

2. CRITICAL SOURCES OF WORKING MEMORY VARIATION

Our work presumes that activation processes vary minimally within and among individuals, thus the critical source of individual and group differences is the efficiency of inhibitory mechanisms and their underlying biology. Inhibitory control appears to vary with age, and the synchrony between an individual's circadian arousal pattern and the time of testing. There are also substantial individual differences within any age group. Inhibitory control is particularly critical in situations to which there are strong but erroneous response tendencies and where there are salient sources of distraction, whether in thought or in the environment.

What we do not yet know is the degree to which the three proposed attentional mechanisms (access, deletion, and restraint) are fully independent or partially overlapping mechanisms. Also unclear is whether the pattern of interdependence or independence remains the same or changes across the adult life span and within circadian arousal patterns at different times of testing. The work of Friedman and Miyake (2004) suggests that access and deletion may be the same for younger adults whereas restraint is a separable process (see Chapter 8). Our ongoing work addresses these issues.

3. OTHER SOURCES OF WORKING MEMORY VARIATION

A major alternative view proposes that the capacity of working memory is the critical determinant of individual differences on a wide range of tasks. Our view stands in sharp contrast to this and suggests instead that individual differences in measures of capacity (e.g., operation span, sentence span) and in the ability of those measures to predict other cognitive functions are actually due to variation in inhibitory control processes.

We agree with Kane et al. (Chapter 2) that the critical aspect of working memory measures is not that they measure capacity but that they measure executive (or, in our view, attentional) control processes. Indeed, we believe they best measure the ability to deal with distraction (past, present, and future). We agree that "executive attention" capabilities are the major source of variation among individuals and that these capabilities are general and critical for a variety of intellectual functions, including controlling interference, memory, problem solving, and fluid intelligence. In our view, however, the central aspects of control are inhibitory in nature; Kane et al.'s view includes excitatory mechanisms for maintaining the activation of representations, including goals. We have reviewed evidence of equivalent activation across the day in younger and older adults and so do not see the need for assuming significant variation in activation processes. In this regard our view differs from that of Munakata et al. (Chapter 7).

(continued)

241

BOX 9.1.   (*continued*)

4. CONTRIBUTIONS TO GENERAL WORKING MEMORY THEORY

Our approach speaks directly to the nature of working memory. It suggests that working memory capacity is not the cognitive primitive it once appeared to be, and instead suggests that the cognitive primitive (if there is one) is inhibitory attentional control. Our studies have included younger and older adults, as well as individuals of this age range who differ in their circadian arousal rhythms. We have also done some work with animal models. All of these studies point toward attentional regulation as a critical determinant of intellectual performance. This conclusion might remind readers of Navon's classic article (1977) on capacity as a theoretical soup stone.

---

evidence to support the role of inhibition (and circadian patterns) in determining long-term memory performance. There are also clear findings that excitatory processes do not change across the day (e.g., Yoon et al., 2000); we and others believe these processes do not change with age (e.g., Duchek et al., 1998). Thus, we see these inhibitory processes, which we argue work together with an individual's goals to determine the contents of consciousness, to be at the heart of what many call working memory. These mechanisms can be thought of as at least partially fulfilling the functions of the executive system of Baddeley's working memory model (1986, 1992, 2003).

Thus, the critical source of working memory variability among (and within) people is inhibition. At the very least, we also know that circadian arousal patterns (and individual differences therein) influence the efficiency of inhibitory control. What we do not know is (a) the degree to which the three proposed inhibitory executive functions (access, deletion, and restraint or suppression) are fully independent or partially overlapping mechanisms, and (b) whether with circadian arousal the pattern of interdependence or independence remains the same or changes across the adult life span and within an age group. Although the research reviewed above in the section Biological Bases for Inhibition Variation indicates that relevant findings are beginning to appear in the literature, we do not know a great deal about the underlying biology of inhibitory control.

We would simply add that the richest explications of the problems of mental control will come from research on a very broad range of participants studied through a broad range of approaches, including self-regulation of motivated behavior (e.g., Muraven & Baumeister, 2000). From our analysis of the overall literature, we suggest that for cognitive efficiency, a narrow, goal-driven focus is ideal for both online performance and subsequent retention of details. To achieve a narrow focus (or to regulate attention effectively), inhibitory processes are required. We argue that there are three such processes (access, deletion, and restraint) and that they vary within an individual, among individuals, and across the life span. Our views are not particularly tied to aging or circadian rhythms, but instead represent a general theory of cognition that suggests that fundamental regulatory mechanisms are inhibitory in nature.

Notes

1. In this chapter we do not discuss the relevant literature on social issues and personality, but note that there is empirical and theoretical overlap among the domains in both tasks and the mechanisms that regulate them (see, e.g., Eysenck, 1995; Muraven & Baumeister, 2000). For example, schizophrenic, creative, and low-span young adults are all more likely to pick up information on the unattended track in a dichotic listening experiment (Conway, Cowan, & Bunting, 2001; Dykes & Mc-Ghie, 1976). Psychosis-prone, creative, and older adults all show less habituation to repeated stimuli (e.g., McDowd & Filion, 1992; Raine, Benishay, Lencz & Scarpa, 1997).

2. In the lab, experimenters typically set goals for participants, whereas in life people set goals for

themselves, sometimes a short-term one (finding a cup of coffee in an unfamiliar city) and sometimes long-term ones (finding first editions of classic psychology texts). Lab and life goals can conflict, setting the stage for poor performance. Sometimes, participants may not adopt the goals set by the experimenters.

3. Although there is a rich literature exploring performance across the day, most of these studies are done without reference to differences in circadian arousal patterns. Although important for the study of younger adults, the failure to take arousal differences into account when comparing across ages is particularly worrisome, given the substantial differences in arousal patterns (see Goldstein et al., 2006).

4. We note that access, too, plays a role in determining both short- and long-term memory performance, including that on working memory tasks, because this process also influences the size of the memory bundles created during encoding. These will be small or large, to the degree that access is or is not efficient, respectively.

5. We note that deletion failures also set the stage for the need for source monitoring, that is, the need to distinguish whether an item or set of items came from the current trial or a previous trial. If items from a previous trial are successfully deleted initially, few source decisions would be required. Further, if items from a previous trial were successfully deleted when that trial was over and the new trial started, source decisions would be easier to make.

References

Alba, J. W., & Hasher, L. (1983). Is memory schematic? *Psychological Bulletin, 93*, 203–231.

Allport, A. (1989). Visual attention. In M. I. Posner (Ed.), *Foundations of cognitive science*, pp 631–682. Cambridge, MA: MIT Press.

Anderson, J. R., & Bower, G. H. (1973). *Human associative memory.* Oxford: V.H. Winston & Sons.

Arbuckle, T. Y., & Gold, D. P. (1993) Aging, inhibition and verbosity. *Journal of Gerontology: Psychological Science, 48*, P225–P232.

Arnsten, A.F.T. (1998). Catecholamine modulation of prefrontal cortical cognitive function. *Trends in Cognitive Sciences, 2*, 436–437.

Aston-Jones, G., Chen, S., Zhu, Y., & Oshinsky, M.L. (2001). A neural circuit for circadian regulation of arousal. *Nature Neuroscience, 4*, 732–738.

Aston-Jones, G., Rajkowski, J., & Cohen, J. (1999). Role of locus coeruleus in attention and behavioral flexibility. *Biological Psychiatry, 46*, 1309–1320.

Baddeley, A. D. (1986). *Working memory.* New York: Oxford University Press.

Baddeley, A. D. (1992). Working memory. *Science, 255*, 556–559.

Baddeley, A. D. (2000). The episodic buffer: a new component of working memory? *Trends in Cognitive Sciences, 4*, 417–423.

Baddeley, A. D. (2003). Working memory: Looking forward and looking backward. *Nature Reviews: Neuroscience, 4*, 829–839.

Baddeley, A. D., & Hitch, G. (1974). Working memory. In G. H. Bower (Ed.), *The psychology of learning and motivation: Advances in research and theory* (Vol. 8, pp. 47–89). New York: Academic Press.

Berridge, C. W., Arnsten, A. F .T., & Foote, S. L. (1993). Noradrenergic modulation of cognitive function: Clinical implications of anatomical, electrophysiological, and behavioural studies in animal models. *Psychological Medicine, 23*, 557–564.

Bodenhausen, G. V. (1990). Stereotypes as judgmental heuristics: Evidence of circadian variations in discrimination. *Psychological Science, 1*, 319–322.

Bowles, R. P., & Salthouse, T. A. (2003). Assessing the age-related effects of proactive interference on working memory tasks using the Rasch model. *Psychology and Aging, 18*, 608–615.

Braver, T. S., & Barch, D. M. (2002). A theory of cognitive control, aging cognition, and neuromodulation. *Neuroscience and Biobehavioral Reviews, 26*, 809–817.

Brush, L. N., & Postle, B. R. (2003). *Neural mechanisms underlying the control of item-specific and item-nonspecific proactive interference in human working memory.* Presented at the Society for Neuroscience 33rd Annual Meeting, New Orleans, November 8–12.

Bunting, M. F. (2006). Proactive interference and item similarity in working memory. *Journal of Experimental Psychology: Learning, Memory & cognition, 32*, 183–196.

Butler, K. M, Zacks, R. T., & Henderson, J. M. (1999). Suppression of reflexive saccades in younger and older adults: Age comparisons on antisaccade task. *Memory & Cognition, 27,* 584–591.

Cabeza, R. (2002). Hemispheric asymmetry in older adults: The HAROLD model. *Psychology and Aging, 17,* 85–100.

Cabeza, R., Dolcos, F., Prince, S. E., Rice, H. J., Weissman, D. H., & Nyberg, L. (2003). Attention-related activity during episodic memory retrieval: A cross-function fMRI study. *Neuropsychologia, 11,* 390–399.

Cameli, L., & Phillips, N. A. (2000). Age-related differences in semantic priming: Evidence from event-related brain potentials. *Brain and Cognition, 43,* 69–73.

Carlson, M. C., Hasher, L., Connelly, S. L., & Zacks, R. T. (1995). Aging, distraction, and the benefits of predictable location. *Psychology and Aging, 10,* 427–436.

Carson, S. H., Peterson, J. B., & Higgins, D. M. (2003). Decreased latent inhibition is associated with increased creative achievement in high-functioning individuals. *Journal of Personality and Social Psychology, 85,* 499–506.

Carstensen, L. L., & Löckenhoff, C. E. (2003). Aging, emotion, and evolution. *Annals of the New York Academy of Science, 1000,* 152–179.

Cermakian, N., & Boivin, D. B. (2003). A molecular perspective of human circadian rhythm disorders. *Brain Research Reviews, 42,* 204–220.

Chiappe, P., Hasher, L., & Siegel, L. S. (2000). Working memory, inhibitory control and reading disability. *Memory & Cognition, 28,* 8–17.

Chiappe, P., Siegel, L. S., & Hasher, L. (2002). Working memory, inhibition, and reading skill. In S. P. Shohov (Ed.), *Advances in psychology research* (Vol. 9, pp. 30–51). Huntington, NY: Nova Science Publishers.

Connelly, S. L., Hasher, L., & Zacks, R. T. (1991) Age and reading: The impact of distraction. *Psychology and Aging, 6,* 533–541.

Conway, A. P. A., Cowan, N., & Bunting, M. F. (2001). The cocktail party phenomenon revisited: The importance of working memory capacity. *Psychonomic Bulletin & Review, 8,* 331–335.

Cowan, N. (1993). Activation, attention, and short-term memory. *Memory & Cognition, 21,* 162–167.

Craik, F. I. M., Govoni, R., Naveh-Benjamin, M., & Anderson, N. D. (1996). The effects of divided attention on encoding and retrieval processes in human memory. *Journal of Experimental Psychology: General, 125,* 159–180.

Csikszentmihalyi, M., Rathunde, K., & Whalen, S. (1993). *Talented teenagers: The roots of success and failure.* New York: Cambridge University Press.

Daneman, M., & Carpenter, P. A. (1980). Individual differences in working memory and reading. *Journal of Verbal Learning and Verbal Behavior, 19,* 450–466.

Daneman, M., & Merikle, P. M. (1996). Working memory and language comprehension: A meta-analysis. *Psychonomic Bulletin & Review, 3,* 422–433.

Deese, J. (1959). On the prediction of occurrence of particular verbal intrusions in immediate recall. *Journal of Experimental Psychology, 58,* 17–22.

Demspter, F. N. (1991). Inhibitory processes: A neglected dimension of intelligence. *Intelligence, 15,* 157–173.

Duchek, J. M., Balota, D. A., & Thessing, V. C. (1998). Inhibition of visual and conceptual information during reading in healthy aging and Alzheimer's disease. *Aging, Neuropsychology, and Cognition, 5,* 169–181.

Dykes, M., & McGhie, A. (1976). A comparative study of attentional strategies of schizophrenic and highly creative normal subjects. *British Journal of Psychiatry, 128,* 50–56.

Dywan, J., & Murphy, W. E. (1996). Aging and inhibitory control in text comprehension. *Psychology and Aging, 11,* 199–206.

Edgar, D. M. (1994). Sleep–wake circadian cycles and aging: Potential etiologies and relevance to age-related changes in integrated physiological systems. *Neurobiology of Aging, 15,* 499–501.

Engle, R. W. (2002). Working memory capacity as executive attention. *Current Directions in Psychological Science, 11,* 19–23.

Engle, R. W., Cantor, J., & Carullo, J. J. (1992). Individual differences in working memory and comprehension: A test of four hypotheses. *Journal of Experimental Psychology: Learning, Memory and Cognition, 18,* 972–992.

Engle, R. W., Tuholski, S. W., Laughlin, J. E., & Conway, A. R. A. (1999). Working memory, short-term memory, and general fluid intelligence: A latent-variable approach. *Journal of Experimental Psychology: General, 128,* 309–331.

Eysenck, H. J. (1995). Creativity as a product of intelligence and personality. In D. Saklofske & M. Zeidner (Eds.), *International handbook of personality and intelligence: Perspectives on individual differences* (pp. 231–247). New York: Plenum Press.

Fernandes, M. A., & Moscovitch, M. (2000). Divided attention and memory: Evidence of substantial interference effects at retrieval and encoding. *Journal of Experimental Psychology: General, 129,* 155–176.

Foote, S. L., Berridge, C. W., Adams, L. M., & Pineda, J. A. (1991). Electrophysiological evidence for the involvement of the locus coeruleus in alerting, orienting, and attending. *Progress in Brain Research, 88,* 521–532.

Friedman, N. P., & Miyake, A. (2004). The relations among inhibition and interference control functions: a latent variable analysis. *Journal of Experimental Psychology: General, 133,* 309–331.

Geisler, M. W., & Polich, J. (1990). P300 and time of day: Circadian rhythms, food intake, and body temperature. *Biological Psychology, 31,* 117–136.

Geisler, M. W., & Polich, J. (1992). P300 and individual differences: Morning/evening activity preference, food, and time-of-day. *Psychophysiology, 29,* 86–94.

Gerard, L., Zacks, R. T., Hasher, L., & Radvansky, G. A. (1991). Age deficits in retrieval: The fan effect. *Journal of Gerontology, 46,* P131–P136.

Gernsbacher, M. A., & Faust, M. E. (1991). The mechanism of suppression: A component of general comprehension skill. *Journal of Experimental Psychology: Learning, Memory, and Cognition, 17,* 245–262.

Giffard, B., Desgranges, B., Kerrouche, N., Piolino, P., & Eustache, F. (2003). The hyperpriming phenomenon in normal aging: A consequence of cognitive slowing? *Neuropsychology, 17,* 594–601.

Goldstein, D., Hahn, C., Hasher, L., & Zelazo, P. (2006). *Circadian arousal and intellectual performance in adolescents.* Manuscript submitted for publication.

Grady, C. L., & Craik, F. I. M. (2000). Changes in memory processing with age. *Current Opinion in Neurobiology, 10,* 224–231.

Greenberg, R., & Underwood, B. J. (1950). Retention as a function of stage of practice. *Journal of Experimental Psychology, 40,* 452–457.

Hamm, V. P., & Hasher, L. (1992). Age and the availability of inferences. *Psychology and Aging, 7,* 56–64.

Harnishfeger, K. K., & Bjorklund, D. F. (1994). A developmental perspective on individual differences in inhibition. *Learning and Individual Differences, 6,* 331–355.

Hartman, M., & Hasher, L. (1991). Aging and suppression: Memory for previously relevant information. *Psychology and Aging, 6,* 587–594.

Hasher, L., Goldstein, D., & May, C. P. (2005). It's about time: Circadian rhythms, memory, and aging. In C. Izawa & N. Ohta (Eds.), *Human learning and memory: Advances in theory and application* (pp. 199–217). Mahwah, NJ: Lawrence Erlbaum Associates.

Hasher, L., Tonev, S. T., Lustig, C., & Zacks, R. T. (2001). Inhibitory control, environmental support, and self-initiated processing in aging. In M. Naveh-Benjamin, M. Moscovitch, & H. Roediger, III (Eds.), *Perspectives on human memory and cognitive aging: Essays in honour of Fergus Craik* (pp. 286–297). Philadelphia: Psychology Press.

Hasher, L., & Zacks, R. T. (1979). Automatic and effortful processes in memory. *Journal of Experimental Psychology: General, 108,* 356–388.

Hasher, L., & Zacks, R. T. (1988). Working memory, comprehension, and aging: A review and new view. In G. H. Bower (Ed.), *The psychology of learning and motivation: Advances in research and theory* (Vol. 22, pp. 193–225). New York: Academic Press.

Hasher, L., Zacks, R. T., & May, C. P. (1999). Inhibitory control, circadian arousal, and age. In D. Gopher & A. Koriat, (Eds.), *Attention and performance XVII: Cognitive regulation of performance: Interaction of theory and application* (pp. 653–675). Cambridge, MA: MIT Press.

Higuchi, S., Liu, Y., Yuasa, T., Maeda, A., & Motohashi, Y. (2000). Diurnal variation in the P300 component of human cognitive event-related potential. *Chronobiology International, 17,* 669–678.

Hofman, M. A. (2000). The human circadian clock and aging. *Chronobiology International, 17*, 245–259.

Horne, J. A., & Ostberg, O. (1976). A self-assessment questionnaire to determine morningness-eveningness in human circadian rhythms. *International Journal of Chronobiology, 4*, 97–110.

Hur, Y., Bouchard, T. J., & Lykken, D. T. (1998). Genetic and environmental influence on morningness-eveningness. *Personality and Individual Differences, 25*, 917–925.

Just, M. A., & Carpenter, P. A. (1992). A capacity theory of comprehension: Individual differences in working memory. *Psychological Review, 99*, 122–149.

Kahneman, D. (1973). *Attention and effort*. Englewood Cliffs, NJ: Prentice-Hall.

Kail, R. (1993). Processing time decreases globally at an exponential rate during childhood and adolescence. *Journal of Experimental Child Psychology, 56*, 254–265.

Kane, M. J., Bleckley, M. K., Conway, A. R. A., & Engle, R. W. (2001). A controlled-attention view of working-memory capacity. *Journal of Experimental Psychology: General, 130*, 169–183.

Kane, M. J., & Engle, R. W. (2000). Working memory capacity, proactive interference, and divided attention: Limits on long-term memory retrieval. *Journal of Experimental Psychology: Learning, Memory, and Cognition, 26*, 336–358.

Kane, M. J., & Engle, R. W. (2003). Working memory capacity and the control of attention: The contributions of goal neglect, response competition, and task set to Stroop interference. *Journal of Experimental Psychology: General, 132*, 47–70.

Kane, M. J., & Hasher, L. (1995). Interference. In G. Maddox (Ed.), *The encyclopedia of aging* (2nd ed., pp. 514–516). New York: Springer-Verlag.

Karlsson, P., Farde, L., & Halldin, C. (2000). *Circadian rhythm in central D1-like dopamine receptors examined by PET*. Presented at the Third International Symposium on Functional Neuroreceptor Mapping, New York, June.

Keppel, G., Postman, L., & Zavortink, B. (1968). Studies of learning to learn: VIII. The influence of massive amounts of training upon the learning and retention of paired-associate lists.

Journal of Verbal Learning and Verbal Behavior, 7, 790–796.

Kerkhof, G. A., & Lancel, M. (1991). EEG slow-wave activity, REM-sleep, and rectal temperature during night and day sleep in morning-type and evening-type subjects. *Psychophysiology, 28*, 678–688.

Kim, S., Dueker, G. L., Hasher, L., & Goldstein, D. (2002). Children's time of day preference: Age, gender, and ethnic differences. *Personality and Individual Differences, 33*, 1083–1090.

Kim, S., Hasher, L., & Zacks, R. T. (in press). A benefit of heightened susceptibility to distraction: An aging study. *Psychonomic Bulletin & Review*.

Laver, G. D. (2000). A speed-accuracy analysis of word recognition in young and older adults. *Psychology and Aging, 15*, 705–709.

Li, K. Z. H., Hasher, L., Jonas, D., Rahhal, T., & May, C. P. (1998). Distractability, circadian arousal, and aging: A boundary condition? *Psychology and Aging, 13*, 574–583

Li, S., & Sikström, S. (2002). Integrative neurocomputational perspectives on cognitive aging, neuromodulation, and representation. *Neuroscience and Biobehavioral Reviews, 26*, 795–808.

Logan, J. M., Sanders, A. L., Snyder, A. Z., Morris, J. C., & Buckner, R. L. (2002). Under-recruitment and nonselective recruitment: Dissociable neural mechanisms associated with aging. *Neuron, 33*, 827–840

Lustig, C., & Hasher, L. (2001). Implicit memory is not immune to interference. *Psychological Bulletin, 127*, 618–628.

Lustig, C., & Hasher, L. (2002). Working memory span: The effect of prior learning. *American Journal of Psychology, 115*, 89–101.

Lustig, C., Hasher, L., & Tonev, S. (in press). Distraction as a determinant of processing speed. *Psychonomic Bulletin & Review*.

Lustig, C., May, C. P., & Hasher, L. (2001). Working memory span and the role of proactive interference. *Journal of Experimental Psychology: General, 130*, 199–207.

Lustig, C. & Meck, W. H. (2001). Paying attention to time as one gets older. *Psychological Science, 12*, 478–484.

Mack, A., & Rock, I. (1998). Inattentional blindness: Perception without attention. In R. D. Wright (Ed.), *Visual attention: Vancouver studies in cognitive science* (Vol. 8, pp. 55–76). New York: Oxford University Press.

MacLeod, C. M., Dodd, M. D., Sheard, E. D., Wilson, D. E., & Bibi, U. (2003). In opposition to inhibition. In B. H. Ross (Ed.), *The psychology of learning and motivation* (Vol. 43, pp. 163–214). San Diego: Academic Press.

Manly, T., Lewis, G. H., Robertson, I. H., Watson, P. C., & Datta, A. K. (2002). Coffee in the cornflakes: Time-of-day as a modulator of executive response control. *Neuropsychologia, 40*, 1–6.

May, C. P. (1999). Synchrony effects in cognition: The costs and a benefit. *Psychonomic Bulletin & Review, 6*, 142–147.

May, C. P., & Hasher, L. (1998). Synchrony effects in inhibitory control over thought and action. *Journal of Experimental Psychology: Human Perception and Performance, 24*, 363–379.

May, C. P., Hasher, L., & Foong, N. (2005). Implicit memory, age and time of day: Paradoxical priming effects. *Psychological Science, 16*, 96–100.

May, C. P., Hasher, L., & Kane, M. J. (1999). The role of interference in memory span. *Memory & Cognition, 27*, 759–767.

May, C. P., Hasher, L., & Stoltzfus, E. R. (1993). Optimal time of day and the magnitude of age differences in memory. *Psychological Science, 4*, 326–330.

May, C. P., Kane, M. J., & Hasher, L. (1995). Determinants of negative priming. *Psychological Bulletin, 118*, 35–54.

May, C. P., Rahhal, T., Berry, E. M., & Leighton, E. A. (2005). Aging, source memory, and emotion. *Psychology and Aging, 20*, 571–578.

May, C. P., Zacks, R. T., Hasher, L., & Multhaup, K. S. (1999). Inhibition in the processing of garden-path sentences. *Psychology and Aging, 14*, 304–313.

McDowd, J. M., & Filion, D. L. (1992). Aging, selective attention, and inhibitory processes: A psychophysiological approach. *Psychology and Aging, 7*, 65–71.

Miller, E. K., & Cohen, J. D. (2001). An integrative theory of prefrontal cortex function. *Annual Review of Neuroscience, 24*, 167–202.

Miyake, A., Friedman, N. P., Emerson, M. J., Witzki, A. H., Howerter, A., & Wager, T. D. (2000). The unity and diversity of executive functions and their contributions to complex "frontal lobe" tasks: A latent variable analysis. *Cognitive Psychology, 41*, 49–100.

Monk, T. H., & Kupfer, D. J. (2000). Circadian rhythms in healthy aging: Effects downstream from the pacemaker. *Chronobiology International, 17*, 355–368.

Moscovitch, M., & Winocur, G. (1995). Frontal lobes, memory, and aging. In J. Gragman, K. J. Holyoak, & B. Boller (Eds.) *Structure and functions of the human prefrontal cortex* (pp. 119–150). New York: New York Academy of Sciences.

Most, S. B., Simons, D. J., Scholl, B. J., Jimenez, R., Clifford, E., & Chabris, C. F. (2001). How not to be seen: The contribution of similarity and selective ignoring to sustained inattentional blindness. *Psychological Science, 12*, 9–17.

Muraven, M., & Baumeister, R. F. (2000). Self-regulation and depletion of limited resources: Does self-control resemble a muscle? *Psychological Bulletin, 126*, 247–259.

Navon, D. (1984). Resources—A theoretical soupstone? *Psychological Review, 91*, 216–234.

Nelson, J. K., Reuter-Lorenz, P. A., Sylvester, C. Y. C., Jonides, J., & Smith, E. E. (2003). Dissociable neural mechanisms underlying response-based and familiarity-based conflict in working memory. *Proceedings of the National Academy of Sciences USA, 19*, 11171–11175.

Nigg, J. T. (2001). Is ADHD a disinhibitory disorder? *Psychological Bulletin, 127*, 571–598.

Park, D. C., Polk, T. A., Mikels, J. A., Taylor, S. F., & Marshuetz, C. (2001). Cerebral aging: Integration of brain and behavioral models of cognitive function. *Dialogues in Clinical Neuroscience, 3*, 151–166.

Park, D. C., Smith, A. D., Lautenschlager, G., Earles, J. L., Frieske, D., Zwahr, M., & Gaines, C. (1996). Mediators of long-term memory performance across the life span. *Psychology and Aging, 11*, 621–637.

Persad, C. C. (2001). The role of inhibition in working memory performance associated with age. *Dissertation Abstracts International: Section B: The Sciences and Engineering, 61*, 4440.

Persad, C. C., Abeles, N., Zacks, R. T., & Denburg, N. L. (2002). Inhibitory changes after age 60 and the relationship to measures of attention and memory. *Journals of Gerontology: Series B: Psychological Sciences and Social Sciences, 57B*, P223–P232.

Phillips, N. A., & Lesperance, D. (2003) Breaking the waves: Age differences in electrical brain activity when reading text with distractors. *Psychology and Aging, 18*, 126–139.

Plude, D. J., & Hoyer, W. J. (1986). Age and the selectivity of visual information processing. *Psychology and Aging, 1*, 4–10.

Polich, J. (1996). Meta-analysis of P300 normative aging studies. *Psychophysiology, 33*, 334–353.

Polich, J., & Kok, A. (1995). Cognitive and biological determinants of P300: An integrative review. *Biological Psychology, 41*, 103–146.

Postle, B. R., Berger, J. S., Goldstein, J. H., Curtis, C. E., & D'Esposito, M. (2001). Behavioral and neurophysiological correlates of episodic coding, proactive interference, and list length effects in a running span verbal working memory task. *Cognitive, Affective, & Behavioral Neuroscience, 1*, 10–21.

Radvansky, G. A., & Curiel, J. M. (1998). Narrative comprehension and aging: The fate of completed goal information. *Psychology and Aging, 13*, 69–79.

Rahhal, T. A., Hasher, L., & Colcombe, S. (2001). Instructional differences and age differences in memory: Now you see them, now you don't. *Psychology and Aging, 16*, 697–706.

Rahhal, T. A., May, C. P., & Hasher, L. (2002). Truth and character: Sources that older adults can remember. *Psychological Science, 13*, 101–105.

Raine, A., Benishay, D., Lencz, T., & Scarpa, A. (1997). Abnormal orienting in schizotypal personality disorder. *Schizophrenia Bulletin, 23*, 101–105.

Ranganath, C., Johnson, M. K., & D'Esposito, M. (2003). Prefrontal activity associated with working memory and episodic long-term memory. *Neuropsychologia, 41*, 378–389.

Raz, N. (2000). Aging of the brain and its impact on cognitive performance: Integration of structural and functional findings. In F. I. M. Craik & T. A. Salthouse (Eds.), *The handbook of aging and cognition* (2nd ed., pp. 1–90). Mahwah, NJ: Lawrence Erlbaum Associates.

Reder, L., & Kusbit, G. W. (1991). Locus of the Moses illusion: Imperfect encoding, retrieval, or

match. *Journal of Memory and Language, 30*, 385–406.

Reuter-Lorenz, P. A. (2002). New visions of the aging mind and brain. *Trends in Cognitive Sciences, 6*, 394–400.

Reuter-Lorenz, P. A., & Lustig, C. (2005). Brain aging: Reorganizing discoveries about the aging mind. *Current Opinion in Neurobiology, 15*, 245–251.

Reuter-Lorenz, P. A., Marschuetz, C., Jonides, J., Hartley, A., & Koeppe, R. (2001). Neurocognitive aging of storage and executive processes. *European Journal of Cognitive Psychology, 13*, 257–278.

Roediger, H. L., III, & McDermott, K. B. (1995). Creating false memories: Remembering words not presented in lists. *Journal of Experimental Psychology: Learning, Memory, and Cognition, 21*, 803–814.

Rokeach, M. (1976). *Beliefs, attitudes and values: A theory of organization and change*. San Francisco: Jossey-Bass.

Rowe, G., Turcotte, J., & Hasher, L. (2006). *Proactive interference in a working memory span tasks*. Manuscript in preparation.

Rowe, G., Valderrama, S., Lenartowicz, A., & Hasher, L. (in press). Attentional disregulation: A benefit for implicit memory. *Psychology and Aging*.

Rubin, D. C. (1999). Frontal-striatal circuits in cognitive aging: Evidence for caudate involvement. *Aging, Neuropsychology, and Cognition, 6*, 241–259.

Salthouse, T. A. (1996). The processing-speed theory of adult age differences in cognition. *Psychological Review, 103*, 403–428.

Shallice, T., & Burgess, P. (1993). Supervisory control of action and thought selection. In A. D. Baddeley & L. Weiskrantz (Eds.), *Attention: Selection, awareness, and control: A tribute to Donald Broadbent* (pp. 171–187). New York: Oxford University Press.

Swick, D., Pineda, J. A., Schacher, S., & Foote, S. L. (1994). Locus-coeruleus neuronal-activity in awake monkeys: Relationship to auditory P300-like potentials and spontaneous EEG. *Experimental Brain Research, 101*, 86–92.

Sylvester, C. Y., Wager, T. D., Lacey, S. C., Hernandez, L., Nichols, T. E., Smith, E. E., & Jonides, J. (2003). Switching attention and resolving interference: fMRI measures of executive functions. *Neuropsychologia, 41,* 357–370.

Tentori, K., Osherson, D., Hasher, L., & May, C. (2001). Wisdom and aging: Irrational preferences in college students but not older adults. *Cognition, 81,* B87–B96.

Tun, P. A., O'Kane, G., & Wingfield, A. (2002). Distraction by competing speech in young and older adult listeners. *Psychology and Aging, 17,* 453–467.

Underwood, B. J. (1957). Interference and forgetting. *Psychological Review, 64,* 49–60.

Underwood, B. J. (1965). False recognition produced by implicit verbal responses. *Journal of Experimental Psychology, 70,* 122–129.

Volkow, N. D., Gur, R. C., Wang, G. J., Fowler, J. S., Moberg, P. J., Ding, Y. S., Hitzeman, R., Smith, G., & Logan, J. (1998). Association between decline in dopamine activity with age and cognitive and motor impairment in healthy individuals. *American Journal of Psychiatry, 155,* 344–349.

Watkins, M. J., & Watkins, O. C. (1976). Cue-overload theory and the method of interpolated attributes. *Bulletin of the Psychonomic Society, 7,* 289–291.

Weinert, D. (2000). Age-dependent changes of the circadian system. *Chronobiology International, 17,* 261–283.

Wenzlaff, R. M., & Wegner, D. M. (2000). Thought suppression. *Annual Review of Psychology, 51,* 59–91.

West, R. L. (1996). An application of prefrontal cortex function theory to cognitive aging. *Psychological Bulletin, 120,* 272–292.

West, R. L. (2000). In defense of the frontal lobe hypothesis of cognitive aging. *Journal of the International Neuropsychological Society, 6,* 727–729.

West, R., Murphy, K. J., Armilio, M. L., Craik, F. I. M., & Stuss, D. T. (2002). Effects of time of day on age differences in working memory. *Journals of Gerontology: Series B: Psychological Sciences and Social Sciences, 57B,* P3–P10.

Winocur, G., & Hasher, L. (1999). Aging and time-of-day on cognition in rats. *Behavioral Neuroscience, 113,* 991–997.

Winocur, G., & Hasher, L. (2002). Circadian rhythms and memory in aged humans and animals. In L. R. Squire & D. L . Schacter (Eds.), *Neuropsychology of memory* (3rd ed., pp. 273–285). New York: Guilford Press.

Winocur, G., & Hasher, L. (2004). Age and time-of-day effects on learning and memory in a non-matching-to-sample test. *Neurobiology of Aging, 25,* 1107–1115.

Wirz-Justice, A. (1984). Dopamine receptor rhythms. *Biological Psychiatry, 19,* 1274–1276.

Wirz-Justice, A. (1987). Circadian rhythms in mammalian neurotransmitter receptors. *Progress in Neurobiology, 29,* 219–259.

Yoon, C., May, C. P., & Hasher, L. (2000). Aging, circadian arousal patterns, and cognition. In D. C. Park & N. Schwarz (Eds.), *Cognitive aging: A primer* (pp. 151–171). Philadelphia: Psychology Press.

Yoon, C., May, C. P., Goldstein, D., & Hasher, L. (in press). Aging, circadian arousal patterns, and cognition. In D. C. Park & N. Schwarz (Eds.), *Cognitive aging: A primer* (2nd ed.). Philadelphia: Psychology Press.

Zacks, R. T., & Hasher, L. (1994). Directed ignoring: Inhibitory regulation of working memory. In D. Dagenbach & T. H. Carr (Eds.), *Inhibitory processes in attention, memory, and language* (pp. 241–264). San Diego: Academic Press.

Zacks, R. T., Hasher, L., & Li, K. Z. H. (2000). Human memory. In F. I. M. Craik & T. A. Salthouse (Eds), *The handbook of aging and cognition* (2nd ed., pp. 293–357). Mahwah, NJ: Lawrence Erlbaum Associates.

Zacks, R. T., Radvansky, G. A., & Hasher, L. (1996). Studies of directed forgetting in older adults. *Journal of Experimental Psychology: Learning, Memory, and Cognition, 22,* 143–156.

Zacks, J. L., & Zacks, R. T. (1993). Visual search times assessed without reaction times: A new method and an application to aging. *Journal of Experimental Psychology: Human Perception and Performance, 19,* 798–813.

Zechmeister, E. G., & Nyberg, S. E. (1982). *Human memory: An introduction to research and theory.* Monterey, CA: Brooks/Cole.

10

The Executive Is Central to Working Memory: Insights from Age, Performance, and Task Variations

PATRICIA A. REUTER-LORENZ and JOHN JONIDES

The model of working memory developed by Alan Baddeley and his colleagues has dominated the landscape of memory research for some time (Baddeley, 1986; Baddeley & Hitch, 1974). According to this model, information is stored in and retrieved from a set of buffers, each specialized for a different kind of information. According to many interpretations of this model, some simple tasks demand only encoding, storage, and retrieval of information from the relevant buffer. An example might be a simple span task in which a set of letters is presented and several seconds later the participant has to recall the letters in the order of presentation. Other tasks, by assumption, require executive processes if the information in a buffer needs to be manipulated prior to the participant's giving a response. An example might be an alphabetic span task in which a set of letters is presented, and several seconds later the participant has to recall the letters in alphabetical order. Executive processes, then, are an added component of the model, and these processes are assumed to be drawn into play when stored information must be transformed.

We maintain that this view of executive processing is too limited. Our argument is that executive processing is required in any working memory task just so long as information must be stored longer than a passive trace is retained. Indeed, the delayed-response task, one of the most widely used tasks to investigate the neural circuitry of working memory in animals, has long pointed to the frontal cortex, the site of the central executive, as crucial to successful working memory performance (see Goldman-Rakic, 1987, for a review). What is debated is whether prefrontal circuitry is the site of working memory storage per se, or whether its contribution is primarily in the form of attentional control (see, e.g., Postle, Druzgal & D'Esposito, 2003, for a review). Attentional control over internal representations figures prominently in our view of the central executive. Although a consensual definition of what constitutes an executive process is lacking, many prominent examples in the literature include filtering irrelevant information, inhibiting competing responses, switching between representations, monitoring ongoing performance, and managing multiple tasks, all of which entail attentional control. A frontal-parietal executive system that includes lateral prefrontal cortex, superior and inferior parietal cortex, and medial frontal cortex, including anterior cingulate and perhaps supplementary motor cortex, is implicated in these forms of attentional control (e.g., Corbetta, Kincade, & Shulman, 2002; Posner & Dehaene, 1994; Posner & Petersen, 1990; Ravizza, Delgado, Chein, Becker, & Fiez, 2004).

By our argument, any attentional process required during working memory engages a good part of the same neural machinery involved when information needs to be manipulated. And it is this engagement of attentional control that is the heart of executive processing, not necessarily the specific manipulations that may be necessary in one task or another (e.g., alphabetizing). Our argument is motivated by data on individual differences in success at working memory tasks, and data on changes in working memory with age, as revealed by neuroimaging experiments. We have found that older adults (and in some cases poor-performing younger adults) recruit executive processes in the service of performance in a working memory task that putatively involves only encoding, storage, and retrieval. We take this finding to indicate that even simple storage tasks have an executive component to them that is stressed in poor-performing young adults and by neural declines that accompany normal aging. When these same participants are then challenged with a task that requires yet further application of attentional control, they are deficient in their performance because their attentional resources are already partly taken up by the basic encoding, storage, and retrieval processes. In short, our view has its genesis in evidence suggesting that working memory may be under the control of a single resource, attentional allocation. This resource can be taxed by high-task demands, by individual differences in performance level, by normal aging, and perhaps by still more individual-difference variables that have yet to be explored. Thus,

rather than viewing executive processing as a module of working memory separate from storage, we view attentional allocation in varying degrees as a necessary component of all working memory storage.

These data have led us to a different view of working memory than that of the canon. The established view is that working memory tasks can be divided into two basic categories: those that require simple storage (e.g., serial span), also referred to as *short-term memory tasks*, and *storage tasks* that also require executive processing (e.g., alphabetic span) (see, e.g., Engle, Tuholski, Laughlin, & Conway, 1999). In the present volume this distinction is captured by the dichotomy between "simple" and "complex" span tasks (Chapter 6), with the former placing minimal if any demands on executive processing. Likewise, according to the view developed by Kane, Conway, Hambrick, and Engle (Chapter 2), complex span tasks measure working memory capacity and entail "short-term memory" plus executive (attentional) processes. Oberauer, Süß, Wilhelm, and Sander (Chapter 3) also distinguish tasks that involve simultaneous storage and processing. Engle et al. (1999) provide the strongest theoretical and empirical elaboration of this view. They are concerned in particular with the extent to which short-term memory and working memory are different constructs that are measurable by different tasks. Using the latent-variable approach, they conclude that these are indeed separate constructs and that it is the "differential reliance on controlled attentional processing that makes these two constructs different theoretically and empirically" (p. 326). The authors go on to agree with Cowan (1995, 1998), who posits that while closely related, short-term and working memory are represented by separate factors and are differentially related to higher-cognitive processes. These conclusions have been echoed by researchers who have taken a life-span approach and determined that across an age range from 20 to 92 years, there is a measurable distinction between short-term memory and working memory (Park et al., 2002). By contrast, our view is that all working memory tasks, including so-called short-term memory or "storage-only" tasks, recruit some degree of attentional control (and therefore executive processing), and so this classification is artificial and misleading. The amount of attentional control called upon by a task alleged to require only storage will depend on the processing demands of that task and on the age and level of working memory skill of the individual. The simplest storage task may recruit attentional control in the hands of a poor performer, and a good performer will need attentional control in some task contexts (i.e., depending on load and retrieval demands). Overall, though, all working memory tasks require attentional control to some degree, much as perceptual processing on incoming sensory information requires attentional control.

While most researchers explicitly acknowledge that no task is pure in its measurement of only storage, or only executive processes, there is a temptation to equate tasks themselves with the underlying constructs. In this chapter, we hope to persuade the reader that this equation should be resisted, if not discarded. Tasks that are described as primarily storage and minimally executive in their demands, activate brain areas associated with executive, and especially attentional, control. Moreover, the same task performed by an older adult or a poor performer can activate control areas to an even greater degree than one finds in the average-performing younger adult.

In the discussion below, we lay out our view of the representational characteristics of working memory, and then review how attentional control is implemented in working memory tasks widely viewed as requiring only storage. With respect to representation, our fundamental view is that there are many cases in which working memory harnesses representations used for perception in the service of storage. In addition, there are also frontal mechanisms that play a role in storage. With respect to executive processing in working memory, we argue that there are varieties of attentional control: those that are used in the service of continued activation of stored information (what is typically called *rehearsal*), and those used in the service of selecting and manipulating information. In both cases, we present the possibility that executive control is simply a

form of attentional allocation, but on mental representations, not on perceptual ones. We are particularly mindful of the role that neuroimaging data have played in furthering our understanding of these characteristics of working memory. After this overall review, we then describe evidence about the recruitment of executive processes in the item recognition task, drawing largely from data comparing older and younger adults.

REPRESENTATION IN WORKING MEMORY

Suppose you need to align two visual objects in a slide of a Powerpoint presentation. You might get the following instructions: click on one of the objects; depress the shift key and click on the other object; go to the menu bar and find the "draw" functions; scroll down to the one labeled "alignment," and then choose the direction in which you want the objects aligned. This is one of a huge number of tasks that require working memory. The memory system that serves these tasks has a small storage capacity, and the information stored there is retained for only a brief duration, measured in seconds. This short duration can be overcome by enlisting rehearsal processes that maintain the strength of the memory trace by refreshing and recycling it. The information in working memory is subject to frequent turnover as well. If, in the above example, you are interrupted in carrying out the directions by a telephone call, you are likely to have lost some or all of the information needed to carry out the alignment. One of the features of working memory that makes it useful is that the information that is stored is rapidly accessible. Another feature is that the information can be manipulated and transformed to meet the needs of various cognitive tasks, from preparing a Powerpoint talk to solving mental arithmetic problems to reasoning deductively. Working memory, in short, is indispensable for normal cognition.

We know a good deal about the psychological processes that underlie working memory. While there are several models of these processes that have been proposed (e.g.,

Baddeley, 1986; Cowan, 1995; Engle, 2002), the model from Baddeley and colleagues has motivated most research. According to this model, memoranda are stored in a set of buffers that differ from one another in the type of information each stores. The most frequently discussed of these buffers includes one for verbal information, one for spatial information, one for visual information that is not spatial, and one for episodic information that is not tied to the modality of coding (Baddeley, 2001). By some accounts, each buffer has a rehearsal process associated with it that allows attention to be paid to the representations stored in the buffer. Information in the buffers is subject to manipulation by executive processes, which in turn allow attention to be paid to relevant representations and shifted from one representation to another as needed for some task. For example, some of the contents of working memory may be critical to some task (e.g., remembering that the "Draw" item in the tool bar is the one that contains the "alignment" tool) whereas others may be irrelevant (e.g., the text tool that allows you to add text to a slide); it is the allocation of attention by executive processes that allows us to focus on the relevant information and gate out what is irrelevant.

There is much to recommend this model of the psychological processes underlying working memory. Even our view of the more ubiquitous role of executive processes shares the assumption that attentional allocation is fundamental to working memory, as the model of Baddeley and colleagues argues. Moreover, the emphasis on attentional control is common to other theorists as well. Engle and colleagues (Engle, 2002; see also Chapter 2, this volume) argue that variation in working memory capacity can be explained by variation in executive attention. Along similar lines, Hasher and colleagues (Chapter 9) emphasize executive processes as a significant source of individual variation, although they stress the inhibitory or gating function of attentional control. Whichever view one takes, it is timely to try to understand the neural implementation of the model's components. What are the sites of storage? What are the mechanisms of rehearsal and is rehearsal

applicable to all of the buffers? How are executive processes represented in the brain? Is there a single executive processor, or are there several that mediate multiple types of executive functions (e.g., inhibiting irrelevant information vs. shifting attention from one representation to another)? In recent years, a good deal of experimental attention has been paid to these questions with good productivity, both from noninvasive studies of humans and from invasive studies of animals other than humans. Consider, for example, some of what we know about the sites of storage (Fig. 10.1, see color insert). By now, there is very good evidence that implicates a network of brain areas that includes sites in occipital, parietal, and frontal cortex in working memory for spatial information. Strong hints about parts of this circuit have come from studies of monkeys storing spatial information in working memory tasks. We can trace the origins of these studies to the classic article by Jacobsen (1935), who found that lesions to dorsolateral prefrontal cortex in monkeys impaired their performance in a spatial delayed-response task. This work has led to studies of single-cell performance in spatial working memory tasks that have uncovered the importance of cells in dorsolateral prefrontal cortex and superior posterior parietal cortex (e.g., Chafee & Goldman-Rakic, 2000). In humans, the network may be even more extensive than this. There are several studies that show activation in superior prefrontal cortex near the superior frontal sulcus tied to the retention interval of a spatial delayed-response task (e.g., Courtney, Petit, Maisog, Ungerleider, & Haxby, 1998; Jonides et al., 1993). We also know from many studies that parietal cortex in the area of the superior parietal lobule and intraparietal sulcus is activated by spatial storage (e.g., Jonides et al., 1993). Furthermore, Awh and Jonides (2001) have shown that there is upward modulation of extrastriate occipital cortex when participants have to store spatial information in contrast to nonspatial storage. This network of frontal, parietal, and occipital sites for the storage of spatial information is reminiscent of the dorsal stream of processing that has been implicated in the perception of spatial features of visual displays (discussed below).

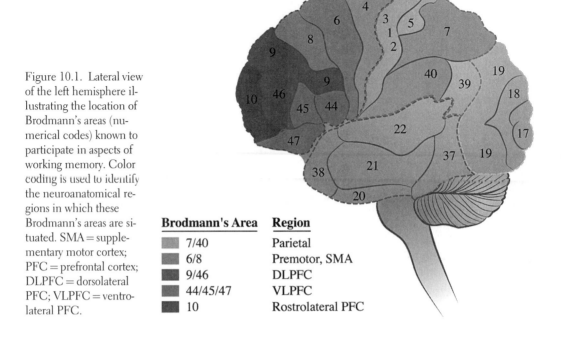

Figure 10.1. Lateral view of the left hemisphere illustrating the location of Brodmann's areas (numerical codes) known to participate in aspects of working memory. Color coding is used to identify the neuroanatomical regions in which these Brodmann's areas are situated. SMA = supplementary motor cortex; PFC = prefrontal cortex; DLPFC = dorsolateral PFC; VLPFC = ventrolateral PFC.

Brodmann's Area	Region
7/40	Parietal
6/8	Premotor, SMA
9/46	DLPFC
44/45/47	VLPFC
10	Rostrolateral PFC

We also have good information about the circuit involved in the storage of visual information that is not spatial in character. Again, some of the footing for our understanding of this circuitry comes from invasive studies of monkeys. Miller and Desimone (1994), for example, have shown that inferotemporal cortex contains cells that are responsive to particular visual stimuli not only when those stimuli are present in the visual environment, but also when the experimental animal is required to store a memory of a stimulus in preparation for a delayed match-to-sample task. These cells seem to be subject to interference from other visual stimulation, however. By contrast, cells in inferior prefrontal cortex in these animals are also selectively responsive to visual stimuli during the delay period of a working memory task, and these cells are less subject to interference effects. Evidence from human studies corroborates the involvement of inferior temporal and inferior frontal sites in memory for visual nonspatial stimuli. Smith et al. (1995) showed this in a PET experiment in which geometric objects were the memoranda. And

several studies have shown that when human faces are the memoranda, there is also activation of inferior temporal regions. Indeed, it appears likely that the very same region involved in the perception of faces in the fusiform gyrus is activated during the retention interval of a task in which faces must be stored (Druzgal and D'Esposito, 2003). So, again there appears to be a parallel between the brain regions responsible for perception of visual information and those responsible for its storage. Although more complex, the same principle may be true for the storage of verbal material. Postle, Berger, and D'Esposito (1999), for example, have shown that there is activation of superior temporal and inferior parietal cortices during the storage of verbal material in working memory. These are areas that are clearly involved in verbal processing for incoming information.

An interesting synthesis of various lines of research on the parallel between perception and storage can be seen in a recent meta-analysis of the working memory literature (Wager & Smith, 2003). In this meta-analysis, the investigators collected activations from over 60 imaging studies of working memory using PET and fMRI. They then conducted a cluster analysis on the peaks of activation that were reported in these various studies to examine a number of issues. One had to do with whether there were differences in activation sites as a function of the type of material stored. In particular, the meta-analysis had a substantial corpus of activation sites for spatial storage and for storage of object information. The clear outcome of this analysis was that spatial storage led to activation of superior posterior sites whereas object storage led to activation of inferior posterior sites. This result summarizes the general point we made above, that there is a seeming parallel between storage and perception. Viewed from an evolutionary point of view, this parallel makes architectural sense. Evolution led to the development of specialized brain mechanisms for the processing of sensory information in an exquisite way. Having evolved, these mechanisms may then have been harnessed for memory purposes as well as perceptual purposes. In principle, what is required for this to happen is the development of hysteresis in the perceptual processing streams, so that the activation of neural structures by a sensory event might then outlast that event. In this way, the very same structures that respond to a sensory event then continue to respond in the absence of that event, at least for a short period of time. This would be an efficient way to construct a system that had both selective perception and selective working memory for environmental events.

Even in the face of this obvious evolutionary advantage, there remains the indisputable fact that not only do posterior regions of cortex show activation in working memory tasks, but so do frontal regions. What might be the functions of these two systems? One possibility is suggested by a classic result documented by Malmo (1942). He showed that the deficit in spatial delayed responding caused by lesions in frontal cortex of monkeys (the result first documented by Jacobsen, 1935) could be eliminated by placing the animals in a darkened environment. That is, in the light, damage to dorso-lateral prefrontal cortex impairs performance in spatial delayed responding, but in the dark, it does not. A ready interpretation of this effect is that the animals have sources of potential visual distraction in a lighted environment that are not present in the dark. So, perhaps the function of the frontal mechanisms of working memory hinge on heightening resistance to distraction. In single-cell studies, Miller and Desimone (1994) confirmed this position by showing that inferotemporal neuronal activation in a working memory task for objects was interrupted by interfering visual events whereas frontal activation was not. Likewise, studies by Constantinidis and Steinmetz (1996) and di Pellegrino and Wise (1993) make the same point about spatial working memory. That is, posterior representations of spatial information are disrupted by interfering information, whereas frontal representations are not. So, the frontal mechanism of working memory may become engaged by resistance to interference while the posterior mechanism may be sensitive to such interference.

This hypothesis has received support from a meta-analysis of patients with deficits in working memory conducted by D'Esposito and Postle (1999). They surveyed the literature to isolate 11 studies of patients who showed impaired working memory in spatial and verbal span tasks. They found that damage to the frontal cortex did not appear to predict working memory impairments for either kind of material, whereas damage to temporal cortex did. By contrast, when patients were confronted with delayed-response tasks in which there was distracting information presented during the retention interval, frontal damage did predict working memory declines. A recent fMRI study by Sakai, Rowe, and Passingham (2002) makes a similar point. When interference was introduced during the retention interval of a working memory task, activation of Brodmann's area 46 differentiated trials in which memory was successful from those in which it was not. Thus studies of monkeys and humans appear to converge on the idea that frontally mediated processes are critical for establishing more resilient representations in working memory.

This view is examined in more detail in the following section.

ATTENTIONAL CONTROL
IN THE SERVICE OF SELECTION
AND ACTIVATION

If regions of posterior cortex participate in storage and if they are sensitive to the effects of interference, there must be a mechanism that works against this interference to create a longer-lasting representation, perhaps the one mediated by frontal cortical sites of working memory. For verbal material, we have known for a long time that this mechanism involves the recycling of a phonological or articulatory code during a retention interval to keep it fresh (see, e.g., Naveh-Benjamin & Jonides, 1984). The brain mechanisms that underlie this recycling appear to depend on a system that includes parietal and frontal components (e.g., Awh et al., 1996; Corbetta et al., 2002; Ravizza et al., 2004). The parietal components are dependent principally on cells in intraparietal sulcus and superior parietal lobule. We know from much work on the processing of spatial displays that this system is a key player in allocating and re-allocating attention to places in space (see Kastner & Ungerleider, 2000). We also know that this same system is not restricted in its attention control function to spatial stimuli; rather, it appears to play a much more general role in allowing us to switch attention from one object to another, whether those objects are perceptual or memorial and whether they are spatial locations, rules, tasks, attributes, or visual objects (Yantis, 2003).

With this evidence in hand, it seems reasonable to hypothesize that the parietal component of verbal rehearsal may be involved in controlling whether our attention is placed on one verbal object or another. It is this control that would allow us to cycle through the individual items in our verbal storage buffer to keep them fresh. The other components of the system are frontal and may include regions that mediate either domain-general or domain-specific processes. One anterior component of the verbal rehearsal circuit appears to be located in left inferior frontal gyrus and possibly left insula cortex. This region is the subject of a good deal of discussion. The classic interpretation of its function includes control of articulation and internal speech (e.g., Paulesu, Frith, & Frackowiak, 1993). By this account, it seems sensible to hypothesize that it is this site that represents verbal information and over which attention has its control as focus is shifted from one item in working memory to another. Another possibility, however, is that a critical function of left inferior frontal gyrus is to control the selection of a piece of information among many (Kan & Thompson-Schill, 2004). By this account, the role of this region in rehearsal may be to select items in turn for attention among the several items held in memory. That is, if the function of this left inferior frontal region is to allow selection of one representation among several alternatives, this would fit the function of rehearsal quite well. By this account, rehearsal amounts to cycling through several representations in turn, requiring selection of which representation is to be the focus of attention in each time epoch. Regardless of whether this site is important for verbal representation or selection, this region unquestionably plays an important role in recycling information in the service of verbal maintenance.

Rehearsal is not restricted to verbal information. Awh and Jonides (2001) have shown that the concept of rehearsal is equally applicable to spatial information. Consider the spatial delayed-response task we discussed above. Several visual locations are marked on a screen, and then a delay interval of a few seconds ensues, during which the locations must be stored. Then a single location is marked, and the observer must decide whether this location is one of those stored in memory. If rehearsal is involved in this task, what exactly is rehearsed? There are data showing that extrastriate and superior parietal cortices play a role in this task (e.g., Jonides et al., 1993). We know that at least a portion of these regions of cortex have a topographical organization such that adjacent locations in the visual world are represented by adjacent locations in the brain. Thus, the spatial topography of a set of locations in space can be preserved by the spatial topography of working memory. Under this model, rehearsal may involve the repeated activation of the re-presented positions in space by activation of their respective neural representations. As with verbal information, control over this cycling of activation of the extrastriate sites may be ex-erted by superior parietal cortex. This link has yet to be firmly established, but what is estab-lished is that there is modulation of extrastriate cortex when spatial information must be stored. Awh and Jonides (2001) have reviewed the rel-evant evidence for this case, and it consists of both behavioral and imaging findings. Behav-iorally, Awh, Jonides, and Reuter-Lorenz (1998) showed that if an observer has to store a location for several seconds, that storage produces a benefit in performing a visual discrimination task at the same location, compared to per-forming one at some other location. Further-more, diverting attention away from the stored location (by having an observer perform a dis-crimination at some other location) reduces performance in the spatial working memory task. Awh et al. (1999) followed up these find-ings with an imaging experiment. They had participants store three locations in working memory for a retention interval during which a visual stimulus was presented. This produced an up-regulation of extrastriate cortex, compared to a control condition in which verbal information had to be stored. A ready interpretation of these results is that rehearsal processes (possibly con-trolled by parietal mechanisms) exert an in-fluence on the activation of the relevant extra-striate regions, keeping them active during the retention interval.

These characterizations of rehearsal for verbal and spatial information share the idea that there is a source of the rehearsal signal and a site for its action. The source may be a common mechanism in parietal cortex that directs attention to relevant memorial repre-sentations. The parietal mechanism is likely to act in concert with prefrontal mechanisms (i.e., in inferior frontal gyrus and superior prefrontal cortex, see below) to select and shift between the relevant representations. The site of acti-vation may vary with the type of information being stored. In the case of verbal information, the source may control an articulatory or phonological representation in inferior frontal cortex; in the case of spatial information, it may control a spatial representation in extra-striate cortex. There may be other sites over which parietal cortex can exert control as well (see research by Yantis, 2003), but our research thus far does not go much beyond verbal and spatial storage.

One important source of information about the hypothesis that attentional mechanisms play a role in rehearsal comes from brain evi-dence on the mechanisms used to control at-tention to spatial locations and the mechanisms that control spatial rehearsal. Kastner and Ungerleider (2000) and Wager, Jonides, and Reading (2004) have surveyed the literature concerned with the allocation of attention. Both groups have found a network of regions that include parietal cortex, superior frontal cortex, and medial frontal cortex that are recruited when subjects face the task of allocating their attention to regions of space and when they have to shift attention from one region to another. Awh and Jonides (1998) examined the literature and discovered that many of the same regions involved in the allocation of attention are also involved in spatial working memory. This parallel allows us to draw the conclusion that spatial working memory has harnessed mecha-nisms of spatial attention to help retain material, presumably by controlling rehearsal processes. What is even more interesting about this argu-ment is that Wager et al. (2004) found that the very same mechanisms, by and large, participate in many shifts of attention, whether to spatial locations, objects, attributes, rules, or tasks. This finding leads to the further hypothesis, as yet untested, that the attention allocation mecha-nism involved in verbal and spatial working memory may also be one involved widely in all sorts of rehearsal.

This review of storage and rehearsal mech-anisms leads us to the following caricature: much of storage involves the very same mech-anisms that are involved in perception, and much of rehearsal involves the mechanisms that are involved in shifts of attention in the visual world. Although probably too broad a con-clusion, it leads one to suppose that what has happened in the evolution of working memory is a co-opting of mechanisms that developed for perceptual purposes. Of course, there are holes in this argument, not the least of which is the importance of frontal mechanisms of storage, especially in the face of interference. Also, we have a good many gaps in our knowledge of storage for information that is not presented visually. Indeed, even auditory presentation has been neglected in imaging studies of storage and rehearsal. But the hypothesis does present a guiding principle that may lead to productive acquisition of more data to fill in the gaps.

WORKING MEMORY CIRCUITRY AND TASK DEMANDS

As we discussed at the start of this chapter, within the working memory literature, and especially in the field of cognitive aging, working memory tasks are considered dichotomously to either emphasize or downplay executive processing. A distinction is often made between rote short-term memory tasks, the so-called storage-only tasks, and working memory tasks that require "storage plus processing." This distinction may be useful as a description of the task design; however, it is often taken to mean more than that, and to refer to neural processing operations that are presumed to underlie the tasks.

Consider, for example, the item recognition task, a canonical storage-only task, in which a number of items are presented to be held in working memory for several seconds. After the completion of the retention interval, a probe item is presented and the participant must decide whether it matches one of the items in memory (Sternberg, 1966). Although the encoding, maintenance, and retrieval required to perform this task are not typically assumed to tax executive processes, the neuroimaging evidence reviewed above indicates that the frontal–parietal executive circuit is actively recruited when item recognition tasks are performed. No matter how seemingly simple the task, working memory tasks involve the selective activation and inhibition of stored information, even if only in the service of maintaining that information. Attentional control over internal

representations is entailed in rehearsal. So, on this count alone, item recognition must involve some degree of executive control. As we review below, there is now ample evidence that a storage task combined with other factors, such as larger memory load, particular task contexts, and the age and performance level of the individual, can further modulate the recruitment of brain regions that mediate executive processes.

Of course, building explicit processing requirements into a task will recruit mental operations to meet such requirements. Consider the more complex 2-back task, which makes obvious demands on storage-plus-processing operations. In this task, a series of single items is presented. For each item, the participant must decide whether it matches the item that appeared two items back in the series. This task also involves rehearsal in that the participant must rehearse the set of items held in memory. However, successful performance on the task requires in addition that the participant drop no-longer relevant items from memory (e.g., the one that is now three items back), add new items as each is presented, and assign the proper "back" tag to the items in memory. By any definition of executive processing, this task involves more than the item recognition task. These examples make clear how different processing requirements can be built into the task to invoke different demands on executive processing.

Nonetheless, it is well documented that seemingly minor variations of a "storage-only" task can recruit executive processing regions. Consider the study by Barch and colleagues (1997), in which the neural consequences of different variations of task difficulty were examined. In their continuous-performance task the subject had to respond to a pre-specified letter sequence, and refrain from responding to non-target sequences. Perceptual difficulty was varied by degrading the visual quality of the letters. Increased memory demands were induced by increasing the delay between consecutive letters. Relative to the short delay, the long-delay condition was associated with greater activation in left dorsolateral prefrontal cortex and left parietal areas 40/7. By contrast, the perceptual degradation did not affect executive recruitment, despite reducing accuracy and response speed. The increased difficulty of perceptual degradation did lead to greater activation of the anterior cingulate. These results indicate that executive recruitment is not a universal response to increased task difficulty, but is a more specific response to increased working memory demands.

A number of studies have manipulated memory load, or the number of items to be retained in working memory in a "storage-only" item recognition task. Without introducing explicit changes in the executive processing demands (e.g., manipulation of the items, or dual-task demands), activity in prefrontal regions associated with executive control increases with increasing set size. For example, Rypma, Prabhakaran, Desmond, Glover, and Gabrieli (1999) compared three- with six-letter memory sets and found greater dorsolateral prefrontal activation during encoding of the larger set. In a 2002 report by Rypma, Berger, and D'Esposito, dorsolateral prefrontal cortex activation was found to be load sensitive during the retention interval. Ventrolateral prefrontal cortex was also affected by load, but only for high-performing subjects. Likewise, for tasks requiring the short-term retention of spatial locations, load effects have been found in dorsolateral, ventrolateral, and medial prefrontal sites, and in parietal cortex (Glahn et al., 2002; Leung, Gore, & Goldman-Rakic, 2002). At least some parietal–frontal components of this executive circuit may be domain general in that they contribute to item recognition of both verbal and nonverbal materials (Ravizza et al., 2004). Speer, Jacoby, and Braver (2003) have further shown that the context in which a particular memory load is experienced can influence the circuitry recruited to perform the task. They presented participants with an item recognition task in which the size of the set of items to be held in memory varied from trial to trial. In one condition, the memory set varied in size from 3 to 6 items, and in the other, from 6 to 11 items. Both conditions included a memory load of six items, and the investigators compared brain activations for this identical memory load depending on the context in which it

occurred. The hypothesis was that executive control strategies would be more preparatory (proactive) in nature when participants expected smaller loads because they would anticipate being able to manage the number of items being presented. However, when they expected larger loads that typically exceed working memory capacity, their strategies would be more reactive. Indeed, the authors found temporal variations in the pattern of prefrontal activation. When the load of six was embedded among smaller loads, these areas were recruited early in the trial, whereas these regions were recruited later in the trial when the six-item load was embedded in trials with longer lists. Taken together these results demonstrate that executive control processes are recruited and play an integral role in the tasks that explicitly require only storage.

By manipulating the context of individual trials in a working memory storage task, our lab has induced different forms of conflict and observed different patterns of prefrontal recruitment in response to these demands. Conflict is created by varying the overlap of items on consecutive trials. Familiarity conflict occurs when a negative probe letter on trial $N + 1$ was a member of the memory set on trial N. Under these circumstances, the probe requires the subject to respond "no" because it is not a member of the current set; however, because the probe was a member of the previous set, it is highly familiar and likely to promote a "yes" response. Indeed, it takes longer to respond "no" to these familiar probes than to probes that are unfamiliar (Jonides, Marshuetz, Smith, Koeppe, & Reuter-Lorenz, 2000; Jonides, Smith, Marshuetz, Koeppe, and Reuter-Lorenz, 1998). Moreover, this additional processing time is associated with the increased activation of ventral prefrontal cortex, Brodmann's areas 44/45 along the inferior frontal gyrus. Although distinct from the more dorsolateral sites in Brodmann's areas 9/46 that are widely viewed as the frontal sites of executive control (e.g., D'Esposito, Postle, Ballard, & Lease 1999; Petrides, 1994), this ventral region is clearly responsive to the increased demand for selection and interference resolution that is evoked by overlapping probes. We find that when the magnitude of familiarity conflict is varied parametrically, for example, when the letter *r* appears in the target set of trial N and trial $N + 1$, and then appears as a negative probe in trial $N + 2$, response time and left inferior frontal gyrus activation increase linearly. Despite these performance and neural signatures, the cognitive demand produced by overlapping probes goes unnoticed by the research participants according to their self-reports. Moreover, this form of conflict does not activate the anterior cingulate gyrus, an area that has been widely associated with increased task difficulty (Nelson, Reuter-Lorenz, Sylvester, Jonides, & Smith, 2003) as well as cognitive control (Botvinick, Braver, Barch, Carter, & Cohen, 2001; Gehring, Goss, Coles, Meyer, & Donchin, 1993). Nonetheless, contextual manipulations of the trials within a task that otherwise demands storage, rehearsal, and retrieval operations clearly recruit executive control processes to mediate the selection among competing codes.

Using a simple variation of the overlap design, a different form of conflict can be engendered that does recruit anterior cingulate. Again, the probe on trial $N + 1$ is a member of the target set on trial N, but in addition this item was a positive probe on that preceding trial and thus is associated with a recent "yes" response. The behavioral effects of this response conflict are indistinguishable from the effects of highly familiar probes. However, these two forms of conflict produce dissociable neural signatures, in that response conflict activates anterior cingulate but does not produce any further increases in the activation of ventral prefrontal cortex. Particularly relevant for the present discussion is the fact that these control processes are recruited merely by the contextual manipulation of a task widely viewed as one that involves only storage.

AGING, WORKING MEMORY, AND ATTENTIONAL CONTROL

The importance of executive processes in canonical storage-only tasks is especially apparent in the neuroimaging evidence from studies of older adults. This evidence challenges a pro-

minent view that emerged from several decades of behavioral research that claimed minimal effects of aging on the performance of working memory tasks, so long as they required simple storage (e.g., Craik, 1977; Craik & Jennings, 1992; Craik, Morris & Gick, 1990; Dobbs & Rule, 1989). This relative preservation of performance on simple storage tasks was in contrast to marked performance declines on executive processing tasks. For example, in a well-cited study by Dobbs and Rule (1989), there were no age differences on the Brown-Peterson short-term memory task, but working memory tasks, similar to the N-back task described above, produced reliable age differences in performance. Data such as these have been taken to imply that storage capacity is less affected by age than the capacity or speed with which executive processing operations can be performed. Indeed, solid support for the conclusion that storage was relatively spared came from a number of empirical reports and a meta-analysis (see Reuter-Lorenz & Sylvester, 2004, for a review; Babcock & Salthouse, 1990). These behavioral results lead naturally to the simple-minded neuroimaging prediction that older and younger adults should show similar activation patterns when performing tasks that emphasize storage, whereas marked age differences should emerge when explicit executive processing demands are entailed in the tasks. Neuroimaging studies comparing older and younger adults reveal a very different picture, however, and argue further for the pervasive nature of executive control in working memory tasks, including those that emphasize storage.

Since 1998, there have been at least 10 published reports describing the effects of age on the activation patterns evoked by working memory tasks that emphasize storage. Although the detailed pictures differ somewhat from one study to the next, in all cases marked age differences in brain activity have emerged even when performance differences have not. One of the most consistent findings is that older adults activate regions of prefrontal cortex that are not significantly activated in the younger group. In some cases this age-related overactivation is accompanied by age-related underactivation in other regions, and in some cases it is not. For example, in one study of spatial working memory from our lab, subjects were required to remember the location of three dots appearing briefly on a computer screen. Younger adults showed lateralized right frontal activation in premotor and supplementary motor cortex, whereas older adults, who performed as accurately as the young adults, activated these same regions bilaterally (Reuter-Lorenz, 2002; Reuter-Lorenz et al., 2000). Older adults also showed activation of left dorsolateral prefrontal cortex, whereas younger adults did not. Likewise, in a study requiring the visual maintenance of gabor patches, which are non-nameable elementary visual stimuli, McIntosh and colleagues (1999) found that older adults showed more activation than younger adults in left dorsolateral prefrontal cortex and less activation in ventral prefrontal regions of the right hemisphere.

Similar patterns are also evident in the verbal domain. We have found that like young adults, older adults activate verbal working memory areas in the left-hemisphere. However, older adults also activate additional regions of ventrolateral and dorsolateral prefrontal cortex in the right hemisphere that are not activated by younger adults performing the same task (Reuter-Lorenz et al., 2000; see also Cabeza et al., 2004). This pattern is evident in Fig 10.2 (see color insert) Although age-related overactivation is not always found for verbal storage tasks (Rypma & D'Esposito, 2001), greater activation of dorsolateral prefrontal cortex is consistently associated with higher performance in the older group, even when young adults show an inverse correlation. A positive correlation between dorsolateral prefrontal cortex activation and performance has also been found during verbal maintenance for older adults (Reuter-Lorenz et al., 2000, Reuter-Lorenz, Marshuetz, Hartley, Jonides, & Smith, 2001). This positive relationship suggests that prefrontal recruitment is beneficial to seniors' performance of storage tasks.

What functions might be subserved by such regions of overactivation in older adults? One possibility that we favor is that older adults rely increasingly on attentional control and other executive processes to manage the memory load on storage tasks. Even in the absence of explicit executive processing task demands, executive recruitment could enhance attention to context, inhibit distraction, and increase cognitive control. We submit that in the aging brain, additional executive resources are needed simply to maintain items in memory. This interpretation makes sense in view of the fact that even in younger adults an increase in working memory demand leads to greater activation of the prefrontal–parietal executive circuitry.

But if the age-related increases in executive processing serve a compensatory function, what are they compensating for? We believe that the answer to this question lies in the more widespread alterations in neural functioning that accompany normal aging (see Reuter-Lorenz & Lustig, 2005 for a review). Aging not only decreases synaptic efficiency (e.g., Kemper, 1994) but also appears to be associated with an increase in neural "noise" (e.g., Li, Lindenberger, & Sikström, 2001). Single-unit recordings in rodents and monkeys indicate that there is a decline in the selectivity of receptive field properties in primary sensory cortices (see Godde, Berkefeld, David-Jurgens, & Dinse, 2002, for a review; Schmolesky, Wang, Pu, & Leventhal, 2000). A breakdown in selectivity means a corresponding decline in the distinctiveness of the neural response to sensory input. Similar effects have recently been documented in humans as well. Through use of fMRI, Park and colleagues (2004) have shown that the specific and localized activity associated with the encoding of such stimuli as faces, places, and letters breaks down in older adults. They found that whereas young adults have discrete and separable regions of localized activity in extrastriate cortex in response to these different classes of stimuli, the activation patterns in older adults lack this selectivity, so that the brain region that responds to places also responds to faces, and vice versa. Thus the older brain is less able to generate distinctive representations of incoming stimuli, and may be less able to reactivate distinct representations stored in memory as well. We submit that this compromise in representational processes leads to an increased reliance on attentional control and other executive processes that normally play an integral

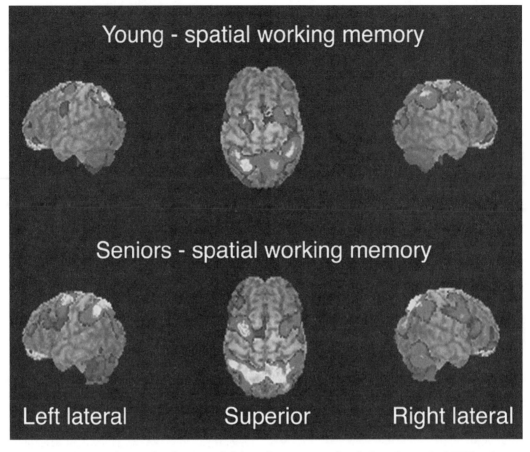

Figure 10.2. Surface-rendered images (left lateral, superior, and right lateral views) of PET activations obtained from younger and older adults performing a verbal working memory task requiring the maintenance only of four letters. The predominance of left-sided activation in the regions of younger adults is evident in contrast to the left- and right-sided activations evident in the older group. For more details see Reuter-Lorenz et al. (2000).

part in working memory but bear an increasing burden in the older brain. That is, age-related increases in the recruitment of attentional processes compensate for declines in the quality of the stored information and in the storage operations themselves (cf. Gutchess et al., 2005).

It is important to point out, however, that an age-related tendency to "over-recruit" executive processes need not imply that these processes are spared the effects of aging. On the contrary, there is strong evidence that prefrontal regions in particular suffer the consequences of normal aging. By measuring gray-matter volumes obtained from structural MRI scans, Raz and

colleagues (e.g., Raz, 2000) have documented that lateral prefrontal cortex is one of the regions that shows the greatest loss of volume in older adults. Although this structural evidence suggests the view that prefrontal overactivation in seniors is a sign of dysfunction in these regions, we find this interpretation unsatisfactory. If age differences in activation were caused by differences in the sheer amount of neural tissue, then we would expect less activation in older than in young adults, rather than more. While it is conceivable that the remaining executive circuitry in these areas has to "work harder" to achieve the same output, this still doesn't explain why the net activation levels would be greater in seniors than in younger adults. Although shrinkage of these areas is correlated with poorer performance on the Wisconsin Card-Sorting Task (Gunning-Dixon & Raz, 2003), a task known to rely on executive processes mediated by lateral prefrontal cortex, it does not predict poorer performance on measures of working memory. We take these results to mean that despite age-related shrinkage, prefrontal regions can contribute to the executive demands of working memory and even do so in a compensatory manner. But what happens in the older brain when executive processes are an explicit part of the task? If older adults rely more on executive processes at lower levels of task demand than young adults, will older adults also reach their resource limit at lower levels of task difficulty compared to young adults? We think this is exactly what happens (see also Reuter-Lorenz & Mikels, 2006).

Consider the age differences that have been found on several tasks that entail the explicit executive processing components required to switch between two tasks. In one study by Di-Giralamo colleagues (2001) the performance of younger and older adults was compared on two classification tasks that were performed separately or intermixed. One task required subjects to decide whether the number of digits appearing in a string was greater or less than five, and the other task required them to decide whether the value of the digits in the string was greater or less than five. The time it takes to make each of these decisions is considerably longer when the tasks are randomly intermixed than when each task is done repeatedly in a block of trials without the requirement to switch back and forth between rules. Indeed, the switching cost, which is a measure of the difference between pure-block and switch-block performance, is greater for older than for younger adults. Neuroimaging measures obtained during pure and switch blocks indicated that younger adults activated dorsolateral prefrontal cortex and medial prefrontal (including anterior cingulate) areas when switching was required. By contrast, older adults activated these regions even in the pure-block conditions, and consequently showed less of an increment

in prefrontal activation in response to the actual switching demand.

We found a comparable outcome in a working memory task that required subjects to encode and retain a short list of unrelated words while verifying a series of mathematical equations (Smith et al., 2001). The best-performing young adults did not need to recruit dorsolateral prefrontal cortex to manage these dual task requirements, but poorer-performing young adults and older adults did recruit this region when performing the task. Older adults also showed significant activation in premotor and parietal regions that was not evident in the younger groups, as would be expected if the attentional circuitry is increasingly taxed by age-related decline. The picture that is emerging, then, is one of older adults being more likely to recruit additional brain regions that are not activated by younger adults performing the same task. Moreover, the additional regions recruited can arguably be linked to the mediation of executive processes, namely attentional control, which may be recruited by this age group even when the task itself does not explicitly make this demand.

Thus far our discussion of aging has focused largely on executive processing generally and attentional control in particular. However, we have said little about inhibitory processing in the aging brain. Hasher, Zacks, and colleagues (see Chapter 9) propose that declines in inhibitory control play a central role in age-related changes in cognition. Their view would predict that older adults should show less activation than young adults in brain regions thought to mediate inhibitory control. As we mentioned previously, a region of left inferior frontal gyrus is activated by younger adults when they confront the need to resolve interference between the tendency to respond "yes" to an item because it is highly familiar and the tendency to respond "no" to the item because it is not part of the current target set (Jonides et al., 1998). Some form of inhibitory control is likely to be critical in resolving the interference produced by these conflicting codes. We have shown that older adults are not only disproportionately challenged when responding during these high-familiarity trials but also fail to activate the region of inferior frontal gyrus recruited by younger adults. This outcome is consistent with the kind of inhibitory deficits proposed by Hasher and Zacks (see also Gazzaley et al, 2005). At the same time, however, these older adults display increased recruitment of what we have referred to as the *executive attentional circuitry* mediated by prefrontal and parietal regions, and this pattern is associated with better performance overall (Reuter-Lorenz et al., 2001). Thus there appears to be a dissociation between older adults' ability to recruit the mechanisms mediating the inhibitory control required to adjudicate between competing codes and their recruitment of attentional control processes engaged during rehearsal and encoding. We are currently investigating whether there are individual differences within older or younger age groups that influence the relationship between an individual's ability to engage interference resolution processes in inferior frontal gyrus and his or her tendency to activate attentional control processes more generally.

We should also note that one of the most prominent "signatures" of neurocognitive aging that we have observed is an increase in bilateral activity under task conditions that evoke lateralized activity in the younger adult. For verbal working memory tasks that typically produce left dominant activation, and for spatial location memory tasks that evoke right dominant activation, older adults show both left *and* right activity in frontal and parietal regions. This increased bilateral activity suggests that there is a breakdown of domain specificity as we age, such that older adults recruit neural resources from both verbal and nonverbal domains to compensate for more general neural declines. This neural pattern predicts that older adults will show greater interference between verbal and spatial tasks in a dual-task situation. However, as Hale, Myerson, Emery, Lawrence, and DuFault report (Chapter 8), domain specificity is preserved in older adults. Although the meaning of this discrepancy between the behavioral and imaging results is unclear, it is clear that resolving it will require a careful mapping of the brain areas engaged by primary and secondary tasks when they are performed separately in each age group, to examine the degree of neural overlap. This overlap can then be used to predict the amount of interference when the two tasks are performed concurrently.

To summarize then, studies of aging have revealed the integrality of attentional and executive processing operations to tasks that are otherwise viewed as requiring only storage. Compensatory recruitment of attentional processes may be especially critical to the extent that representational mechanisms are compromised with age (Li et al., 2001; Park et al., 2004). Our studies of aging bring home the messages conveyed throughout this chapter. Clearly, brain imaging shows that there is no simple one-to-one mapping of tasks onto brain circuits. Indeed, equivalent performance levels can recruit different circuitry, and the critical dimension along which variation occurs is in recruitment of resources for attentional control.

CONCLUSIONS AND DISCUSSION OF FOUR THEMATIC QUESTIONS

QUESTION 1: OVERARCHING THEORY OF WORKING MEMORY

What we have reviewed is the basis for a somewhat different view of working memory than the traditional one attributed to Baddeley and colleagues and widely held in the cognitive and aging fields. Their work is largely guided by a distinction between working memory tasks that engage storage mechanisms alone and those that engage storage mechanisms plus executive processing. We argue instead that all working memory is best conceived as requiring storage and the sort of attentional control processes that define the central executive. Our view is based on both animal neurophysiology and human neuroimaging evidence indicating the recruitment of a frontal–parietal executive attention system in tasks presumed to emphasize only storage.

Specifically, we base our argument on three major sources of evidence. First, neuroimaging studies reveal a clear overlap in the brain regions required for attentional selection of sensory percepts and the maintenance of the corresponding representations in working memory. Put boldly, it seems possible that the very same mechanisms that control attention to incoming sensory information control attention to pieces of information in working memory. Prefrontal sites, in particular, that are linked to executive control play an essential role in establishing representational stability in the face of distraction. Second, executive processes are recruited by increases in load or retention interval, or minor modifications in the context of a task that otherwise requires only storage. Thus alterations in functional circuitry can occur without any explicit changes in the nature of what gets stored, and they require no knowledge or explicit strategy changes on the part of the subject. Third, comparison of adults of different ages and performance levels indicates that executive processes are readily recruited in tasks that are nominally only storage tasks. Executive control operations are thus integral to the circuitry of most working memory tasks, and the explicit structure of the task itself is but one of the factors that determines their recruitment.

Of course, we see the possibility that executive control operations are not all of a type. For example, they may be differentiable by the type of information on which they operate. Evidence about the mutual non-interference between visual and verbal working memory tasks bring this issue to the fore (e.g., Duncan, Martens, & Ward, 1997; Luck & Vogel, 1997). If this is the case, then executive processes would be mischaracterized by calling them all examples of attentional allocation. At present, there is simply too little evidence to draw a conclusion about the differentiability of executive processes by type of material or by any other taxonomy. On the one hand, it does appear that working memory for different types of material may be less mutually interfering than working memory for the same type of material, a pattern suggesting at the very least a fractionation of executive processing by type of

material. On the other hand, if one looks to the recent literature on attentional processes in perceptual cases, it appears that there may be a single set of mechanisms that control attention, regardless of whether the attention is allocated to spatial locations, objects, or auditory material (see Yantis, 2003). By analogy to this literature, one might draw a parallel to attentional operations on working memory to propose that they are also mediated by a single mechanism. This issue is by no means settled, and it certainly warrants further investigation.

One might question whether the tasks that have appeared prominently in the literature have simply been too taxing to avoid executive operations, even as conceived in the canonical model of Baddeley and colleagues. That is, even according to this model, when the capacity of working memory is exceeded, participants must employ strategies that will recruit executive processing to satisfy task requirements. For example, they might temporally group items to increase their capacity. With this in mind, one might ask whether neuroimaging studies of working memory have all, by happenstance, stretched the limits of working memory too much to see evidence of a "pure" storage process with no executive component. While possible, we find this view unlikely. Even the most elementary working memory paradigm, an item recognition task with four or fewer items, yields activation in superior parietal and/or medial frontal regions that are emblematic of attentional engagement (e.g., Smith, Jonides, & Koeppe, 1996). Thus, there appears to be evidence that even the simplest cases of working memory require some degree of attentional control.

QUESTION 2: CRITICAL SOURCES OF WORKING MEMORY VARIATION

We have focused on aging as a critical source of variation in working memory. However, we have departed from the major thrust of this volume in that our focus has been less on explaining performance differences and more on the underlying neural mechanisms and how their recruitment varies with performance level and age. Neuroimaging reveals that the same level of performance can be achieved in different ways: older and younger adults can perform an item recognition task with equal levels of accuracy while relying on different neural circuitry. Much of our discussion about aging has been focused on the source and function of this neural variation and how it might serve to *minimize* differences in performance. In fact, the neuroimaging data turn the variance to be explained on its head, so to speak. Here, we have aimed to understand the basis for the variations in neural activation patterns and what these patterns tell us about how the task is being performed.

QUESTION 3: CONSIDERATION OF OTHER SOURCES OF WORKING MEMORY VARIATION

Although the data we have to support these claims are limited, we can speculate that the source of performance variations differs in younger and older adults, even though executive processing recruitment figures prominently in both age groups. In younger adults it is most advantageous to rely minimally on executive control, whereas for older adults, greater reliance on executive processes is beneficial to performance. While we cannot say for certain what causes this interaction of performance and age, we believe that different factors are at work across these age ranges (cf. Rypma, Berger, & D'Esposito, 2002; Rypma & D'Esposito, 2001; Rypma, Prabhakaran, Desmond, & Gabrieli, 2001). At the very least we can suggest that for older adults the increased reliance on executive processes essentially compensates for declining storage and representational processes by "cleaning up" and ensuring the durability of the stored representations. In younger adults who are low performers, greater recruitment of executive resources may reflect lower efficiency than that of their higher-performing counterparts. Thus in both age groups the efficiency of executive processing resources is likely to prove an important source of performance variation.

Others are now beginning to recognize the importance of individual-difference variables in accounting for working memory performance (cf., the other chapters in the other chapters in this volume). For example, Braver and colleagues (Chapter 4) conducted a set of studies showing that variation in fluid intelligence, as measured by the Raven's Test of Progressive Matrices, indicates some important performance differences in working memory paradigms. By their account, the critical conceptual dimension captured by fluid intelligence is whether a person is more proactive or more reactive in dealing with potential sources of interference from unwanted information. Proactive types can prepare themselves more readily for upcoming interference and fend off some of its consequences; reactive types wait for the interference to be upon them before dealing with it. Of course, in situations where interference cannot be predicted, both types must be reactive. In one set of studies, Gray, et al., (2003) showed that a difference in fluid intelligence predicts whether individuals will prepare themselves for the proactive interference like that which invades the item recognition task we have investigated. Thus, this approach blends nicely with the data we have accumulated to suggest a further understanding of the differential recruitment of attentional control by different populations and the other cognitive skills that may be correlated with this. We might expect, for example, that the greater the executive recruitment in older adults, the more likely they would be to exert proactive control.

Our view also interleaves well with the emphasis on inhibitory declines in aging, expressed by Hasher and colleagues (Chapter 9). To the extent that the deletion of irrelevant items from working memory is compromised, there will be an increased need for attentional control to manage a larger memory load and increased effects of proactive interference. We have shown that some aspects of inhibitory control and interference resolution may be compromised with age, leading perhaps to an increased need for compensatory recruitment of other executive processes, including attentional control.

QUESTION 4: CONTRIBUTIONS TO GENERAL WORKING MEMORY THEORY

There is little doubt about the groundbreaking conceptual contribution of the differentiation between storage and executive processing. This distinction has motivated a great deal of valuable research on basic characteristics of working memory. We hope we have added to this conceptual contribution by suggesting that what has been called *executive processing* (what we have called *attentional control*) may be even more ubiquitous than previously imagined. There may be precious few situations in which some level of attentional control is not needed

---

BOX 10.1.   SUMMARY ANSWERS TO BOOK QUESTIONS

1. THE OVERARCHING THEORY OF WORKING MEMORY

We agree with Baddeley's original model of working memory that postulates storage and executive components. However, we take issue with the tendency in the field to minimize the importance of executive operations, specifically attentional control, in the performance of tasks classified as "short-term" rather than "working memory" tasks. These so-called storage-only tasks reveal pervasive recruitment of executive processes that is accentuated in older adults and poorer-performing young adults, and when there are minor changes in the tasks that do not explicitly require item manipulation or other processes that typically characterize working memory tasks.

2. CRITICAL SOURCES OF WORKING MEMORY VARIATION

While we see aging as a critical source of variation in working memory performance, our focus has been less on explaining performance differences per se and more on the underlying neural mechanisms and how their recruitment varies with performance level and age. In particular, our data and data from other labs have shown that the same level of task performance in younger and older adults is associated with recruitment of different neural circuitry. Our efforts have been directed toward trying to understand what accounts for this variation in neural activation patterns and what these variations tell us about the cognitive operations underlying these tasks.

3. OTHER SOURCES OF WORKING MEMORY VARIATION

In a general sense, we see the reliance on attentional control as an important source of variation in working memory performance. Our working hypothesis is that, to the extent that attentional control is recruited at lower levels of task demands, the availability of control processes will be limited when higher levels of demand are imposed. When this limit is reached, performance will suffer. The individual-difference variables that are critical for predicting the availability of attentional control include age, as mentioned above, and, as others in the volume have noted, Gf.

4. CONTRIBUTIONS TO GENERAL WORKING MEMORY THEORY

By challenging the tendency to reify the distinction between storage and processing tasks, we hope to emphasize the utility of neural evidence for clarifying the nature of psychological constructs. By revealing the involvement of executive brain regions in "storage" tasks, neuroimaging evidence argues against a simple equation of tasks with underlying processes. Such evidence can guide a more precise taxonomy of the representational and cognitive operations that mediate working memory performance. Ultimately, it will be crucial to arrive at a fine-grained characterization of the central executive, which will in turn provide a more accurate vocabulary for specifying the cognitive demands of the tasks we employ.

when working memory is called onto the field. Thus, rather than distinguishing between tasks needing attentional control from tasks that do not, we think it is more productive to ask how attentional control may play a role in any working memory task. This perspective opens up the study of working memory tasks to a finer-grained analysis of the role of attentional control as it participates with representational processes to mediate what is a vital human skill.

Acknowledgments

Preparation of this chapter was supported by grants AG18286 and MH60655. The authors thank Laura Zahodne for her editorial assistance with this chapter.

References

Awh, E., and Jonides, J. (1998). Spatial selective attention and spatial working memory. In R. Parasuraman (Ed.), *The attentive brain*. (pp. 353–380). Cambridge, MA: MIT Press, 1998.

Awh, E., & Jonides, J. (2001). Overlapping mechanisms of attention and spatial working memory. *Trends in Cognitive Sciences 5*, 119–126.

Awh, E., Jonides, J., & Reuter-Lorenz, P. A. (1998). Rehearsal in spatial working memory. *Journal of Experimental Psychology: Human Perception and Performance 24*, 780–790.

Awh, E., Jonides, J., Smith, E. E., Buxton, R. B., Frank, L. R., Love, T., Wong, E. C., & Gmeindl, L. (1999). Rehearsal in spatial working memory: Evidence from neuroimaging. *Psychological Science 10*, 433–437.

Awh, E., Jonides, J., Smith, E. E., Schumacher, E. H., Koeppe, R. A., & Katz, S. (1996). Dissociation of storage and rehearsal in verbal working memory: Evidence from PET. *Psychological Science 7*, 25–31.

Babcock, R. L., & Salthouse, T. A. (1990). Effects of increased processing demands on age differences in working memory. *Psychology and Aging, 5*, 421–428.

Baddeley, A. D. (1986). *Working memory*. Oxford: Clarendon Press.

Baddeley, A. D., & Hitch, G. J. (1974). Working memory. In G. H. Bower (Ed.), *The psychology of learning and motivation: Advances in research and theory* (Vol. 8, pp. 47–89). New York: Academic Press.

Baddeley, A. D. (2001). Is working memory still working? *American Psychologist, 56*, 851–864.

Barch, D. M., Braver, T. S., Nystrom, L. E., Forman, S. D., Noll, D. C., & Cohen, J. D. (1997). Dissociating working memory from task difficulty in human prefrontal cortex. *Neuropsychologia, 35*, 1373–1380.

Botvinick, M.M., Braver, T.S., Barch, D.M., Carter, C.S., Cohen, J.D. (2001). Conflict monitoring and cognitive control. *Psychological Review, 108*, 624–652.

Cabeza, R., Daselaar, S. M., Dulcos, F., Prince, S. E., Budde, M., & Nyberg, L. (2004). Task-independent and task-specific age effects on brain activation during working memory visual attention and episodic retrieval. *Cerebral Cortex, 14*, 364–375.

Chafee, M. V., & Goldman-Rakic, P. S. (2000). Inactivation of parietal and prefrontal cortex reveals interdependence of neural activity during memory-guided saccades. *Journal of Neurophysiology, 83*, 1550–1566.

Constantinidis, C., & Steinmetz, M. A. (1996). Neuronal activity in posterior parietal area 7a during the delay periods of a spatial memory task. *Journal of Neurophysiology, 76*, 1352–1355.

Corbetta, M., Kincade, J. M., & Shulman, G. L. (2002). Neural systems for visual orienting and their relationships to spatial working memory. *Journal of Cognitive Neuroscience 14*, 508–523.

Courtney, S. M., Petit, L., Maisog, J. M., Ungerleider, L. G., & Haxby, J. V. (1998). An area specialized for spatial working memory in human frontal cortex. *Science, 279*, 1347–1351.

Cowan, N. (1995). *Attention and memory: An integrated framework*. Oxford: Oxford University Press.

Cowan, N., Wood, N.L., Wood, P.K., Keller, T.A., Nugent, L.D., & Keller, C.V. (1998). Two separate verbal processing rates contributing to short-term memory span. *Journal of Experimental Psychology: General, 127*, 141–160.

Craik, F. I. M. (1977). Age differences in human memory. In J. E. Birren & K. W. Schaie (Eds.), *Handbook of the psychology of aging* (pp. 384–420). Englewood Cliffs, NJ: Prentice-Hall.

Craik, F. I. M., & Jennings, J. M. (1992). Human memory. In F. I. M. Craik & T. A. Salthouse (Eds.), *Handbook of aging and cognition* (pp. 51–109). Hillsdale, NJ: Lawrence Erlbaum Associates.

Craik, F. I. M., Morris, R. G., & Gick, M. L. (1990). Adult age differences in working memory. In G. Vallar & T. Shallice (Eds.) *Neuropsychological impairments of short-term memory* (pp. 247–267). New York: Cambridge University Press.

D'Esposito, M., & Postle, B. R. (1999). The dependence of span and delayed-response performance on prefrontal cortex. *Neuropsychologia, 37*, 1303–1315.

D'Esposito, M., Postle, B. R., Ballard, D., & Lease, J. (1999). Maintenance versus manipulation of information held in working memory: An event-related fMRI study. *Brain and Cognition, 41*, 66–86.

DiGirolamo, G. J., Kramer, A. F., Barad, V., Cepeda, N. J., Weissman, D. H., Milham, M. P., Wszalek, T. M., Cohen, N. J., Banich, M. T., Webb, A., Belopolsky, A. V., & McAuley, E. (2001). General and task-specific frontal lobe recruitment in older adults during executive processes: A fMRI investigation of task-switching. *Neuroreport, 12*, 2065–2071.

di Pellegrino, G., & Wise, S. P. (1993). Effects of attention on visuomotor activity in premotor and prefrontal cortex of a primate. *Sensorimotor and Motor Research, 10*, 245–262.

Dobbs, A. R., & Rule, B. G. (1989). Adult age differences in working memory. *Psychology and Aging, 4*, 500–503.

Druzgal, T. J., & D'Esposito, M. (2003). Dissecting contribution of prefrontal cortex and fusiform face area to face working memory. *Journal of Cognitive Neuroscience, 15*, 771–784.

Duncan, J., Martens, S., & Ward, R. (1997). Restricted attentional capacity within but not between modalities. *Nature, 387*, 808–810.

Engle, R. W. (2002). Working memory capacity as executive attention. *Current Directions in Psychological Science, 11*, 19–24.

Engle, R. W., Tuholski, S. W., Laughlin, J. E., & Conway, A. R. A. (1999). Working memory, short-term memory, and general fluid intelligence: A latent-variable approach. *Journal of Experimental Psychology: General, 128*, 309–331.

Gazzaley, A., Cooney, J.W., Rissman, J. & D'Esposito, M.D. (2005). Top-down suppression deficit underlies working memory impairment in normal aging. *Nature Neuroscience, 8* (10), 1298–1302.

Gehring, W. J., Goss, B., Coles, M. G. H., Meyer, D. E., & Donchin, E. (1993). A neural system of error detection and compensation. *Psychological Science, 4*, 385–390.

Glahn, D. C., Kim, J., Cohen, M. S., Poutanen, V.-P., Therman, S., Bava, S., Van Erp, T. G. M., Manninen, M., Huttunen, M., Lönnqvist, J., Standertskjöld-Nordenstam, C. G., & Cannon, T. D. (2002). Maintenance and manipulation in spatial working memory: Dissociations in the prefrontal cortex. *NeuroImage, 17*, 201–213.

Godde, B., Berkefeld, T., David-Jurgens, M., & Dinse, H. R. (2002). Age-related changes in primary somatosensory cortex of rats: Evidence for parallel degenerative and plastic-adaptive processes. *Neuroscience and Biobehavioral Reviews, 26*, 743–752.

Goldman-Rakic, P. S. (1987). Circuitry of the primate prefrontal cortex and the regulation of behavior by representational memory. In F. Plum (Ed.), *Handbook of physiology, the nervous systems, higher functions of the brain*. Section I, Vol. V (pp. 373–417). Bethesda, MD: American Physiological Society.

Gray, J.R., Chabris, C.F., Braver, T.S. (2003). Neural mechanisms of general fluid intelligence. *Nature Neuroscience, 6*, 316-322.

Gunning-Dixon, F. M., & Raz, N. (2003). Neuroanatomical correlates of selected executive functions in middle-aged and older adults: A prospective MRI study. *Neuropsychologia, 41*, 1929–1941.

Gutchess, A. H., Welsh, R.C., Hedden, T., Bangert, A., Minear, M., Liu, L.L., & Park, D.C. (2005). Aging and the neural correlates of successful picture encoding: Frontal activations for decreased medial temporal activity. *Journal of Cognitive Neuroscience, 17*, 84–96.

Jacobsen, C. F. (1931). The functions of frontal association areas in monkeys. *Comparative Psychology Monographs, 13*, 1–60.

Jacobsen, C. F. (1935). Functions of the frontal association area in primates. *Archives of Neurology and Psychiatry, 33*, 558–569.

Jonides, J., Marshuetz, C., Smith, E. E., Reuter-Lorenz, P. A., & Koeppe, R. A. (2000). Age differences in behavior and PET activation reveal differences in interference resolution in verbal working memory. *Journal of Cognitive Neuroscience, 12*, 188–196.

Jonides, J., Smith, E. E., Koeppe, R. A., Awh, E., Minoshima, S., & Mintun, M. A. (1993). Spatial working memory in humans as revealed by PET. *Nature 363*, 623–625.

Jonides, J., Smith, E. E., Marshuetz, C., Koeppe, R. A., & Reuter-Lorenz, P.A. (1998). Inhibition in verbal working memory revealed by brain activation. *Proceedings of the National Academy of Sciences USA 95*, 8410–8413.

Kan, I. P., & Thompson-Schill, S. L. (2004). Selection from perceptual and conceptual representations. *Cognitive, Affective, and Behavioral Neuroscience, 4*, 466–482.

Kastner, S., & Ungerleider, L. G. (2000). Mechanisms of visual attention in the human cortex. *Annual Review of Neuroscience, 23*, 315–341.

Kemper, T. L. (1994). Neuroanatomical and neuropathological changes during aging and dementia. In M. L. Albert & J. E. Knoefel (Eds.), *Clinical neurology of aging* (2nd ed.) (pp. 3–67). New York: Oxford University Press.

Leung, H. C., Gore, J. C., & Goldman-Rakic, P. S. (2002). Sustained mnemonic response in the human middle frontal gyrus during on-line storage of spatial memoranda. *Journal of Cognitive Neuroscience, 14*, 659–671.

Li, S., Lindenberger, U., & Sikström, S. (2001). Aging cognition: From neuromodulation to representation. *Trends in Cognitive Sciences, 5*, 479–486.

Luck, S. J., & Vogel, E. K. (1997). The capacity of visual working memory for features and conjunctions. *Nature, 390*, 279–281.

Malmo, R. (1942). Interference factors in delayed response in monkeys after removal of frontal lobes. *Journal of Neurophysiology, 5*, 295–308.

McIntosh, A. R., Sekuler, A. B., Penpeci, C., Rajah, M. N., Grady, C. L., Sekuler, R., & Bennett, P. J. (1999). Recruitment of unique neural systems to support visual memory in normal aging. *Current Biology, 9*, 1275–1278.

Miller, E. K., & Desimone, R. (1994). Parallel neuronal mechanisms for short-term memory. *Science, 263*, 520–522.

Naveh-Benjamin, M., & Jonides, J. (1984). Maintenance rehearsal: A two-component analysis.

Journal of Experimental Psychology: Learning, Memory, and Cognition 10, 369–385.

Nelson, J. K., Reuter-Lorenz, P. A., Sylvester, C. Y., Jonides, J., & Smith, E. (2003). Dissociable neural mechanisms underlying response-based and familiarity-based conflict in working memory. *Proceedings of the National Academy of Science USA, 100*, 11171–11175.

Park, D. C., Lautenschlager, G., Hedden, T., Davidson, N. S., Smith, A. D., & Smith, P. K. (2002). Models of visuospatial and verbal memory across the adult life span. *Psychology and Aging, 17*, 299–320.

Park, D. C, Polk, T. A., Park, R., Minear, M., Savage, A., & Smith, M. R. (2004). Aging reduces neural specialization in ventral visual cortex. *Proceedings of the National Academy of Sciences USA, 101*, 13091–13095.

Paulesu, E., Frith, C. D., & Frackowiak, R. S. J. (1993). The neural correlates of the verbal component of working memory. *Nature, 362*, 342–343.

Petrides, M. (1994). Frontal lobes and working memory: Evidence from investigations of the effects of cortical excisions in nonhuman primates. In F. Boller & J. Grafman (Eds.), *Handbook of neuropsychology* (Vol. 9, pp 59–82). Amsterdam: Elsevier.

Postle, B. R., Berger, J. S., and D'Esposito, M. (1999). Neuroanatomical double dissociation of mnemonic and executive control processes contributing to working memory performance. *Proceedings of the National Academy of Science USA, 96*, 12959–12964.

Postle, B. R., Druzgal, T. J., & D'Esposito, M. (2003) Seeking the neural substrate of working memory storage. *Cortex, 39*, 927–946.

Posner, M. I., & Dehaene, S. (1994). Attentional networks. *Trends in Neuroscience, 17*, 75–79.

Posner, M. I., & Petersen, S. E. (1990). The attention systems of the human brain. *Annual Review of Neuroscience, 13*, 25–42.

Ravizza, S. M., Delgado, M. R., Chein, J. M., Becker, J. T., & Fiez, J. T. (2004). Functional dissociations within the inferior parietal cortex in verbal working memory. *NeuroImage, 22*, 562–573.

Raz, N. (2000). Aging of the brain and its impact on cognitive performance: Integration of structural and functional findings. In F. I. M. Craik and T. A. Salthouse (Eds.) *Handbook of aging and* cognition–II. (pp. 1–90) Mahwah, NJ: Lawrence Erlbaum Associates.

Reuter-Lorenz, P. A. (2002). New visions of the aging mind and brain. *Trends in Cognitive Sciences*, 6, 394–400.

Reuter-Lorenz, P. A., Jonides, J., Smith, E. E., Hartley, A., Miller, A., Marshuetz, C., & Koeppe, R. A. (2000). Age differences in the frontal lateralization of verbal and spatial working memory revealed by PET. *Journal of Cognitive Neuroscience*, 12, 174–187.

Reuter-Lorenz, P.A. and Lustig, C. (2005). Brain aging: reorganizing discoveries about the aging mind. *Current Opinion in Neurobiology*, 15 (4) 245–251.

Reuter-Lorenz, P. A., Marshuetz, C., Hartley, A., Jonides, J., & Smith, E. E. (2001). Neurocognitive ageing of storage and executive processes. *European Journal of Cognitive Psychology*, 13, 257–278.

Reuter-Lorenz, P.A. & Mikels, J. A. (2006). The Aging Brain: The implications of enduring plasticity for behavioral and cultural change. In Baltes, P., Reuter-Lorenz, PA., & Roesler, F. (Eds.), *Lifespan development and the brain: The perspective of biocultural co-constructivism* (pp. 255–277). New York: Cambridge University Press.

Reuter-Lorenz, P. A., & Sylvester, C. Y. (2004). The cognitive neuroscience of aging and working memory. In R. Cabeza, L. Nyberg, & D. Park (Eds.), *The cognitive neuroscience of aging* (pp. 186–217). New York: Oxford University Press.

Rypma, B., Berger, J. S., & D'Esposito, M. (2002). The influence of working-memory demand and subject performance on prefrontal cortical activity. *Journal of Cognitive Neuroscience*, 14, 721–731.

Rypma, B., & D'Esposito, M. (2001). Age-related changes in brain–behavior relationships: Evidence from event-related functional MRI studies. *European Journal of Cognitive Psychology*, 13, 235–256.

Rypma, B., Prabhakaran, V., Desmond, J. E., & Gabrieli, J. D. E. (2001). Age differences in prefrontal cortical activity in working memory. *Psychology and Aging*, 6, 371–384.

Rypma, B., Prabhakaran, V., Desmond, J. E., Glover, G. H., & Gabrieli, J. D. E. (1999). Load-dependent roles of frontal brain regions in the maintenance of working memory. *NeuroImage*, 9, 216–226.

Sakai, K., Rowe, J. B., & Passingham, R. E. (2002). Active maintenance in prefrontal area 46 creates distractor-resistant memory. *Nature Neuroscience* 5, 479–484.

Schmolesky, M. T., Wang, Y., Pu, M., & Leventhal, A. G. (2000). Degradation of stimulus selectivity of visual cortical cells in senescent rhesus monkeys. *Nature Neuroscience*, 3, 384–390.

Smith, E. E., Geva, A., Jonides, J., Miller, A., Reuter-Lorenz, P. A., & Koeppe, R. A. (2001). The neural basis of task-switching in working memory: Effects of performance and aging. *Proceedings of the National Academy of Sciences USA*, 98, 2095–2100.

Smith, E. E., Jonides, J., & Koeppe, R. A. (1996). Dissociating verbal and spatial working memory using PET. *Cerebral Cortex* 6, 11–20.

Smith, E. E., Jonides, J., Koeppe, R. A., Awh, E., Schumacher, E. H., & Minoshima, S. (1995). Spatial vs. object working memory: PET investigations. *Journal of Cognitive Neuroscience* 7, 337–356.

Speer, N. K., Jacoby, L. L., & Braver, T. S. (2003). Strategy-dependent changes in memory: Effects on brain activity and behavior. *Cognitive, Affective, & Behavioural Neuroscience*, 3, 155–167.

Sternberg, S. (1966). High-speed scanning in human memory. *Science*, 153, 652–654.

Wager, T. D., Jonides, J., & Reading, S. (2004). Neuroimaging studies of shifting attention: A meta-analysis. *NeuroImage*, 22, 1679–1693.

Wager, T. D., & Smith, E. E. (2003). Neuroimaging studies of working memory: A meta-analysis. *Cognitive, Affective, & Behavioral Neuroscience*, 3, 255–274.

Yantis, S. (2003). Cortical mechanisms of attention shifts: Space, features, and objects. *Abstracts of the Psychonomic Society*, 8, 47.

11

Specialized Verbal Working Memory for Language Comprehension

DAVID CAPLAN, GLORIA WATERS, and GAYLE DEDE

The concept of working memory (WM) was popularized in, if not introduced into, contemporary cognitive psychology by Baddeley and Hitch (1974), who argued that a short-duration, capacity-limited, "working memory" system was used in a variety of cognitive tasks. This system, which both maintained representations and performed computations on them, was thought to be responsible, at least in part, for limitations on human performance in a wide range of cognitive tasks. The linking of the maintenance of a limited amount of information for a short period of time with computational operations on that information constituted a significant change from the then-prevailing view that the function of "short-term memory" was to allow entry of information into "long-term memory." In the 30 years since Baddeley and Hitch's article, the concept of WM has evolved. In some researchers' formulations, it has come almost full circle, to the view that WM capacity is largely a measure of attentional control that is related to the encoding and activation of representations in long-term memory. We will return to some of these more recent formulations in the discussion section of this chapter, but we begin with what we take to be the original Baddeley and Hitch concept of WM as a capacity-limited, short-duration store in which computations are performed in the service of task goals.

If WM is characterized this way, language comprehension requires WM. Regardless of whether language is written or spoken, the input becomes available over time and temporally discontinuous parts of the input must be related to one another for language to be understood. The need for WM applies to the construction of all levels of language—segmental and lexical phonological representations, morphology, intonational structure, syntax, and discourse.

Our work has focused on the WM requirements of syntactic processing. We begin this chapter by illustrating the WM requirements associated with syntactic processing, and then document the existence of variability in subjects' efficiency in handling these WM demands. We then explore the relationship between subjects' efficiency in handling syntactic WM demands and individual differences in WM capacity due to normal variation in healthy college students, aging, and various types of neuropathology. We then briefly review other types of data (e.g., neuroimaging) that we have collected that are consistent with the results from these populations.

To anticipate, we have not found that efficiency in handling syntactic WM demands is predicted by individual differences in WM capacity using standard tests of this function, such as the reading span test. On the other hand, we have replicated other researchers' findings of a relationship between other aspects of language processing, such as text memory and comprehension, and standard tests of WM. These findings have led us to argue for a fractionation of the WM system used in language processing into a specialized verbal WM system (svWM) that supports specific aspects of language processing that we refer to as *interpretive processing*, and a more general verbal working memory system (gvWM) that supports other aspects of language processing that we refer to as *post-interpretive processing* (Caplan & Waters, 1999a, 1999b, 2002). We conclude with a discussion of the implications of these results, couched in terms of answers to the four questions that serve as themes for this volume.

WORKING MEMORY AND SYNTAX

It is clear that sentences differ in terms of how easy they are to understand. Virtually all readers or listeners can understand sentences such as (1) and (2) below. However, very few readers or listeners can understand sentences such as (3), even though such sentences are grammatically acceptable.

1. The mouse that the dog bit ran away.
2. The dog that the cat scratched bit the mouse.
3. The mouse that the dog that the cat scratched bit ran away.

Sentences 1 and 2 each have one embedded clause (1: that the dog bit, 2: that the cat scratched), while Sentence 3 has two embedded clauses (that the dog bit, that the cat scratched). The inability of most language users to understand sentences such as (3) is thought to result from limitations in WM capacity, making it difficult for them to structure the sentence syntactically (Gibson, 1998; Just & Carpenter, 1992; Lewis, 1996).

There is also considerable evidence that even syntactic structures that can be understood by most or all language users differ in the ease with which they can be understood. This is true whether sentence processing is measured using an "off-line" task, in which subjects are asked to make a judgment after hearing a sentence, or "on-line tasks," in which the amount of time required to process each word or phrase is measured on-line. A prototypical example of sentences that differ in terms of how easily they can be understood, despite the fact that they contain the same lexical items, are sentences with subject- and object-extracted relative clauses (often referred to as subject and object relatives). Subject-extracted sentences are syntactically simpler than object-extracted sentences. In subject-extracted sentences, the subject of the relative clause has been extracted from the clause; in object-extracted sentences the object has been extracted. These are illustrated in Sentences 4 and 5:

4. The scout warmed the cabin that contained the firewood. (Subject-extracted)
5. The cabin that the scout warmed contained the firewood. (Object-extracted)

The WM demands of object-extracted sentences are thought to be greater than those of subject-extracted sentences because they involve more storage or reference to more items held in memory (i.e., keeping track of partially processed syntactic dependencies that are awaiting their second element for the sentence to be grammatical) and more integration of or more computations on items held in memory (connecting a newly input word into the structure that has been built so far) (Gibson, 1998).

In off-line tasks in which subjects are asked to judge the acceptability of sentences such as

(4) and (5) that are intermixed with unacceptable sentences (e.g., "The criminal cursed the judge who astonished the verdict"), even college students take longer to judge the acceptability of sentences with object-extracted clauses than for subject-extracted clauses (e.g., Waters, Caplan, & Hildebrandt, 1987). Moreover, performance on on-line tasks, such as self-paced reading or listening, in which the sentences are divided into words or phrases and subjects press a button for the successive presentation of each segment, has shown that reading and listening times are longer at the very regions of object-extracted sentences where WM load is thought to be higher. The assumption underlying these tasks is that reading or listening times to words or phrases presented one at a time reflect the time it takes to integrate lexical items into an accruing syntactic and semantic structure and are therefore longer when this integration is more difficult. Thus, longer reading or listening times for a particular part of the sentence are thought to be a reflection of increased WM or processing demands.

Typical results from a self-paced listening study of ours are shown in Figure 11.1. The on-line sentence-processing paradigm we used in this study was the auditory moving windows paradigm (Ferreira, Henderson, Anes, Weeks, & McFarlane, 1966), in which sentences are recorded as a whole with normal prosody, digitized, and segmented into words or phrases, and subjects press a button to receive successive items.[1] The stimuli consisted of three different pairs of sentences, illustrated in Table 11.1, in which one member of each pair consisted of a syntactic structure that contained a subject-extracted relative clause and the other member contained a more difficult object-extracted relative clause. Each pair of sentences contained the same words and differed only in the order of the words. The sentences were intermixed with unacceptable sentences and subjects were asked to pace their way through each sentence as quickly as possible and then to make a judgment about whether the sentence was an acceptable sentence in English. Figure 11.1 shows the segment listening times for acceptable sentences that were correctly judged as such. As can be seen, listening times were

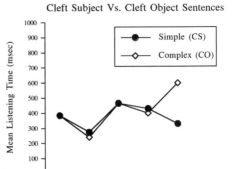
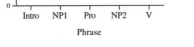
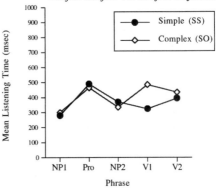
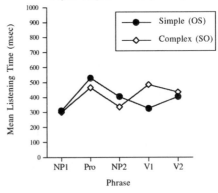

Figure 11.1. Word-by-word listening times for college students on three pairs of syntactically simple and complex sentences. Intro = introductory phrase; NP1 = first noun phrase; Pro = pronoun; NP2 = second noun phrase; V = verb.

TABLE 11.1. Examples of the Three Pairs of Sentences Used in the Auditory Moving Windows Task

Sentence Type					
Subject Relative	*Cleft Subject (CS)*				
PhraseIntro	NP1	Pro	V1	NP2	Continuation
It was/	the book/	that/	interested/	the teenager/	because it was a romance.
Object Relative	*Cleft Object (CO)*				
PhraseIntro	NP1	Pro	NP2	V1	Continuation
It was/	the teenager/	that/	the book/	interested/	because it was a romance
Subject Relative	*Subject Subject (SS)*				
PhraseNP1	Pro	V1	NP2	V2	NP3
The law/	that/	favored/	the millionaire/	frustrated/	the workers.
Object Relative	*Subject Object (SO)*				
PhraseNP1	Pro	NP2	V1	V2	NP3
The law/	that/	the millionaire/	favored/	frustrated/	the workers.
Subject Relative	*Object Subject (OS)*				
PhraseNP1	V1	NP2	Pro	V2	NP3
The millionaire/	favored/	the law/	that/	frustrated/	the workers.
Object Relative	*Subject Object (SO)*				
PhraseNP1	Pro	NP2	V1	V2	NP3
The law/	that/	the millionaire/	favored/	frustrated/	the workers.

Intro = introductory phrases; NP1 = first noun phrase; Pro = pronoun; V1 = first verb; V2 = second verb; NP2 = second noun phrase; continuation = final phrase.

virtually identical for the two members of each pair, for all segments other than the verb.

Why do processing times increase at the verb in object-extracted sentences? Processing difficulty occurs at points in sentences where a larger amount of information must be integrated and where such integration must occur over longer distances (Gibson, 1998; King & Just, 1991; MacDonald, Pearlmutter, & Seidenberg, 1994). All procedural models of parsing recognize both a higher memory load and a higher computational load at the verb in object-relativized clauses than at any point in subject-relativized clauses. The increase in listening time seen at the verb is taken as being due to the difficulty associated with integrating the verb of the object-relativized clause into the accruing representation of the structure and the meaning of the sentence, since it involves reference to more items held in memory and more compu-

tations on those items than is the case at the corresponding points in subject-relativized clauses.

One other potential source of the increase in listening time at the verb in object-relativized clauses is that the verb in these structures also corresponds to the final word of the clause or in some cases to the final word of the sentence. Numerous studies have documented longer reading times at the end of clauses (Balogh, Zurif, Prather, Swinney, & Finkel, 1998). The increase in reading time at the end of a clause is referred to as a *wrap-up effect*. Therefore, an additional comparison that can be made to ensure that the increase in listening time at the verb in object-relativized sentences is due to the WM load imposed at this point is to compare listening time at this point (V1) with the word that is the last word of the clause in the subject-relativized sentence (i.e., the second noun phrase, or NP2, which is the clause final word). If the effect is truly one due to the WM load at the verb, then listening times at the verb in object-relativized clauses should be longer than both those at the verb and the second noun phrase of the corresponding subject-relativized sentence. Thus, the increase in listening time seen at the verb in both comparisons is likely due to the greater WM demands at the embedded verb of an object-relativized sentence than at the corresponding points in a subject-relativized sentence.

How much do individuals vary in their abilities to meet these WM needs? Table 11.2 shows the mean listening time (corrected for the length of the segment) at two different points in subject- and object-relativized sentences—one in which there should be no difference in processing load or integration costs (the first noun phrase, NP1) and one in which processing and integration should be more difficult in the object-relativized sentence (the first verb, V1). Table 11.2 shows that, even in college students, there is considerable individual variability in listening times for words and phrases in sentences containing subject- and object-extracted relative clauses. This variability (as shown by the standard error and coefficient of variability) is much greater in object-extracted (cleft object, CO, and subject

object, SO) than in subject-extracted (cleft subject, CS; object subject, OS; and subject subject, SS) sentences and at the embedded verb of object-extracted relative clauses (V1) than at the verb of subject-extracted relative clauses. Table 11.3 shows that the greatest variability in listening time differential between matched segments in object- and subject-extracted relative clauses is in the difference between listening times for the embedded verb of object-extracted relative clauses (V1) and the corresponding embedded verb (V1) and relative-clause final noun (NP2) in subject-extracted relative clauses. Variability across these segments is much greater than across control segments (NP1) that should not differ in integration costs or processing load. These data show that there is considerable individual variability in the efficiency with which subjects deal with the local WM demands (i.e., WM demands at the point of difficulty) of the object-extracted relative-clause construction. We shall refer to this as variability in WM utilization.

Table 11.4 shows the correlation between the difference scores for different sentence pairs and comparisons that we take to be good measures of syntactic WM utilization in this paradigm for the data from the group of college students shown in Figure 11.1. The fact that there are high, significant correlations between

TABLE 11.2. Variability in Segment Listening Times in College Students

Segment	Mean	Standard Error	Coefficient of Variability	Minimum	Maximum
CS NP1	279.8	17.5	.43	−14.2	590.9
CO NP1	241.9	20.3	.58	−88.5	608.7
CS V1	331.8	16.9	.35	76.6	580.3
CO V1*	604.5	47.6	.54	119.6	1714.3
SS NP1	280.8	19.1	.47	−52.0	537.1
SO NP1	299.3	19.2	.44	22.4	613.3
SS V1	323.1	14.8	.32	130.6	530.8
SOV1*	484.9	41.1	.59	145.4	1775.4
OS NP1	308.8	17.1	.38	16.1	577.1
SO NP1	299.3	19.2	.44	22.4	613.3
OS V1	326.9	16.6	.35	108.3	607.1
SOV1*	484.9	41.1	.59	145.4	1775.4

CS = cleft subject; CO = cleft object; SS = subject subject; OS = object subject; SO = subject object; V1 = first verb; NP1 = first noun phrase; NP2 = second noun phrase.
*indicates segment at which processing load is high.

Data from Waters and Caplan (2005).

TABLE 11.3. Difference in Listening Time between Matched Segments of Sentences with Subject- and Object-Relative Clauses

Segment	Difference	Standard Error	Minimum	Maximum
CO NP1–CSNP1	−37.9	7.5	−149.7	84.6
CO V1–CSV1*	272.7	40.3	−253.2	1218.7
COV1–CSNP2*	171.6	43.9	−322.8	1368.4
SO NP1–SSNP1	18.5	10.4	−164.3	248.3
SOV1–SSV1*	161.8	35.3	−41.7	1373.5
SOV1–SSNP2*	116.8	32.6	−138.7	1362.6
SO NP1–OSNP1	−9.5	13.1	−381.5	304.2
SOV1–OSV1*	158.0	36.2	−127.3	1460.0
SOV1–OSNP2*	78.3	31.7	−179.9	1214.9

CS = cleft subject; CO = cleft object; SS = subject subject; OS = object subject; SO = subject object; V1 = first verb; NP1 = first noun phrase; NP2 = second noun phrase.

*indicates contrast at which processing load difference between sentence types is high.

Data from Waters and Caplan (2005).

all of the difference scores supports the hypothesis that individual differences in syntactic WM utilization that are measured in this paradigm are stable and reliable. The question we shall explore in the next sections of this chapter is whether this variability is related to WM capacity as measured by standard tests of this function.

Before reviewing our work on this topic, we note two important methodological and interpretive issues regarding the relationship between gvWM and syntactic processing. First, the effort to relate individual differences in gvWM capacity to individual differences in the efficiency of syntactic processing requires that

there be an equally reliable way to measure gvWM in individual subjects. One of the most widely used WM tasks is the Daneman and Carpenter (1980) reading or listening span task in which participants read aloud or listen to increasingly longer sequences of sentence and then recall the final words of all of the sentences in each sequence. Working memory span is taken to be the longest list length at which recall of the sentence final words is correct on the majority of trials. Despite widespread use of the reading span task, several basic psychometric properties of this task remain incompletely characterized or inadequate. For example, we found that the task's

TABLE 11.4. Correlation between Measures of Syntactic Working Memory use across Three Different Sets of Sentences

	COV1–CSV1	COV1–CSNP2	SOV1–SSV1	SOV1–SSNP2	SOV1–OSV1	SOV1–OSNP2
Difference Score						
COV1–CSV1	—	.96	.69	.67	.67	.65
COV1–CSNP2	—	—	.71	.69	.72	.69
SOV1–SSV1	—	—	—	.94	.97	.94
SOV1–SSNP2	—	—	—	—	.92	.92
SOV1–OSV1	—	—	—	—	—	.93
SOV1–OSNP2	—	—	—	—	—	—

Note: All correlations are significant. CS = cleft subject; CO = cleft object; SS = subject subject; OS = object subject; SO = subject object; V1 = first verb; NP1 = first noun phrase; NP2 = second noun phrase.

Data from Waters and Caplan (2005).

test–retest reliability and the stability of categorization of subjects into WM groups over
short time periods through use of the reading
span task were extremely poor (Waters & Caplan, 1996b, 2003). The approach we have
taken to resolve this problem in our research
has changed over time. In some of our earlier
studies we used our own variant of the task,
which required participants to make a plausibility judgment about each sentence before
recalling the final words of all of the sentences
in a set (Waters & Caplan, 1996b). This version has somewhat better test–retest reliability
and stability of subject classification than the
task by Daneman and Carpenter. In our more
recent studies, we have used a composite WM
score that is based on four different WM
measures (alphabet span, Craik, 1986; subtract
2 span, Salthouse, 1988; two versions of reading span, Waters & Caplan, 1996b) that confirmatory factor analysis suggests reflect a
common factor. We found these measures to
have the best test–retest reliability and stability of
subject classification over a 6-week period (Waters & Caplan, 2003).

Another important issue concerns the type
of results that would provide evidence of any
cognitive operation relying on gvWM. Most
studies have used off-line tasks, such as making
judgments at the end of a sentence. However,
off-line tasks do not measure syntactic complexity effects as they occur and thus give only
an indirect view of syntactic processing abilities. Furthermore, end-of-sentence measures
are likely to include effects of syntactic complexity associated with reviewing sentences to
satisfy task requirements such as making plausibility or grammaticality judgments or matching sentences to pictures (i.e., post-interpretive
processes). For these reasons, most researchers
believe that on-line tasks are necessary to characterize first-pass syntactic processing (see
MacDonald et al., 1994, for a review).

In addition, gvWM may affect performance
on both off-line and on-line tasks for a number
of reasons (Waters & Caplan, 1996b). Therefore, evidence that gvWM has a specific effect
on a linguistic (e.g., syntactic) operation requires that both off-line and on-line measures
be more affected by linguistically more de-

manding (syntactically more complex) structures (i.e., that group differences increase when
the demands made by structure-building and
interpretive operations increase). If on-line measures are taken at multiple points in a sentence,
as in self-paced reading or listening, it is therefore necessary to compare points of high and
low demand across sentences. Support for a role
of gvWM in syntactic processing would come
from the finding of a greater effect on performance in subjects with low gvWM at the complex parts of complex sentences (such as at the
verb in object-relativized sentences in the examples outlined above) than at other positions (such
as at the first noun phrase in the examples outlined above).

SYNTACTICALLY BASED SENTENCE COMPREHENSION AND WORKING MEMORY IN YOUNG SUBJECTS

In this chapter, we focus on research into the
WM demands of syntactic processing that has
capitalized on the differences in the WM demands associated with processing sentences
with subject-extracted and object-extracted
relative clauses. Studies with other syntactic
structures have yielded similar results and conclusions (see Waters & Caplan, 1996b, for a
review). However, because of space limitations
we will focus on work with sentences with relative clauses.

The first experiment in the literature to investigate the ability of college students who
differ in WM capacity to process sentences with
subject- and object-extracted clauses was carried
out by King and Just (1991, Experiment 1).
They reported self-paced word-by-word reading times for high- and low-span subjects for
these two sentence types in a Daneman and
Carpenter–type sentence span task. In this
study, King and Just (1991) present a graph indicating that the biggest reading time differences between high- and low-span subjects are
in the syntactically critical area of the object-
relative sentences. However, no statistical analyses were reported to support the contention that
the difference in reading times between high-
and low-span subjects is specifically localized

to the region of object-relative sentences where there is the greatest processing load (Waters & Caplan, 1996b). In addition, the data presented by King and Just (1991) did not isolate performance on sentences in which the subjects did not have to retain the sentence-ending words (no analyses were reported by King and Just on the sentences in the zero-load condition alone).

Our first experiment examined the relationship between working memory capacity as measured using our variant of the reading span task and on-line syntactic processing, as measured using the auditory moving windows task, in a group of 100 college students (Waters & Caplan, 2004). In this study, subjects were tested on two of the three pairs of sentences shown in Table 11.1 (cleft-subject [CS] vs. cleft-object [CO] and object-subject [OS] vs. subject-object [SO]). The stimuli in this study differed from those in Table 11.1 in that different lexical items were used in the matched pairs of sentences and the effects of lexical frequency were regressed out. In addition, the CS/CO sentences did not contain an extra phrase at the end (continuation in Table 11.1). Acceptable sentences were intermixed with unacceptable sentences and subjects made a judgment about acceptability at the end of each sentence. The use of these two pairs of sentences allowed for two separate tests of the hypothesis that there is a relationship between working memory capacity and on-line sentence processing efficiency using different sets of stimulus materials.

Subjects were classified as high, medium, or low WM span on the basis of their performance on the Waters and Caplan (1996a) reading span task. Figure 11.2 shows the mean listening time for each phrase of the two types of subject- and object-extracted sentences for the three span groups. Comparison of listening times at each phrase showed that there were the predicted increases in these times at the more capacity-demanding phrases of the more complex sentences. For the cleft subject–cleft object sentences this increase occurred at the verb. For object subject–subject object sentences the increase occurred at both verbs and was carried through the end of the sentence. As can be seen in Figure 11.2, all three groups of

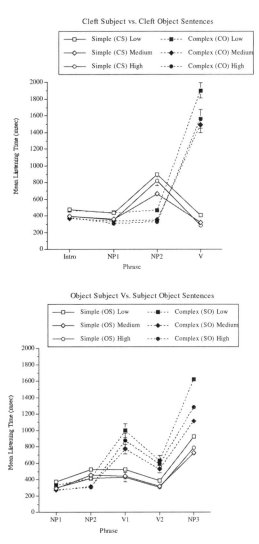

Figure 11.2. Word-by-word listening times for college students who differ in WM capacity on syntactically simple and complex sentences. Intro = introductory phrase; NP1 = first noun phrase; NP2 = second noun phrase; V1 = first verb; V2 = second verb; NP3 = third noun phrase.

subjects showed the expected pattern. Furthermore, listening times were also longer on the verb of the more complex object-extracted sentences than on the final noun phrase (NP2) of the subject-extracted sentences, indicating that the increase at the verb is not simply due to its clause-final position. Examination of the reaction time and error data on the plausibility judgment at the end of the sentence showed that, as expected, all subjects took longer to make judgments about sentences with object-extracted forms than sentences with subject-extracted forms. However, these effects were not larger in low-span subjects. Together, these results suggest that subjects who differ in WM capacity as measured by the reading span test do not differ in their ability to structure sentences syntactically.

Because of our concern about the reliability of WM span measures outlined above, we carried out a second study of 48 college students in which subjects were tested on four measures of working memory capacity. These measures consisted of two versions of the reading span task used in the experiment outlined above (one in which the stimuli consisted of syntactically simple sentences and one in which they consisted of syntactically complex sentences); an alphabet span task (Craik, 1986) in which subjects were presented with a list of words in random order and required to repeat them back in alphabetical order; and the subtract 2 span task (Salthouse, 1988), in which subjects were presented with digits and required to repeat them back after subtracting 2 from each. These tasks were chosen because they represent a range of processing operations that overlap computationally to different degrees with the on-line comprehension task and because our previous study showed that a composite WM score based on these four tasks resulted in the best test–retest reliability ($r = .85$). In this experiment, all subjects were tested up to a common span size on the working memory measures, and the number of items recalled in correct serial order was used as the measure of working memory capacity in correlational analyses.

The stimulus materials were also modified in this experiment. To eliminate end-of-sentence effects on critical phrases (the verb in CO sentences), an additional (continuation) phrase was added at the end of CS and CO sentences. Sample stimuli from this study are shown in Table 11.1. A third type of sentence used in a number of other studies (e.g., King & Just, 1991), subject subject (SS), was added in this study. The subject subject–subject object comparison is thought to be a purer test of the difference between object and subject

relativization than the object subject–subject object comparison because, in both subject-object and subject-subject sentences, the second verb (the main verb) must be connected to the first noun over the intervening relative clause, which is not the case in object-subject sentences. For example, in the examples in Table 11.1 in both the subject-subject and subject-object sentences the second verb *frustrated* must be connected to the first noun phrase *the law*, whereas in the object-subject sentence there is no intervening material between *the law* and *frustrated*. To control for lexical effects, the subject-subject, object-subject and subject-object sentences were developed in triplets using the same words.

In addition, in this study all subjects were also tested on a more global test of language comprehension, the Nelson Denny Reading Test. This test is one of the most common criterion tasks used in studies of the relationship between working memory and language comprehension, and several previous studies have indicated that it is related to working memory capacity. The use of the Nelson Denny Reading Test serves to determine whether the relationship that is usually found between working memory and general measures of comprehension is found in the subjects studied here.

The on-line data for this study are those seen in Figure 11.1. As outlined above, these subjects showed the typical pattern of on-line effects seen in studies of sentences with subject- and object-extracted relative clauses. Examination of the WM data for the subjects in this study showed that they differed widely in terms of their working memory capacities as measured by the four WM tasks. Using the same criteria used to classify subjects into discrete memory-span groups as in Experiment 1, 12 were classified as low span, 20 as medium span, and 16 as high span on the basis of their scores on the reading span task with cleft subject sentences.

The relationship between on-line performance and WM capacity was addressed in correlational analyses in this study. Pearson Product Moment Correlation Coefficients were computed between working memory, measured in percent of items correctly recalled in the correct serial order, and the six difference scores described above that we think reflect WM utilization in syntactic processing (see Tables 11.3 and 11.4). Since a positive score indicates that subjects took longer to process the verb of the more complex object-relativized sentence than the corresponding verb or the last noun phrase of subject-relativized sentences, one would expect to find significant negative correlations between these scores and the WM measures if gvWM is related to on-line syntactic processing. None of the correlations between the on-line measures and any of the WM measures were significant (Pearson's r ranged from $-.13$ to $.18$). The failure to find these correlations can not be due simply to the unreliability of the difference scores used as a measure of on-line performance, since there were strong correlations between the difference scores themselves (Table 11.4). However, we did find significant correlations between performance on the reading comprehension measure of the Nelson-Denny Reading Test and performance on the WM measures ($r = .29$ for alphabet and subtract 2 span; .36 and .28 for the two measures of reading span; .36 for a composite WM measure based on performance on all four WM tasks). These latter findings replicate others in the literature and support the view that WM capacity as measured by standard tests is related to aspects of language processing that we refer to as *post-interpretive*.

These results replicate other work we have carried out using a different on-line measure—the continuous lexical decision task—to measure on-line processing of subject- and object-relativized sentences in college students who differed in gvWM capacity (Caplan & Waters, 1999a). In this task, sequences of words and non-words are presented sequentially and subjects must indicate for each successive string whether it is a word or non-word. On some trials the sequences consist entirely of real words, and processing time for each word is measured as in the auditory moving windows task. In one study, sentences were presented auditorily and in another, in written form. In both studies we replicated previous findings of an increase in lexical decision times at the capacity-demanding portion of more complex object-relativized sentences. However, the magnitude of this effect did not differ in subjects with different gvWM capacities.

Thus, our data across several studies in which different groups of subjects, tasks, and modalities of presentation were used are consistent in suggesting that gvWM capacity is not related to the on-line construction of syntactic form.

SYNTACTICALLY BASED SENTENCE COMPREHENSION AND WORKING MEMORY IN AGING

Most studies have found that gvWM capacity declines with age (see Carpenter, Miyake, & Just, 1994, for a review), so the study of age-related changes in sentence comprehension provides indirect evidence about the effect of changes in working memory capacity on this function. Elderly subjects perform more poorly overall than younger subjects in many tests of sentence comprehension (e.g., Feir & Gerstman, 1980). In addition, some studies have reported a correlation between measures of gvWM and off-line measures of sentence comprehension in aging (e.g., Kemper, 1986). However, as noted above, these correlations do not provide evidence for the relationship between WM capacity and the on-line construction of syntactic form.

A limited number of studies have examined on-line syntactic processing in the elderly. Baum (1991) and Waldstein and Baum (1992) used the word-monitoring paradigm to investigate the sensitivity of younger and older adults to local and long-distance ungrammaticalities. In the word-monitoring paradigm, subjects listen to a sentence while monitoring for a particular word. Sentences were ungrammatical at either a "local" (e.g., the boy *were*...) or "long-distance" (the boy who the girl liked *were*...) position. For the elderly group, processing times and accuracy in detecting ungrammaticality were higher overall than those of the younger subjects, but elderly subjects were not more reliant on sentential context or less sensitive to ungrammaticalities than young subjects. Baum (1991) argued that her data did not provide evidence for age differences, and hence for the role of gvWM, in syntactic processing. Kemtes and Kemper (1997) found that older and younger subjects did not differ in the on-line interpretation of sentences in a study investigating the effect of syntactic ambiguity on word-by-word reading times. Kemtes (1999) measured younger and older adults' on-line grammaticality decisions for two types of complex sentences and their performance on various measures of gvWM and perceptual speed. Increased age was associated with poorer performance on measures of gvWM and perceptual speed, but these factors did not affect on-line grammaticality decisions. Age differences were not larger for syntactically complex sentence regions than for simple ones, and individuals who differed in gvWM did not differ in terms of on-line grammaticality decisions or in off-line question accuracy. Finally, Stine-Morrow, Loveless, and Soederberg (1996) showed that older adults were as sensitive as younger adults to the syntactic demands of a text in a self-paced reading study.

Three studies have found results that have been taken to support a role for gvWM in on-line syntactic processing in older subjects. Using the cross-modal lexical naming paradigm, in which participants listen to sentences and are asked to name words that appear on a computer screen at particular points during the presentation of the sentence, Zurif, Swinney, Prather, Wingfield, and Brownell (1995) found that older subjects were delayed at establishing the connection between a trace in a relative clause and the head of the clause. However, the delay was relative to performance of younger subjects on a different set of materials; a comparison young group was not tested on the same materials as the older subjects. In addition, gvWM was not tested in the elderly subjects. Therefore, Zurif et al.'s data are difficult to interpret in connection with the relationship of either age or gvWM to on-line syntactic processing. Kemper and Kemtes (1999) found that among elderly, but not young, subjects, those with lower gvWM capacities had longer reading times for ambiguous sections of questions such as *to paint* in *"Who did John ask to paint?"* However, gvWM also affected reading times for both young and old subjects in the unambiguous portions of these sentences, making the results inconclusive with respect to the effect of the combination of gvWM and age specifically on syntactic processing. Stine-Morrow, Ryan, and Leonard (2000) used a self-paced reading task to test younger and older subjects' ability to process sentences with subject- and object-extracted relative clauses. They found that older subjects showed *less of an effect* of object extraction at the verb than younger subjects. They argued that this result arose because subjects were not able to assign a syntactic structure and so abandoned the effort to process the sentence. They interpreted this result as evidence for impaired syntactic processing in aging due to gvWM decline. However, overall, most studies have not found differences in on-line syntactic processing as a function of age or gvWM.

We have carried out several studies, using the same methods and materials outlined in the studies of college students above, that have investigated the effects of age on on-line processing of sentences with subject-extracted and object-extracted relatives clauses. In our first study (Waters & Caplan, 2001), we tested a total of 139 individuals divided into the five age groups, seen in Figure 11.3, using the same methods and materials as in the study of 100 college students outlined above. All subjects were also tested on a battery of seven working memory measures. There were significant effects of age on all of the WM measures, with performance decreasing across the five age groups. As can be seen in Figure 11.3, older subjects had longer on-line processing times than those of younger subjects. All subjects also showed the predicted on-line effects of increased processing at the verb of object-extracted sentences. However, this effect was not any larger in older subjects than in younger subjects. In addition, there were no significant correlations between the WM measures and difference scores that reflected the increase in processing time seen at the verb of object-extracted sentences.

We carried out a second study in which we compared 48 elderly subjects to the 48 young subjects shown in Figure 11.2 (Waters & Caplan, 2005). These data are shown in

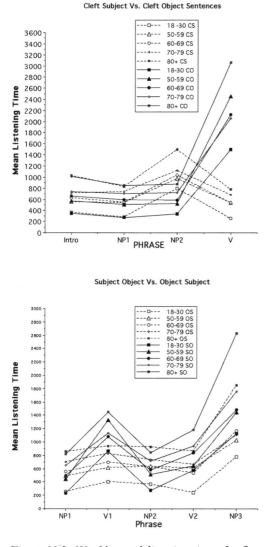

Cleft Subject Vs. Cleft Object Sentences

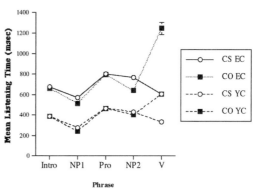

Object Subject Vs. Subject Object Sentences

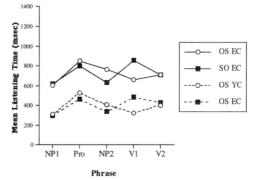

Subject Subject Vs. Subject Object Sentences

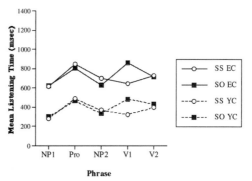

Figure 11.3. Word-by-word listening times for five groups of subjects who differ in age on syntactically simple and complex sentences. Intro = introductory phrase; NP1 = first noun phrase; NP2 = second noun phrase; V1 = first verb; V2 = second verb; NP3 = third noun phrase.

Figure 11.4. Word-by-word listening times for 48 young (YC) and 48 elderly (EC) subjects. Intro = introductory phrase; NP1 = first noun phrase; Pro = Pronoun; NP2 = second noun phrase; V1 = first verb; V2 = second verb.

Figure 11.4. Once again, listening times were longer overall for the elderly subjects than for the young subjects. As in the previous study, listening times were consistently longer at the capacity-demanding regions of the harder than the matched simpler sentence types for all subjects. However, once again, this effect was not larger in the older subjects or in subjects who had reduced gvWM. Table 11.5 shows the correlation between the composite WM score based on four WM tasks and the on-line measures, as well as measures taken at the end of sentence (i.e., reaction time and errors in

TABLE 11.5. Correlation between Composite Working Memory Measure and Language Measures

Type of Measure	Working Memory
On-line Measures	
COV1–CSV1	−.23*
COV1–CSNP2	−.11
SOV1–SSV1	.02
SOV1–SSNP2	.00
SOV1–OSV1	.01
SOV1–OSNP2	.11
End-of-Sentence Measures	
CO–CS response time	.05
SO–OS response time	.11
SO–SS response time	.07
CO–CS accuracy	.23*
SO–OS accuracy	.26*
SO–SS accuracy	.06
Discourse Measure	
Nelson Denny comprehension	.27*
Nelson Denny rate	.25*

*$p<.05$ CS = cleft subject; CO = cleft object; SS = subject subject; OS = object subject; SO = subject object; V1 = first verb; NP1 = first noun phrase; NP2 = second noun phrase.

Data from Waters and Caplan (2005).

making acceptability judgments to more complex object-relativized sentences compared to simple subject-relativized sentences). In this case, there was a significant correlation between WM and processing times at the verb of cleft-object sentences. However, the fact that the correlation was not significant when the verb in cleft-object sentences was compared to the final noun phrase in cleft-subject sentences suggests that the effect is an end-of-clause effect, rather than a syntactic effect. In addition, for the cleft subject–cleft object comparison and for the object subject–subject object comparison, subjects who made more errors on the acceptability judgment task for the more complex object-relativized sentences tended to have lower WM scores, as shown by the significant correlation between WM and these end-of-sentence measures. Finally, as in our study of young subjects, there were significant cor-

relations between the WM measures and performance on the Nelson-Denny Reading Comprehension Test.

Taken together, the results of our studies and those of others show that, although older individuals perform more poorly on standard tests of working memory, this decrement in working memory capacity is not related to a decrement in the on-line construction of syntactic form. Standard measures of working memory are related, however, to on-line measures that are likely due to clause-final "wrap-up" processes, to off-line measures taken at the end of sentences, and to more global measures of language comprehension in both young and elderly individuals. These findings suggest that gvWM is involved in operations that occur after the initial processing of a sentence has taken place.

STRUCTURAL EQUATION MODELING

We have further explored the relationship between WM capacity and interpretive and post-interpretive processing through the use of structural equation modeling. We modeled both the relationship between WM measures and on-line language processing (LP in Fig. 11.5) and between WM measures and global language processing (ND in Fig. 11.5) in a group of young and elderly subjects. Working memory measures included alphabet span (Alph), backward digit span (Back), subtract 2 span (Subt), running item span (Run), and a sentence span measure formed by combining performance on the final-word recall component of two sentence span tasks (WM comp). On-line language processing was measured by the increase in processing time at the capacity-demanding portion of the complex compared to the simple sentence types (V CO-CS and V1 SO-OS in Fig. 11.5). Global language processing was measured with the Nelson Denny Reading Comprehension Test. In both cases we were able to find a good fit for the model. In the model of on-line sentence processing, all parameter estimates were significant other than those between memory and language

**Working Memory Span Measures
and On-line Language Processing**

**Working Memory Span Measures
and Nelson Denny Comprehension**

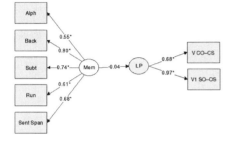
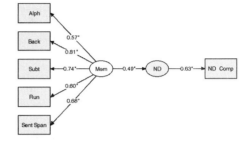

Model Fit Indices
Probability of $\chi^2(10) = .30$
NFI = .92
CFI = .97
RMSEA = 0.07
All parameter estimates
significant at p<.05 except the one
between Mem and LP.

Model Fit Indices
Probability of $\chi^2(9) = .22$
NFI = .94
CFI = .99
RMSEA = 0.05
All parameter estimates significant at
p<.05

Figure 11.5. Structural equation models of the relationship between working memory span measures and measures of on-line and global language processing. Alph = alphabet span; Back = backward digit span; Subt = subtract 2 span; Run = running item span; Sent Span = sentence span; Mem = working memory span measures; LP = language processing; ND = Nelson Denny Reading Comprehension Test.

processing. In contrast, in the model with Nelson Denny Reading Comprehension, all parameter estimates were significant, including those between memory and comprehension. In subsequent models, we have replicated this result using measures of on-line language processing that are not confounded by end-of-clause wrap-up effects (i.e., COV–CS NP1; SOV–OS N1) (DeDe, Caplan, Kemtes, & Waters, 2004). These data are consistent with the view dividing language processing into two functional areas that are and are not related to WM as measured by standard tests.

SENTENCE COMPREHENSION AND WORKING MEMORY IN PATIENTS WITH ALZHEIMER DEMENTIA

Patients with Alzheimer dementia (AD) provide an excellent population in which to examine the effects of a reduction in gvWM on sentence comprehension. Patients with AD have impairments in the central executive component of gvWM, as shown by performance on both span and other tasks (Morris, 1984). The central executive is thought to play a critical role in the storage and processing of items in gvWM and has been argued to play a very important role in standard WM tests (Just & Carpenter, 1992). The gvWM limitations seen in AD patients are often severe and are stable. Thus, if gvWM as measured by standard WM tests plays an important role in structuring sentences syntactically, then patients with AD should perform very poorly on sentence comprehension tasks that require them to structure sentences syntactically.

We tested 26 AD patients in the mild-to-moderate stages of the disease and 26 age- and education matched controls on the six WM tasks outlined above in the structural equation modeling work. All of the AD patients were able to perform all of the tasks, although the tasks ranged in terms of difficulty. Several patients were able to perform the sentence-processing and word recall components of the reading span task alone but were unable perform the two tasks together. General verbal WM spans of the patients were significantly lower than those of controls on all of the tasks. Internal consistency was high for all of the tasks. Test–retest reliability for a composite measure based on performance on six of the span measures for the patients was high ($r = .95$ for Time I and Time II). These data show that the working memories of AD patients are considerably more reduced than those of matched normal subjects. The problem of reliably classifying subjects with respect to gvWM does not arise with AD patients, particularly when a composite measure based on several different gvWM tests is used.

Given the severity of the WM decrements seen in AD, if AD patients with gvWM impairments do not show impairments in syntactic processing, this would provide strong evidence that this functional ability does not rely on the gvWM system. Conversely, evidence from AD could show that gvWM is involved in syntactic processing. This argument requires two steps. First, AD patients must be shown to have disproportionate impairments on syntactically more complex sentences (see above). Second, these impairments must be related to the gvWM limitations of the patients, either through correlational analyses or other experimental manipulations (such as contrasting visual pre-

sentation of entire sentences with auditory presentation; see Caplan & Waters, 1990, for discussion).

Studies of the sentence comprehension abilities of AD patients have been inconsistent. Some authors have asserted that sentence comprehension is impaired (e.g., Kontiola, Laaksonen, Sulkava, & Erkinjuntt, 1985) and others that it is preserved (e.g., Schwartz, Marin, & Saffran, 1979). Careful examination of the results of these studies suggests that AD patients may have performed poorly in many studies because of deficiencies in their ability to access semantic knowledge, to enact responses, and to accomplish other post-interpretive requirements of many of these tasks (see Rochon, Waters, & Caplan, 1994, for discussion). Some studies have reported that comprehension is differentially impaired in AD on syntactically more complex sentence structures, providing evidence for a syntactic processing deficit (e.g., Grober & Bang, 1995), while other have not found this to be the case (e.g., Rochon et al., 1994; Waters, Caplan, & Rochon, 1995).

However, the relationship between poorer performance on syntactically more complex sentences and reductions in gvWM in AD is not clear. For example, Grober and Bang (1985) reported that AD patients performed more poorly on syntactically complex sentences in a sentence picture–matching test, but they argued that the impairment was not related to an impairment in gvWM, since the syntactic deficit persisted even when a written sentence and a picture were in view simultaneously. Grossman, Mickanin, Onishi, and Hughes (1995) found that AD patients had an impairment in tasks assessing quantifier–noun agreement but argued that the deficit could not be explained by their short-term memory deficits. Small, Kemper, and Lyons (2000) reported that AD patients were worse at repeating syntactically complex sentences and they attributed the impairment to reduced gvWM in the patients, but the correlations between gvWM and performance were not greater for the syntactically complex than for the syntactically simple sentences. Our own work using off-line tasks has found that AD patients are not disproportionately affected by increased syntactic complexity in sentence–picture matching or acceptability judgment compared to elderly controls. We showed that AD patients perform more poorly overall on several off-line measures, such as sentence–picture matching and sentence acceptability judgment, when the stimuli consist of syntactically simple sentences (subject relatives) and complex sentences (object relatives) (Rochon et al., 1994; Waters et al., 1995). However, we have consistently found that they do not do disproportionately more poorly on the more complex sentence structures.

As elsewhere, more persuasive evidence regarding AD patients' capacities would come from on-line measures. Although it initially seemed possible that AD patients might not be able to perform on-line tasks, several research groups have shown such measures can be obtained in AD. These studies show surprisingly good on-line performance in some syntactic comprehension tasks, and little effect of gvWM on performance in this population. For instance, MacDonald and colleagues used an on-line cross-modal naming task, and found that Alzheimer patients showed the same increase in reading times for violations of subject–verb agreement and verb transitivity as that of normal controls (Kempler, Almor, Tyler, Andersen, & MacDonald, 1998). Moreover, the difference in reading times for the grammatical and ungrammatical continuations did not correlate with a composite measure of gvWM in these studies. In other work, these investigators have used a task in which subjects had to read aloud a sentence containing a heteronym (e.g., *dove, bow, wind*) whose correct pronunciation depended on prior syntactic or semantic information (Stevens et al., 1998). The performance of the AD patients and elderly controls was similar and showed that both groups relied on the semantic and syntactic context to resolve the ambiguity. Almor, MacDonald, Kempler, Andersen, and Tyler (2001) reported that AD patients and controls showed the same sensitivity to violations in subject–verb number agreement in a short-sentence condition and similar degradation of this sensitivity in a long-sentence condition. Performance in neither

condition was related to gvWM. These results suggest that many aspects of on-line syntactic processing are normal in Alzheimer patients.

Two additional studies by MacDonald and colleagues suggest, however, that while the memory impairment seen in AD does not interfere with on-line grammatical processing within sentences, it may affect on-line processing across sentences. In one study (Almor, Kempler, MacDonald, Andersen, & Tyler, 1999), AD patients and controls heard an introductory two-sentence passage and the beginning of a third sentence, followed by a written pronoun that was either contextually appropriate or inappropriate. Both AD patients and controls had longer reading times for inappropriate than appropriate pronouns, but the magnitude of the effect was smaller in AD patients and was correlated with a measure of gvWM. One feature of this study that bears noting is that the control subjects answered questions about the appropriateness of the pronoun after every passage whereas the patients only answered questions after every fourth passage, which may have led to the greater sensitivity of the controls to the pronouns' appropriateness. A second experiment (Almor et al., 2001) showed that AD patients were less sensitive than controls to pronoun–antecedent number agreement violations across sentences, and that their performance was correlated with measures of gvWM.

Altogether, two studies show that AD patients have difficulties with pronominal coreference in short discourses, and the literature otherwise indicates that AD patients in the early to middle stages of the disease show normal on-line syntactic processing. However, to date, very few on-line studies have been done.

We tested 20 AD patients and 20 controls on six tests of gvWM and on the auditory moving windows task outlined above in which the stimuli consisted of pairs of sentences seen in Table 11.1 (Waters & Caplan, 2001; see also Waters & Caplan, 1997). Patients had lower gvWM scores than controls, with the average reading span of the patients being only 1.2 compared to 3.1 for the controls. The patients performed more poorly than the controls on the end-of-sentence acceptability judgments. However, patients were not more affected than controls by the syntactic complexity of a sentence in these judgments. Figure 11.6 shows that AD patients and elderly controls showed similar effects of syntactic structure in the listening time data. Table 11.6 shows the correlation between the on-line and end-of-sentence measures and the composite WM measures. These results are very similar to those in the study of young vs. elderly subjects outlined above. There was a significant correlation between listening time at the verb of cleft subject sentences and WM. However, as in the study of normals, this effect seemed to be an end-of-clause effect rather than a syntactic effect. In addition, there was also some evidence for a relationship between WM and accuracy in making judgments at the end of the sentence in this group of elderly subjects. These results indicate that early-stage AD patients are not impaired in their ability to assign syntactic structure and to use it to determine aspects of sentence meaning, despite their reduced working memories.

STUDIES OF APHASIC PATIENTS WITH REDUCED RESOURCES FOR SYNTACTIC PROCESSING

The studies outlined to this point have all relied upon data from normal individuals or from patients who have impairments in gvWM. However, there are other patients who seem to have impairments in the svWM system that is used for syntactic processing. Patients with aphasia provide such cases. Research into the nature of the sentence comprehension impairments seen in patients who are aphasic subsequent to a left hemisphere stroke has shown that many such patients have disturbances affecting their ability to use syntactic form to determine the meaning of a sentence (see Berndt, Mitchum, & Haendiges, 1996, for review). Several aspects of the performance of these patients suggest that one reason for this impairment is a reduction in the processing resources that a patient can apply to this task. One piece of evidence that favors this

view is that groups of patients have been shown to have difficulty understanding sentences with more complex syntactic structures (Caplan, Baker, & Dehaut, 1985). Second, factor analyses have shown that a single factor on which all sentence types load accounts for about two-thirds of the variance in many syntactic comprehension tasks in aphasic groups (Caplan et al., 1985). Third, cluster analysis shows that patients tend to be grouped according to their overall level of performance in these tasks, with performance in more impaired clusters showing greater effects of syntactic complexity (Caplan et al., 1985). Finally, some patients have been able to interpret sentences when either of two syntactic features was present, but not when both were found in a sentence (Hildebrandt, Caplan, & Evans, 1987). These patterns of performance are consistent with the hypothesis that the problem in syntactic processing in sentence comprehension that is seen in many aphasic patients results in part from reductions in their ability to allocate processing resources to the syntactic comprehension task.

Study of these patients has allowed us to approach the question of the relationship between working memory capacity and syntactic processing in sentence comprehension from another angle, by examining the effect of a concurrent memory load on syntactic comprehension in patients in whom there is evidence for a reduction in the resources available for syntactic processing in sentence comprehension. The rationale for such studies is that, if syntactic processing relies on svWM, a concurrent gvWM load would not further reduce syntactic processing performances in individuals whose syntactic processing is already compromised by reduced svWM; if syntactic processing relies on gvWM, a concurrent gvWM load *would* further reduce syntactic processing performances. These studies are relevant here because they use variability in WM, in this case svWM, as a source of data about the structure of the central executive. We examined the effect of a concurrent digit load on the sentence comprehension performance of aphasic patients (Caplan & Waters, 1996). Over 100 aphasic patients were screened to ensure that we only tested patients who

Cleft Object vs. Cleft Subject Sentences

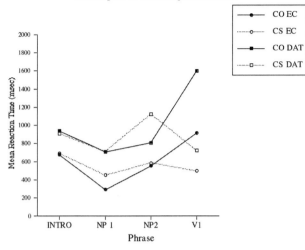

Object Subject vs. Subject Object Sentences

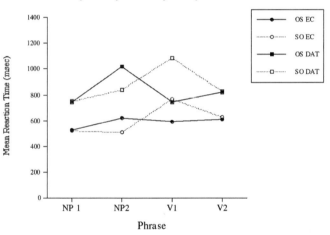

Subject Subject vs. Subject Object Sentences

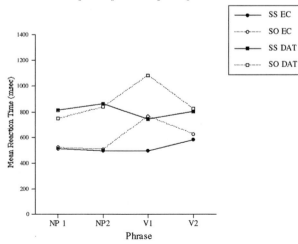

Figure 11.6. Word-by-word listening times for patients with Alzheimer dementia (DAT) and for elderly controls (EC). Intro = introductory phrase; NP1 = first noun phrase; NP2 = second noun phrase; V1 = first verb; V2 = second verb.

TABLE 11.6. Correlation between Composite Working Memory Measure and Language Measures for Elderly Controls, Patients with Alzheimer Dementia, and Combined Group of Subjects (All)

	Elderly Controls	Alzheimer Group	All
On-line Measures			
COV1–CSV1	−.28	−.21	−.44*
COV1–CSNP2	−.17	.11	−.10
SOV1–SSV1	.01	−.06	−.07
SOV1–SSNP2	−.02	.16	.13
SOV1–OSV1	−.03	.01	−.14
SOV1–0SNP2	−.12	.19	.15
End-of-Sentence Measures			
CO–CS response time	−.48*	−.24	−.11
SO–OS response time	.01	.21	.17
SO–SS response time	.05	.25	.21
CO–CS accuracy	.28	.24	.12
SO–OS accuracy	.49*	.06	.15
SO–SS accuracy	.35	.09	−.09

CS = cleft subject; CO = cleft object; SS = subject subject; OS = object subject; SO = subject object; V1 = first verb; NP1 = first noun phrase; NP2 = second noun phrase.

Data from Waters and Caplan (2002).

showed effects of syntactic complexity on a sentence picture–matching task, whose performance was below ceiling and above chance on that task, and whose abilities to repeat single words permitted them to be tested on a digit span task. We selected 10 patients who met these criteria, and tested them on a sentence picture–matching task in no-interference and concurrent load conditions (repeating a string of digits that was equivalent to their span or to their span −1). The data in Figure 11.7 show the typical pattern seen in aphasic patients (when tested without any concurrent load) of decreasing levels of performance as the syntactic complexity of the sentence increases. Although aphasic patients showed large effects of syntactic complexity when tested without a concurrent load, these effects were not exacerbated by the addition of a memory load. Their performance on the concurrent memory task was poorer with larger digit loads, but the effect of syntactic complexity was not exacerbated. These results provide striking evidence for the separation of the resources used in syntactic processing in sentence comprehension and those required for span tasks.

STUDIES OF THE NEURAL BASIS OF SYNTACTIC COMPREHENSION

A last approach to investigating the possibility that svWM, not gvWM, underlies syntactic processing is to examine neural responses to svWM and gvWM load. We have used the first of these approaches, and tested subjects who differ in either gvWM or svWM to see if their neurovascular responses to svWM load differ.

Our approach to the study of the functional neuroanatomy of syntactic processing in sentence comprehension has been to compare PET activity associated with processing syntactically more complex objected-extracted sentences to that with simpler subject-extracted sentences as in examples (4) and (5) outlined above. Experimental controls and counterbalances were used to ensure that the two conditions differed only along the syntactic dimension. Behavioral data (reaction times and accuracy) were collected on a plausibility judgment task in all PET runs. Established methods were used for PET acquisition, image reconstruction, normalization, and statistical

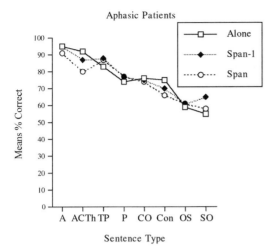

Figure 11.7. Performance of aphasic patients on a sentence picture–matching task with no concurrent interference task, while remembering a sequence of digits equal to their span minus 1, and while remembering a sequence of digits at span. Sentences on ordinate are listed in order of increasing syntactic complexity. A = active; ACTh = active conjoined theme; TP = truncated passive; P = passive; CO = cleft object; Con = conjoined; OS = object subject; SO = subject object.

analysis. Our work with young subjects showed a replicable pattern of increased regional cerebral blood flow (rCBF) in Broca's area when subjects made plausibility judgments about the more complex object-extracted sentences compared to that with the simpler subject-extracted sentences (Caplan, Alpert, & Waters, 1998; Caplan, Alpert, Waters, & Olivieri, 2000; Stromswold, Caplan, Alpert, & Rauch, 1996).

We followed up these findings with a study of young subjects who were matched for language-processing efficiency but who differed in gvWM (Waters, Caplan, Alpert, & Stanczak, 2003). We studied nine pairs of subjects who differed in their verbal gvWM as measured by a composite score on the tests outlined above that have been found to be the most reliable measures of gvWM. The groups were closely matched for age and sex and for level of performance on a screening test of syntactic processing in which reaction times and errors in making plausibility judgments about sentences were measured. Analysis of the high- and low-gvWM subjects'

behavioral responses showed no differences in accuracy or reaction times on the plausibility judgments made during scanning. High- and low-gvWM subjects both activated the same areas in the left and right inferior frontal cortex, as well as midline structures. We then reviewed the gvWM and syntactic processing screen performances of the subjects and regrouped them to form two new groups, each containing eight subjects, who were matched for gvWM and who differed in proficiency of syntactic processing on a screening test. As in previous studies, high-proficiency subjects activated the inferior frontal cortex, and low-proficiency subjects activated posterior structures. The results demonstrate that individual differences in the gvWM system measured by standard gvWM tests are not associated with differences in neural hemodynamic responses to syntactic processing, while differences in proficiency of processing are. Taken together, the results of this study provide converging evidence for the notion that individual differences in gvWM capacity are not related to syntactic processing ability.

SUMMARY OF THE EMPIRICAL DATA

To summarize the empirical data, we have found the following:

- Standard measures of WM capacity are not related to the efficiency with which subjects assign syntactic structures on-line.
- Patients with reduced ability to use WM in syntactic comprehension are not further affected by a concurrent verbal memory load.
- Regional CBF effects in sentence comprehension are modulated by the proficiency of syntactic processing but not by WM capacity.

We have interpreted the failure to find significant interactions between age (or gvWM), syntactic complexity, and region in our on-line studies as evidence for a specific WM resource used in the interpretation of syntactically complex sentences. However, there are several methodological and theoretical issues that must be considered in relation to accepting the null hypothesis.

Salthouse and Coon (1994) have pointed out that postulation of a separate process on the basis of the lack of significant interactions between age and an experimental manipulation requires evidence that the measure presumed to reflect the added process (V in object-extracted sentences) have at least a moderate amount of variance that is independent of the variance in the original measure (V in subject-extracted sentences) assumed to reflect the operation of all other processes involved in the task. Our data seem to meet this criterion. As seen in Table 11.2, comparison of matched segments in object- and subject-extracted sentences shows that there is much more variability in listening times for the verbs than for other segments.

A related issue is the extent to which the failure to find a relationship between gvWM and syntactic processing reflects a lack of statistical power, rather than a true absence of such a relationship. One issue concerns whether sufficient numbers of subjects were tested to provide adequate power. The self-paced studies measuring listening times for subject and object relatives were initially carried out on 100 college students and 130 individuals ranging from 18 to 80+ years of age. They were subsequently replicated with a new set of stimulus materials in a study of 48 college students and 48 elderly individuals and a study of 20 AD patients and 20 matched controls. In these studies, listening times at the most capacity-demanding portion of the syntactically more complex sentence are typically twice as long as those seen on the same word when it appears in a syntactically simpler sentence. Thus, these are very large effects. In addition, all of these studies have tested subjects on two and in some cases three pairs of sentences that provide a test of the hypothesis. The results of these studies with several hundred subjects and dozens of comparisons have been overwhelmingly consistent with the view that the increase in processing time at the verb in more

complex sentences is not associated with gvWM.

Another issue is whether gvWM measures are reliable enough to classify subjects and whether the division of subjects into arbitrary gvWM groups based on span measures may mask finer distinctions in gvWM among subjects who are members of the same group (Miyake, Emerson, & Friedman, 1999). In all of our on-line studies, we have measured gvWM using a variety of gvWM measures (Waters & Caplan, 2001), and in our more recent studies we have classified subjects on the basis of a composite score that reflects performance on several different gvWM measures and that has good test–retest reliability (Waters & Caplan, 2003, 2004, 2005). In addition, in several studies we have tested all subjects on all span sizes from 2 to 8 on the gvWM measures and have used the total number of items recalled in correct serial position, rather than span, in correlational analyses with the listening time measures (Waters & Caplan, 2004, 2005). This approach is more likely to detect relationships among measures, if they exist, than factorial analyses with group as a factor. The results of all of these analyses have been consistent and have not suggested a relationship between gvWM and on-line syntactic processing.

A related question is whether the measures of gvWM that we and other researchers have used are measuring the wrong WM construct. While tests that have been developed to measure WM have generally invoked the Baddeley and Hitch concept of WM that emphasizes the storage and computation functions of WM, many of them seem to us to be better measures of the Engle-type WM that emphasize the storage and divided-attention components of WM. For instance, complex span tasks (e.g., reading span) all require ongoing division of attention across two often completely unrelated tasks, and many do not include a measure of the computations in the task in the measure of WM. Other working memory tasks (e.g., alphabet span, subtract 2 span) require the memory and processing components of the task to be related to each other, as they are in naturally occurring tasks that require working memory, and are more naturally related to the Baddeley and Hitch notion of WM. Measurements of WM that use the latter type of task do not show relationships with syntactic processing.

DISCUSSION

Our discussion of these findings is organized in terms of the four questions posed to all contributors to this volume. An overview of our answers to the four questions is presented in Box 11.1.

Theory of Working Memory

The theoretical framework we operate within is that of Baddeley and Hitch (1974), which postulates the existence of a short-duration, capacity-limited, memory system that is capable of both maintaining representations and performing computations on them. Our focus within this framework is on the central executive component of WM. Our work suggests that there is a specialization within the central executive for the assignment of the syntactic structure of a sentence and the use of that structure in conjunction with the meanings of the words in the sentence to determine aspects of the propositional meaning of the sentence. Several points need to be made about this putative specialization.

First, if it exists, it is likely to apply only to the initial assignment of syntactic structure. Revisions of that structure, as occur in garden path effects, are not necessarily independent of working memory capacity as usually measured.

Second, if this specialization exists, we suggest that it is unlikely that its application is restricted to this one aspect of comprehension. Rather, we hypothesize that a specialized WM system supports a wider set of processes that accomplish the initial, automatic, on-line, obligatory, unconscious processes that assign the structure and the literal, preferred, discourse-congruent meaning of utterances. We have called these *interpretive* processes. We suggest

that processes that take as input the products of interpretive processes— specifically, that take as input the propositional content of sentences and the relations between propositions in the preferred interpretation of a discourse—and operate on these representations in the service of functions such as reasoning, entry into semantic memory, etc., do not use this specialized WM system.

One question that arises about this hypothesis is what the set of operations is that falls within the scope of svWM. There are three aspects to our answer to this question. The first point is that the answer requires commitment to a theory of linguistic structure and its processing. For instance, the studies in Fodor and Ferreira (1998) present a variety of models of features of the structure of sentences and discourse that do and do not trigger controlled revisions. Each of these models yields a slightly different characterization of interpretive processes. Second, we think that progress can be made by examining phenomena for which there is good evidence that they involve automatic first-pass processing. Third, we note that the major contrast we propose is between assignment of initial meaning and the use of that meaning to accomplish tasks. It is therefore possible to test our model by varying task demands, as well as by contrasting initial automatic and controlled sentence processing. Overall, though there are unquestionably gray areas where it is not clear whether a process that is relevant to establishing meaning is automatic or controlled, the theory seems to us to be sufficiently well articulated to be tested in many uncontroversial ways.

A second question relates to the notion of automaticity. There are two issues here. First, automaticity of a process is usually said to preclude its having resource demands, but this cannot be an appropriate way to conceptualize automaticity if processes such as on-line comprehension can be shown to require such resources but are to be considered to be automatized. We believe that the notion of automaticity needs to be revised to exclude the idea that automatic processes are resource-free. Second, one could see the data as indicating that syntactic processing is so automatized that it requires very little in the way of WM resources, rather than as pointing to the existence of a separate WM system dedicated to syntactic comprehension (and, by hypothesis, related aspects of comprehension).

Though the "automatized" view is possible, we are inclined toward the "separate system" view because of two features of the results. First, the sentence types we have used to measure WM use are at the limit of human comprehension abilities. Most listeners cannot understand object-extracted relative clauses that contain one more embedding than those used in our materials, such as Sentence 6:

6. The boy that the baby that the girl hugged kissed slipped.

Second, some subjects, such as AD patients, who showed normal effects of syntactic WM demand in these structures have extremely reduced WM capacity.

Taken together, these two facts indicate that individuals with extremely reduced WM have normal capacity to handle the greatest WM demands associated with syntactic processing that can ordinarily be handled. Though this could occur if syntactic processing were so automatized that the largest universally tractable WM demands it imposed were within the capacity of a WM system that is reduced as much as is ever seen, it seems to us to shift the burden of argument onto those who favor the "automatized" view.

Sources of Variability in Working Memory

Our results indicate that variability in utilization of WM in on-line first-pass syntactic processing is not related to overall WM capacity as measured by standard tests, or to age. We comment briefly on both these findings.

One consideration regarding the finding that "standard" WM capacity does not predict WM utilization in syntactic processing is that "standard" WM measures are measures of WM capacity and the measures of on-line processing are measures of utilization. A relationship

between the two would not be expected if resource demands do not affect processing when they fall within the range of resource availability. If there is only one resource available to meet the WM demands of syntactic processing, this conclusion would entail that these demands are minimal, which raises the issues considered immediately above in our discussion of automaticity. If there is a specialized WM system for syntactic processing, the WM demands made on this system by the sentences we have used are within subjects' capacity, since the reaction time measures we use are based on sentences that subjects responded to correctly and error rates were relatively low. It still may be the case that individual differences in utilization of this putative WM resource are related to individual differences in this specialized resource's capacity. To see if this is the case, we need a measure of the capacity of this specialized resource, something like a measure of span rather than a measure of its utilization.

Using the example of span (or complex span), such a measure would indicate the level of syntactic WM load at which sentence comprehension fails for each individual. This would require that subjects be tested for comprehension of sentences that differ by small increments in their peak WM load, and the point at which they fail to reliably understand the sentences be determined. Ideally, their on-line performances would also be measured to ensure that comprehension failure is associated with abnormal on-line processing at points of peak load. The psychometric properties of the measure would have to be established. Eventually, if the data have the hoped-for properties, a measure based on comprehension data could be used as a measure of syntactic WM capacity. This is a daunting research program, although its scope is certainly not greater than that of research programs into constructs such as "fluid intelligence." Until a sufficient part of it is accomplished to have a preliminary measure of this sort, the question of whether individual differences in the utilization of a putative WM resource for syntactic processing are related to individual differences in this resource's capacity remains unanswered.

In addition to asking whether individual differences in utilization of a putative specialized WM resource are related to individual differences in the resource's capacity, we can also ask whether they are related to the utilization, rather than the capacity, of a "standard" WM resource. To answer this question, we need a measure of WM utilization, not WM capacity. Perhaps a measure can be found in some chronometric value, such as the duration of the initial pause before list production in recall or the duration of inter-item pauses in recall trials. The operational problem we see here is that a "standard WM resource" involves many types of operations (attention, inhibition, search, etc.) and it may be necessary to measure different ones differently.

Turning to the age variable, the fact that age does not predict utilization of this putative specialized WM system indicates that syntactic processing groups with measures of crystallized intelligence, like vocabulary size, not fluid intelligence, like performance on the Raven's matrices, with respect to its relationship to age. Operationally, syntactic processing seems to lie between doing the Raven's test and retaining vocabulary. It resembles the Raven's test and is distinguished from vocabulary retrieval insofar as it involves computations that relate different items. It differs from the Raven's insofar as the computations it requires for the most part involve a relatively small set of highly overpracticed operations.[2] The Raven's test requires new computations, at least in its mid- and late items. Syntactic processing seems to lie between prototypical tasks that are weighted toward crystallized intelligence and those weighted toward fluid intelligence. We return to this point in relationship to Question 3.

What, then, does determine individual variability in use (and maybe capacity) of svWM? We see two main possibilities. One is that exposure and practice leads to the development of reliance on an independent resource and that these effects of experience and practice asymptote relatively early in the life cycle. However, in addition to exposure and practice, we think that an innateness factor is needed to account for the highly idiosyncratic nature of the representations constructed in parsing and that there are very

likely to be genetic factors that partially determine variability in svWM use. The relative roles of these two factors are unknown. (Disease also affects svWM use, as seen in aphasic cases).

Extending our perspective, considerations regarding both experience and innate endowment are consistent with the speculation that svWM, if it exists, supports interpretive processing and not just syntactic comprehension. Considering exposure and practice, extracting the literal, preferred, discourse-congruent meaning of an utterance involves constructing a limited number of types of representations using a limited number of operations, and constructing these representations using these operations constitutes one of the most overpracticed sets of related cognitive functions that humans undertake. After it has been recovered from an utterance, literal, preferred, discourse-congruent propositional meaning engages different cognitive operations as a function of the purpose of listening—entry into semantic memory; use in immediate planning of action, etc.—and these operations are far less practiced than the extraction of this representational set from the signal, simply because the number of times they are engaged is a proper subset of the number of times interpretive operations are engaged. However, practice patterns alone cannot explain the fact that interpretive operations co-occur the way they do. Why, for instance, is phonological form automatically converted into lexical and lexical semantic representations but not automatically entered into long-term memory? Again, innately specified, genetically and/or epigenetically determined processes seem to be involved to delineate the basic architecture of processes that use linguistic representations.

Other Sources of Variability in Working Memory and Connection to Other Work Reported in this Volume

Our work suggests that the central executive is fractionated, and suggests that variability in subparts of the central executive may not be shared with that in other parts. It also provides clues as to lines along which the central executive may be explored and fractionated.

Models of WM—whether they be the original Baddeley and Hitch model that postulated the existence of the central executive but did not characterize it or more recent models that link performance on WM tasks to processes that are supported by the central executive (e.g., attentional control)—seem to us to generally understate the "processing" that the central executive accomplishes. Many models emphasize the role of attention, inhibition and other aspects of control in central executive function without much emphasis on the processing that occurs once attention has been deployed or inhibition achieved. Some models specify processing, but characterize it at a relatively general level. For instance, Oberauer et al. (Chapter 3) characterize processing as "binding" but say little about what binding consists of; Cowan refers to "search" as an operation that takes place during pauses between retrieval of words in span tasks, but search is surely only one of many processing operations that the central executive accomplishes. In part this emphasis may stem from the attempt to characterize performance on WM tasks or, in the case of complex span tasks, on the recall measures in such tasks, which do not involve complex computational processes. However, even in work that varies processing load in the non-recall task in complex span tasks, what subjects have to do to meet the processing load is rarely as relevant to the issues explored as that the processing load is varied. A considerable amount of work in this volume also attempts to predict general intellectual capacity (fluid intelligence) using factor analyses of task performance, rather than mechanistic descriptions of the operations that subjects use to perform tasks, as a measure of this construct. We think these approaches, while important, miss one potentially equally important aspect of central executive function—how tasks are accomplished. This is the middle ground that lies between fluid and crystallized intelligence referred to earlier, that is occupied by models of tasks such as syntactic comprehension.

There are some papers that consider tasks in relation to WM theory that provide much more elaborate descriptions of the processes that go on in accomplishing those tasks (Kieras Meyer,

Mueller, and Seymour, 1999). These papers and our orientation fit well into the general framework developed by Ericsson and his colleagues (Ericsson & Delaney, 1999), that emphasizes the importance of activated knowledge and operational routines in long term memory in determining how tasks are accomplished. Unlike the expert performances that Ericsson and colleagues have studied, which involve highly trained specialized domains such as chess playing, our interest has been in a domain in which expertise is widespread in neurologically intact individuals who have had normal exposure to language and normal opportunity for its use. Despite this difference in how expertise is acquired and some rather fascinating differences in the ability to expand the skill,[3] skilled performances in these different domains all involve highly efficient utilization of complex, domain-specific, operations and knowledge. We think that many aspects of ordinary cognitive functioning in which normal individuals show highly skilled performance (e.g., visual categorization, reaching and throwing, and so on) involve similar domain-specific knowledge and operations and, in some cases, application of such knowledge and operations to representations that have been activated at temporally discontinuous points; i.e., a WM system in the sense we started with. We believe our work points to a need to include detailed models of the processing requirements of tasks—especially everyday ecologically utilitarian tasks—into models of the central executive.

Additionally, along these lines, our results suggest that the central executive may be fractionated along lines that are defined by the nature of these processes, not just the nature of the representations to which the processes apply. That is, within the domain of verbal functions, processes related to syntactic comprehension appear to dissociate with respect to WM utilization from processes that underlie performance on other verbally mediated tasks. While one can characterize the processes that are needed in each domain in broad terms such as "binding," the actual operations that take place and the representations that are constructed in each domain have important individual features.

This is clearly seen in the area of syntax, where the particular structures that are constructed are unlike those seen in any other cognitive domain. These operations may define components of the central executive.

While our work is closely aligned with that of Ericsson, Kieras, Meyer and others, it is not easy to relate it to other work presented in this volume; specifically, to research into the importance of the domain-general operations such as attentional control, inhibition, search and others in WM. For instance, Engle and colleagues (Engle, Kane, & Tuholski, 1999) emphasize the role of attentional control in performing WM tasks and the importance of this ability in explaining the predictive value of WM for fluid intelligence. It is not easy to see how attentional control (or inhibition, or search) is related to handling the WM demands imposed by syntactic processing. While sentence comprehension requires that sentences be attended to, it is unclear that any variation in attentional control occurs as a function of local syntactic WM load. Rather, once attended to, initial sentence processing proceeds as best it can, limited by factors that we do not understand. In this sense, if the notions "automatic" and "uncontrolled" apply to any cognitive function beyond perceptual identification, many aspects of the comprehension of a sentence—the ones we are focusing on—are automatic and uncontrolled once a sentence is attended. One can, of course, reformulate the notion of "attention" or "attentional control" to include whatever underlies coping with local variation in WM demand in sentences. This would be consistent with the tradition of conceiving of "attention" as a "resource," as in Kahneman (1973). If one takes this approach, the difference between the Baddeley and Hitch and Engle models evaporates. In that case, our model would have to be reformulated as claiming that there is a specialized attentional resource subcomponent.

Other researchers (not represented in this volume) go further, and deny the existence of working memory (or WM limitations) altogether. MacDonald and Christiansen (2002) argue that procedure-based symbol-manipulating models impose limits on the combination of computational activity and memory storage by artificial means; in their view, a limited WM capacity is a Deus ex Machina. They claim that connectionist models provide a more realistic computational mechanism for cognitive processes and that, in such models, limits on computational capacity are determined by the experience of the system. We strongly disagree with this view. Connectionist models are limited by their intrinsic, a priori, architectures (cf., the added power associated with hidden units), which are, at present, just as arbitrary as WM capacity limits on symbolic manipulations. There are three issues that need to be explored. What are the limits on human information processing? Are these limits domain-specific (and, if so, what are the domains)? Why do these limits arise? Denying the existence of limits is not an option.

There are also empirically based challenges to the need for WM, if not to the concept itself. Salthouse, for instance, has argued that age-related variation in processing speed accounts for age-related variation in WM (see Salthouse, 1996, for a review). An important question is whether processing speed reduction, or other similar mechanisms such as sensory threshold elevation, are alternatives to working memory accounts of reduced processing efficiency. One mechanism that Salthouse (1996) has suggested whereby processing speed might affect performance levels is if the temporal course of the activation of representations is slowed beyond a point that allows incoming material to be integrated into a developing set of representations (sensory threshold elevation could operate through a similar mechanism). However, this will only happen if incoming and/or constructed materials cannot be adequately stored in a memory system, which leads directly back to WM limitations. Our research could be recast as demonstrating domain-specific decrements in processing speed; it is less easy to see how our results could be consistent with elevated sensory thresholds being responsible for decreasing processing efficiency, given that sensory thresholds apply ubiquitously to stimuli and we have documented domain-specific decrements in processing.

Contribution to General Working Memeory Theory

Our answer to this question can be brief because it is contained in our previous discussion. We think that our work makes a contribution in that it argues for the existence of at least one specialization within the central executive. It suggests that operational domains in the central executive may be defined computationally as well as according to types of representation (verbal, visual). Our work also suggests that characterization of the actual operations required to perform a task is an important part of characterizing the nature of the central executive. Attention, inhibition, search, etc. all must apply to representations that are subject to computations; an understanding of the central executive requires understanding these representations and computations. Indeed, to go out on a bit of a limb, it seems worthwhile to ask whether the sometimes not inconsiderable variance in composite measures of fluid intelligence and factors like "g" that remains unaccounted for after variance due to attention, inhibition, search, etc. is removed might not reflect individual differences in the ability to deal with task-specific computations on particular types of representations.

BOX 11.1.   SUMMARY ANSWERS TO BOOK QUESTIONS

1. THE OVERARCHING THEORY OF WORKING MEMORY

We operate within a Baddeley and Hitch–type framework in which there is a short-duration, capacity-limited, verbal working memory system capable of maintaining representations and performing computations on them. Our focus is on the central executive component of WM. We hypothesize that the central executive is divided into at least two components—one that is involved in the initial assignment of meaning, and one that uses that meaning to accomplish tasks.

2. CRITICAL SOURCES OF WORKING MEMORY VARIATION

Variability in use of WM in the domain of syntactic comprehension that we are interested in is not related to overall WM capacity as measured by standard tests, or to age. There seem to be two main possibilities for what determines individual variability in use (and maybe capacity) of svWM. One is that exposure and practice lead to the development of reliance on an independent resource that asymptotes relatively early in the life cycle. In addition, an innateness factor likely accounts for the highly idiosyncratic nature of the representations constructed in parsing and a genetic factor likely helps determine variability in svWM utilization. The relative roles of these factors are unknown.

3. OTHER SOURCES OF WORKING MEMORY VARIATION

In our view, the central executive is fractionated. This fractionation may occur along lines defined by the nature of the representations and/or by the nature of the processes involved in a task. Variability in subparts of the central executive may not be shared with that in other parts.

4. CONTRIBUTIONS TO GENERAL WORKING MEMORY THEORY

Our work argues for the existence of at least one specialization within the central executive. It suggests that operational domains in the central executive may be defined computationally as well as according to types of representation (verbal, visual). Characterization of the actual operations required to perform a task may be an important part of characterizing the nature of the central executive.

Notes

1. Ferreira and colleagues have shown that this paradigm is sensitive to the same sorts of linguistic variables, and yields similar results, as the widely used self-paced reading paradigm (Ferreira et al., 1996).

2. Note that this is an area in which the choice of parsing model makes an enormous difference. The characterization of parsing as using a small number of overpracticed operations is predicated upon parsing being a matter of assigning higher-order categories and links between these categories to lexical syntactic categories and features that are activated as part of lexical access. If parsing consists of word-to-word associations, as posited by some connectionist modelers (e.g., Christiansen and Chater, 1999), most sentences would require novel operations, much more akin to those required by the Raven's test.

3. Skills seem to asymptote at higher levels in specialized domains. Even extensive practice (in anyone) does not seem to improve the ability to deal with multiply embedded object extractions anywhere near as much as practice (in some people) improves the ability to look ahead in chess.

References

Almor, A., Kempler, D., MacDonald, M. C., Andersen, E. S., & Tyler, L. K. (1999). Why do Alzheimer's patients have difficulty with pronouns? Working memory, semantics, and reference in comprehension and production of Alzheimer's disease. *Brain and Language, 67*, 202–228.

Almor, A., MacDonald, M. C., Kempler, D., Andersen, E. S., & Tyler, L. K. (2001). Comprehension of long distance number agreement in probable Alzheimer's disease. *Language and Cognitive Processes, 16*, 35–63.

Baddeley, A. D., & Hitch, G. (1974). Working memory. In G. H. Bower (Ed.), *The psychology of learning and motivation: Advances in research and theory* (Vol. 8, pp. 47–89). New York: Academic Press.

Balogh, J., Zurif, E. B., Prather, P., Swinney, D., & Finkel, L. (1998). Gap filling and end of sentence effects in real-time language processing: Implications for modeling sentence comprehension in aphasia. *Brain and Language, 61*, 169–182.

Baum, S. (1991). Sensitivity to syntactic violations across the age span: Evidence from a word-monitoring task. *Journal of Clinical Linguistics and Phonetics, 5*, 317–328.

Berndt, R., Mitchum, C. C., & Haendiges, A. N. (1996). Comprehension of reversible sentences in "agrammatism": A meta-analysis. *Cognition, 58*, 289–308.

Caplan, D., Alpert, N., & Waters, G. S. (1998). Effects of syntactic structure and propositional number on patterns of regional cerebral blood flow. *Journal of Cognitive Neuroscience, 10*, 541–552.

Caplan, D., Alpert, N., Waters, G., & Olivieri, A. (2000). Activation of Broca's area by syntactic processing under conditions of concurrent articulation. *Human Brain Mapping, 9*, 65–71.

Caplan, D., Baker, C., & Dehaut, F. (1985). Syntactic determinants of sentence comprehension in aphasia. *Cognition, 21*, 117–175.

Caplan, D., & Waters, G. (1990). Short-term memory and language comprehension: A critical review of the neuropsychological literature. In T. Shallice and G. Vallar (Eds.), *The neuropsychology of short-term memory* (pp. 337–389). Cambridge, UK: Cambridge University Press.

Caplan, D., & Waters, G. S. (1996). Syntactic processing in sentence comprehension under dual-task conditions in aphasic patients. *Language and Cognitive Processes, 11*, 525–551.

Caplan, D., & Waters, G. S. (1999a). Verbal working memory and sentence comprehension. *Behavioral and Brain Sciences, 22*, 77–94.

Caplan, D., & Waters, G. S. (1999b). Verbal working memory and sentence comprehension [discussion]. *Behavioral and Brain Sciences, 22*, 95–126.

Caplan, D., & Waters, G. S. (2002). Working memory and connectionist models of parsing: A response to MacDonald and Christiansen. *Psychological Review, 109*, 66–74.

Carpenter, P. A., Miyake, A., & Just, M. A. (1994). Working memory constraints in comprehension: Evidence from individual difference, aphasia and aging. In M. A. Gernsbacher (Ed.), *Handbook of psycholinguistics* (pp. 1075–1122). New York: Academic Press.

Christiansen, M. H. and Chater, N. (1999). Toward a connectionist model of recursion in human linguistic performance. *Cognitive Science, 23*: 157–205.

Craik, F. I. M. (1986). A functional account of age differences in memory. In F. Klix & H. Hagendorf (Eds.), *Human memory and cognitive capabilities* (pp. 409–421). New York: Elsevier.

Daneman, M., & Carpenter, P. (1980). Individual differences in working memory and reading. *Journal of Verbal Learning and Verbal Behavior, 19,* 450–466.

DeDe, G., Caplan, D., Kemtes, K., & Waters, G. S. (2004). The relationship between age, verbal working memory and language comprehension. *Psychology and Aging, 19,* 601–616.

Engle, R. W., Kane, M. J., & Tukholski, S. W. (1999). Individual differences in working memory capacity and what they tell us about controlled attention, general fluid intelligence, and functions of the pre-frontal cortex. In A. Miyake & P. Shah (Eds.), *Models of working memory: Mechanisms of active maintenance and executive control* (pp. 102–134). New York: Cambridge University Press.

Ericsson, A., & Delaney, P. F. (1999). Long-term working memory as an alternative to capacity models of working memory in everyday skilled performance. In A. Miyake & P. Shah (Eds.), *Models of working memory* (pp. 257–297). New York: Cambridge University Press.

Fier, C. D., & Gerstman, L. J. (1980). Sentence comprehension abilities throughout the adult life span. *Journal of Gerontology, 35,* 722–728.

Ferreira, F., Henderson, J. M., Anes, M. D., Weeks, P. A., & McFarlane, D. K. (1996). Effects of lexical frequency and syntactic complexity in spoken language comprehension: Evidence from the auditory moving window technique. *Journal of Experimental Psychology: Learning, Memory, and Cognition, 22,* 324–335.

Fodor, J. D., & Ferreira, F. (1998). *Reanalysis in sentence processing.* Boston: Kluwer.

Gibson, E. (1998). Linguistic complexity: Locality of syntactic dependencies. *Cognition, 68,* 1–76.

Grober, E., & Bang, S. (1995). Sentence comprehension in Alzheimer's disease. *Developmental Neuropsychology, 11,* 95–107.

Grossman, M., Mickanin, J., Onishi, K., & Hughes, E. (1995). An aspect of sentence processing in Alzheimer's disease: Quantifier-noun agreement. *Neurology, 45,* 85–91.

Hildebrandt, N., Caplan, D., & Evans, K. (1987). The man left without a trace: A case study of aphasic processing of empty categories. *Cognitive Neuropsychology, 4,* 257–302.

Just, M. A., & Carpenter, P. A. (1992). A capacity theory of comprehension: Individual differences in working memory. *Psychological Review, 99,* 122–149.

Kahneman, D. (1973). *Attention and effort.* Englewood Cliffs, NJ: Prentice Hall.

Kemper, S. (1986). Imitation of complex syntactic constructions by elderly adults. *Applied Psycholinguistics, 7,* 277–287.

Kemper, S., & Kemtes, K. (1999). Limitations on syntactic processing. In S. Kemper & R. Kliegl (Eds.), *Constraints on language: Aging, grammar, and memory* (pp. 79–105). Boston: Kluwer.

Kempler, D., Almor, A., Tyler, L. K., Andersen, E. S., & MacDonald, M. C. (1998). Sentence comprehension deficits in Alzheimer's disease: A comparison of off-line vs. on-line sentence processing. *Brain and Language, 64,* 297–316.

Kemtes, K. (1999). *Decomposing adults' sentence comprehension: The role of age, working memory, inhibitory functioning, and perceptual speed.* Unpublished doctoral dissertation, University of Kansas, Lawrence, KS.

Kemtes, K., & Kemper, S. (1997). Younger and older adults' on-line processing of syntactically ambiguous sentence. *Psychology and Aging, 12,* 362–371.

Kieras, D. E., Meyer, D. E., Mueller, S., & Seymour, T. (1999). Insights into working memory from the perspective of the EPIC architecture for modeling skilled perceptual-motor and cognitive human performance. In A. Miyake & P. Shah (Eds.), *Models of working memory: Mechanisms of active maintenance and executive control* (pp. 183–223). New York: Cambridge University Press,

King, J. W., & Just, M. A. (1991). Individual difference in syntactic processing: The role of working memory. *Journal of Memory and Language, 30,* 580–602.

Kontiola, P., Laaksonen, R., Sulkava, R., & Erkinjuntt, T. (1985). Patterns of language impairment is different in Alzheimer disease and multi-infarct dementia. *Brain and Langauge, 38*, 364–383.

Lewis, R.I. (1996). Interference in short-term memory: The magical number two (or three) in sentence processing. *Journal of Psycholinguistic Research, 25*, 93–115.

MacDonald, M. E., & Christiansen, M. H. (2002). Reassessing working memory: A reply to Just and Carpenter and Waters and Caplan. *Psychological Review, 109,*

MacDonald, M. C., Pearlmutter, N. J., & Seidenberg, M. S. (1994). Lexical nature of syntactic ambiguity resolution. *Psychological Review, 101*, 676–703.

Miyake, A., Emerson, M. J., & Friedman, N. P. (1999) Good interactions are hard to find. *Behavioral and Brain Sciences, 22*, 108–109.

Morris, R.G. (1984). Working memory in Alzheimer-type dementia. *Neuropsychology, 8*, 544–554.

Rochon, E., Waters, G. S., & Caplan, D. (1994). Sentence comprehension in patients with Alzheimer's disease. *Brain and Language, 46*, 329–349.

Salthouse, T. A. (1988). The role of processing resources in cognitive aging. In M. L. Howe & C. J. Brainerd (Eds.), *Cognitive development in adulthood* (pp. 185–239). New York: Springer-Verlag.

Salthouse, T. A. (1996). The processing-speed theory of adult age differences in cognition. *Psychological Review, 3*, 403–428.

Salthouse, T. A., & Coon, V. E. (1994). Interpretation of differential deficits: The case of aging and mental arithmetic. *Journal of Experimental Psychology: Learning, Memory, and Cognition, 20*, 1172–1182.

Schwartz, M. F., Marin, O. S., & Saffran, E. M. (1979). Dissociations of language function in dementia. A case study. *Brain and Language, 7*, 277–306.

Small, J., Kemper, S., & Lyons, K. (2000). Sentence repetition and processing resources in Alzheimer's disease. *Brain and Language, 75*, 232–258.

Stevens Dagerman, K., Almor, A., MacDonald, M.E., Kempler, D., & Andersen, E. (1998). Preserved use of semantic and syntactic context in Alzheimer' disease. *Brain and Language, 65*, 87–132.

Stine-Morrow, E., Loveless, M. K, & Soederberg, L. M. (1996) Resource allocation in on-line reading by younger and older adults. *Psychology and Aging. 11*, 475–486.

Stine-Morrow, E. A. L., Ryan, S., & Leonard, J. S. (2000). Age differences in on-line syntactic processing. *Experimental Aging Research, 26*, 315–322.

Stromswold, K., Caplan, D., Alpert, N., & Rauch, S. (1996). Localization of syntactic comprehension by positron emission tomography. *Brain and Language, 52*, 452–473.

Waldstein, R., & Baum, S. (1992). The influence of syntactic and semantic context on word monitoring latencies in normal aging. *Journal of Speech Language Pathology and Audiology, 6*, 217–222.

Waters, G. S., & Caplan, D. (1996a). The measurement of verbal working memory capacity and its relation to reading comprehension. *Quarterly Journal of Experimental Psychology, 49A*, 51–75.

Waters, G. S., & Caplan, D. (1996b). The capacity theory of sentence comprehension: Critique of Just and Carpenter (1992). *Psychological Review, 103*, 761–772.

Waters, G. S., & Caplan, D. (1997). Working memory and on-line sentence comprehension in patients with Alzheimer's disease. *Journal of Psycholinguistic Research, 26*, 377–400.

Waters, G. S., & Caplan, D. (2001). Age, working memory and on-line syntactic processing in sentence comprehension. *Psychology and Aging, 16*, 128–144.

Waters, G. S., & Caplan, D. (2002). Working memory and on-line syntactic processing in Alzheimer's disease: Studies with auditory moving windows presentation. *Journal of Gerontology B: Psychological Sciences and Social Sciences, 57*, P298–311.

Waters, G. S., & Caplan, D. (2003). The reliability and stability of verbal working memory measures. *Behavior Research Methods, Instruments & Computers, 35*, 550–564.

Waters, G. S., & Caplan, D. (2004). Verbal working memory and on-line syntactic processing: Evidence from self-paced listening. *Quarterly Journal of Experimental Psychology, 57*, 129–164.

Waters, G. S., & Caplan, D. (2005). The relationship between age, processing speed, working memory capacity, and language comprehension. *Memory, 13*, 403–413.

Waters, G. S., Caplan, D., Alpert, N., & Stanczak, L. (2003) Individual differences in rCBF correlates of syntactic processing in sentence comprehension: Effects of working memory and speed of processing. *NeuroImage, 19,* 101–112.

Waters, G. S., Caplan, D., & Hildebrandt, N. (1987). Working memory and written sentence comprehension. In M. Coltheart (Ed.), *Attention and Performance XII: The psychology of reading* (pp. 531–555). Hillsdale, NJ: Erlbaum.

Waters, G. S., Caplan, D., & Rochon, E. (1995). Processing capacity and sentence comprehension in patients with Alzheimer's disease. *Cognitive Neuropsychology, 12,* 1–30.

Zurif, E., Swinney, D., Prather, P., Wingfield, A., & Brownell, H. (1995). The allocation of memory resources during sentence comprehension: Evidence from the elderly. *Journal of Psycholinguistic Research, 24,* 165–182.

Author Index

Subject Index

Note: Page numbers followed by f and t refer to figures and tables, respectively.

315